T0333691

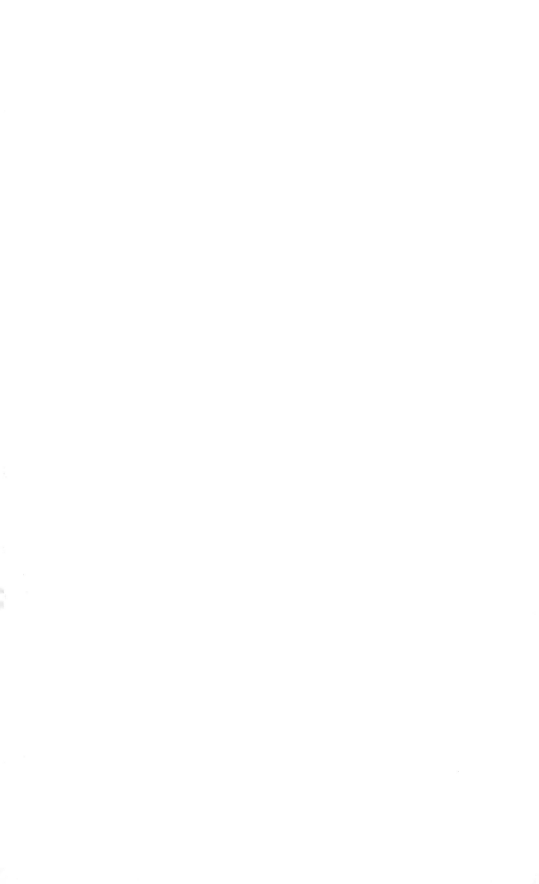

Evidence for Child Welfare Practice

The purpose of this book is to provide a "work-in-progress" that seeks to capture the micro (direct service) and macro (managerial) perspectives related to identifying evidence for practice within the practice domain of public child welfare. It is divided into two categories; namely, evidence for direct practice and evidence for management practice. In Part I, the articles are categorized in the areas of child welfare assessment and child welfare outcomes. Expanded versions of the chapters can be accessed at www.bassc.net.

In Part II, the focus is on organizational issues that relate to evidence for management practice. This section includes an overview of evidence-based practice from an organizational perspective along with evidence related to the experiences of others in implementing evidence-based practice.

This book pushes the discussion of evidence-based practice in several new directions regarding: 1) the use of structured reviews to complement the systematic reviews of the Cochrane and Campbell Collaboratives, 2) the process of viewing the call for evidence-based practice as a goal or future vision of practice and evidence for practice provides a more immediate approach to promote evidence-informed practice, and 3) a recognition that evidence-informed practice is part of building agency-based knowledge sharing systems that involve the tacit and explicit knowledge needed to improve the outcomes of social services.

This book was previously published as a special issue of the *Journal Of Evidence-Based Social Work.*

Michael J. Austin is the Milton and Florence Krenz Mack Professor of Nonprofit Management at the School of Social Welfare, University of California, Berkeley. He is the former dean of the University of Pennsylvania School of Social Work, and teaches in the area of non-profit and public sector management, community planning and the social environment dimensions of human behavior and the social environment.

Evidence for Child Welfare Practice

Edited by Michael J. Austin

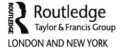
Routledge
Taylor & Francis Group
LONDON AND NEW YORK

First published 2010 by Routledge
270 Madison Avenue, New York, NY 10016

Simultaneously published in the UK
by Routledge
2 Park Square, Milton Park, Abingdon, Oxon, OX14 4RN

Routledge is an imprint of the Taylor & Francis Group, an informa business

© 2010 Edited by Michael J. Austin

Typeset in Times by Value Chain, India
Printed and bound in Great Britain by MPG Books Group

British Library Cataloguing in Publication Data
A catalogue record for this book is available from the British Library

ISBN10: 0-7890-3814-5 (hbk)
ISBN10: 0-7890-3815-3 (pbk)
ISBN13: 978-0-7890-3814-2 (hbk)
ISBN13: 978-0-7890-3815-9 (pbk)

CONTENTS

CHILD WELFARE OUTCOMES

PART II

EVIDENCE FOR MANAGEMENT PRACTICE

Introduction

Michael J. Austin, PhD

The growing interest in evidence-based practice has generated discussion in a wide variety of journals related to such questions as to "how do you define it?," "how to do it?," "how to teach it?," and "how do you evaluate its feasibility and outcomes?". Those who support it draw heavily on the pioneering work of Sackett and colleagues who define evidence-based practice as a "conscientious, explicit, and judicious use of current best evidence in making decisions about individuals" along with special attention to the values and expectations of clients (Sackett, Straus, & Richardson, 1997).

This book builds upon these questions and definitions within the context of child welfare practice by attempting to step back from the challenges of implementing evidence-based practice by raising a slightly different set of questions. These include:

1. What do we mean by "best evidence" in the social services and particularly in public child welfare?
2. What do we mean by "practice" that features evidence-based decision-making, especially in the context of child welfare that includes direct services to individuals, inter-agency collaboration, and the management of organizational processes?
3. Given the complexity of engaging in evidence-based practice, to what extent should it be viewed as a future goal or vision of practice rather than something that can be implemented tomorrow?

Michael J. Austin is Mack Professor of Nonprofit Management, School of Social Welfare, University of California, Berkeley.

In seeking to address these questions, this book reflects some preliminary conclusions based on a collaboration between universities and eleven county social service agencies that are part of a Bay Area Social Services Consortium (BASSC) founded in 1987. Given the limited and uneven support of child welfare research in the U.S. over the past half century, it is increasingly clear that evidence-based child welfare continues to be a goal or vision of future practice. While the search for "best evidence" is a challenge even in the most highly funded areas of health care research, it is even more challenging in the field of child welfare with its limited number of studies based on random control trials (RCTs). While we now have international databases in health (Cochrane Collaborative) and social sciences (Campbell Collaborative) designed to feature the results of systematic reviews of RCTs and other types of study designs, there are large holes in the databases related to the limited number of RCTs in the social welfare component of the social sciences. It is clear that more expanded research funding is needed in social welfare (and child welfare in particular) in order to use the most rigorous research methods as well as other methods to address complex service delivery issues. In the meantime, however, it is increasingly clear that we need to "spread the net" as widely as possible to capture a wide range of research that may reflect less rigor than is found in RCTs.

In addition to the interests in the research community related to rigorous research methods, another source of interest in evidence-based practice emerged in the social service practice community. As practitioners noticed that their colleagues in mental health and health care are being called upon by their accrediting bodies, government accountability mandates, and the pressures of managed care to engage in more evidence-based practice, it became clear that those in the public social services would soon be called upon to do the same. The federal standards for child welfare outcomes are only the beginning of this movement to raise questions about the evidentiary foundation of current practice. In addition, dependency court judges are increasingly interested in seeing if the court reports of child welfare workers might also include relevant research, in addition to expert professional judgment. In response to these new realities, social service agency directors are interested in finding ways to support their staff members (and those with whom they contract for services) with an increased understanding of evidence-based practice. And finally, since changes in professional education often follow innovations is practice, university faculty members and agency trainers are also challenged to find ways to help students and staff assess research in a way that would inform practice.

In the light of these challenges, the contents of this book (developed between 2004 and 2006 with funding from BASSC, the Zellerbach Family Fund, and the VanLobenSels/RembeRock Foundation) place more emphasis on "evidence for practice" than on evidence--based practice. The strategy involves structured literature reviews (made transparent by the explicit use of search terms, database identification, and inter-rater reliability checks on the description and interpretation of findings in searches that yielded large numbers of studies) in contrast to the use of systematic reviews conducted for the international collaboratives related to evidence-based practice. Structured reviews include the assessment of multiple types of research (evidence resulting from qualitative and quantitative studies) that are relevant to direct practice with clients and the management of social services. Each structured review in this book began with a general question; such as "what does research tell us about the disproportionate number of children of color entering the public child welfare system?" or "what does research tell us about the challenges of disseminating and utilizing research findings in daily practice?" The goal of each review was to provide a synthesis of the most rigorous and relevant research (when available), the identification of major themes, and the specification of preliminary implications for practice. While structured reviews are quite common, the unique features of these reviews are that they are driven by the needs of practice and reflect an attempt to summarize available research within a short timeframe for a practice audience. Vulnerable child welfare populations have urgent and immediate needs and practitioners are increasingly being pressed to identify and implement evidence-based interventions. Another key aspect of these structured reviews is the identification of the many gaps in the research and the need for more and more rigorous research.

In addition to our approach to structured reviews in order to provide evidence for practice, it is also important to identify research that would inform the future implementation of evidence-base practice. While considerable attention has been given in the UK to training staff to engage in evidence-based practice, it became increasingly clear that attention would also need to be given to the organizational and managerial supports for staff engaged in evidence-based practice. While some argue that line staff should be trained to identify, select, assess, and incorporate research findings, the magnitude of such an endeavor in the light of heavy agency service delivery demands is so great as to overwhelm the most talented among us. Therefore, we take the view that researchers located in our universities are in the best position to conduct the reviews while agency practitioners are in the best position to: (1) identify topics or questions to guide a search, (2) assess the utility of structured reviews, and (3) to identify potential uses of such reviews provided they are given the organizational supports needed to engage in evidence-based practice on a daily basis. In essence, without managerial support, this new form of practice would be difficult to implement.

This line of inquiry led us to explore the idea of evidence for management practice with a focus on how research is used to inform managerial decision-making. Since the bulk of the research appears in the literature of the for-profit sector, it became clear that we were searching in the area of knowledge management. We began with the following questions: (1) how is research disseminated and utilized?, (2) what is the impact of an organizational change (like evidence-based practice) on the organization's culture, (3) which human service agencies in the U.S. have implemented evidence-based practice and what has been their experience?, and (4) what is the difference between tacit practitioner knowledge and explicit research-based knowledge and how are these two managed?

In the light of these questions, the chapters in this book are organized in two categories; namely, evidence for direct practice and evidence for management practice. In Part I, the chapters are divided into two categories. The first relates to the complex area of child welfare assessment where we identify research findings related to the use of various assessment instruments; namely, child risk and safety, family functioning, and child and youth well-being. In addition, we looked at some of the outcomes of risk assessment to learn more about the disproportional number of children from communities of color who enter the child welfare system. In the second section of Part I, we focus on the other end of the continuum of service where outcomes are assessed; namely, outcome measurement, outcomes of parent education programs (a frequent referral source in child welfare), and outcomes of substance abuse treatment programs. Most of the chapters in Part I are brief versions of larger reports that can be accessed on the BASSC Website <www.bassc.net>.

In Part II, the focus is on organizational issues that relate to evidence for management practice. This section includes an overview of evidence-based practice from an organizational perspective along with evidence related to the experiences of others in implementing evidence-based practice. The remaining chapters draw heavily upon social science research related to the dissemination and utilization of research, research on organizational change and its impact on organizational culture, and research on sharing tacit and explicit knowledge within the context of knowledge management.

The purpose of this book is to capture the micro (direct services) and macro (managerial) perspectives that relate to identifying evidence for practice within the practice domain of public child welfare. While it emerged out of local interests in the San Francisco Bay Area, it should have relevance throughout the country because it draws upon national databases. While our research team attempted to locate all relevant sources of data, it is quite possible that some were missed or have appeared following our search. Our primary approach to electronic database searching means that hand-searching of documents was quite limited with the exception of selected book chapters.

It should also be noted that the vast majority of work reflected in these pages was conducted by a very talented group of current and former doctoral students and I want to acknowledge the project leadership roles carried out so effectively by Amy D'Andrade, PhD (Assistant Professor, School of Social Work, San Jose State University), Kathy Lemon Osterling, PhD (Assistant Professor, School of Social Work, San Jose State University), and Michelle A. Johnson, soon-to-be PhD (School of Social Welfare, University of California, Berkeley). In addition, Susan Stone, PhD (Assistant Professor, School of Social Welfare, University of California, Berkeley) and Barbara Needell, PhD (Senior Research Specialist, Center for Social Welfare Research, School of Social Welfare, University of California, Berkeley) each played a significant role in helping us conceptualize several of the structured reviews.

Our collective efforts represent an attempt to push the discussion of evidence-based practice in several new directions regarding: (1) the use of structured reviews to complement the systematic reviews of RCTs and related designs carried out by the Cochrane and Campbell Collaboratives, (2) the process of viewing the call for evidence-based practice as a goal or future vision of practice that includes both micro and macro practice implications, and (3) a recognition that evidence-based practice is not simply a set of important activities carried out by individual practitioners but rather a part of a larger knowledge management system of sharing tacit and explicit knowledge to improve the outcomes of social services.

REFERENCE

Sackett, D.L., Straus, S.E., & Richardson, W.S. (1997). Evidence-based medicine: How to practice and teach EBM. NY: Churchill Livingston.

PART I

EVIDENCE FOR DIRECT PRACTICE

Understanding and Addressing Racial/Ethnic Disproportionality in the Front End of the Child Welfare System

Kathy Lemon Osterling, PhD
Amy D'Andrade, PhD
Michael J. Austin, PhD

SUMMARY. Racial/ethnic disproportionality in the child welfare system is a complicated social problem that is receiving increasing amounts of attention from researchers and practitioners. This review of the literature examines disproportionality in the front-end of the child welfare system and interventions that may address it. While none of the interventions had evidence suggesting that they reduced disproportionality in child welfare front-end processes, some of the interventions may im-

Kathy Lemon Osterling is Doctoral Research Assistant, Amy D'Andrade is BASSC Research Director, and Michael J. Austin is Professor, Bay Area Social Services Consortium, Center for Social Services Research, School of Social Welfare, University of California, Berkeley.

prove child welfare case processes related to disproportionality and outcomes for families of color.

KEYWORDS. Racial/ethnic disproportionality, child welfare, interventions, front-end processes

INTRODUCTION

Racial/ethnic disproportionality in the child welfare system is a complicated social problem that is receiving increasing amounts of attention from researchers and practitioners. While disproportionality and disparities in outcomes exist throughout the child welfare system, a substantial portion is introduced through front end processes such as referral, investigation, substantiation and placement into care. Little is known about what kinds of interventions might be effective in reducing disproportionality at these decision points. This review of the literature examines the nature of disproportionality in the front-end of the child welfare system and the interventions that may address it.

Disproportionality In The Front End Of The Child Welfare System Research suggests that children of color tend to be disproportionately represented in the child welfare system as a whole, as well as at various decision points or stages within the system (Hines, Lemon, Wyatt & Merdinger, 2004; Kemp & Bodonyi, 2002; Needell, Brookhart & Lee, 2003; Wells & Guo, 1999). There is also evidence to suggest that children of color, and in particular African American children, tend to have longer stays in out-of-home care, receive less comprehensive services and are less likely to reunify than white children (Courtney, Barth, Berrick, Brooks, Needell, & Park, 1996; Hines, Lee, Drabble, Snowden, & Lemon, 2002; Jones, 1998; Wells & Guo, 1999).

Figures 1 and 2 show that African American and Native American children are over-represented in the child welfare system, while white children tend to be under-represented, both nationally and within California. Hispanic/Latino children are neither over- nor under-represented in the child welfare system nationally, but in California they are somewhat under-represented, as are Asian American children (Needell, Webster, Cuccaro-Alamin, Armijo, Lee, & Lery, 2004; U.S. Department of Health and Human Services, 2002).

To better understand disproportionality in the child welfare system, it can be helpful to consider the various case decision points throughout

FIGURE 1. Racial/Ethnic Disproportionality in the U.S. Child Welfare System

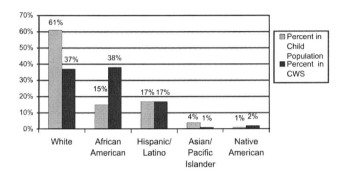

FIGURE 2. Racial/Ethnic Disproportionality in the California Child Welfare System

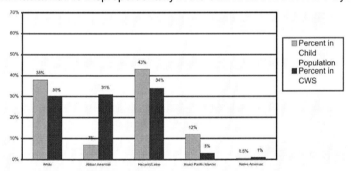

the system separately (Derezotes & Poertner, 2005). This article focuses on the four major decision-making points in the front-end of the system. First, a community resident or mandated reporter decides whether to make a referral to the child welfare system. Once a referral is made, child welfare workers must decide: (1) whether to investigate the report, (2) if investigated, whether to substantiate the allegation of maltreatment or dismiss the case, and (3) if substantiated, whether to place a child in out-of-home care.

Some research suggests that children of color are referred, investigated, substantiated, and placed in care at a higher rate than white children. California data, for instance, reflect dramatic differences in rates of referral. The incidence of referral per 1,000 children in the population for African Americans is 100.6, compared to 45.5 for white children,

45.6 for Hispanic children, 18.2 for Asian American children and 56.4 for Native American children (see Figure 3) (Needell et al., 2004).

In other studies, referrals of children of color have been found to be investigated at a higher rate than referrals involving white children (Fluke, Yuan, Hedderson & Curtis, 2003; Wells, Fluke & Brown, 1995); to have an elevated likelihood of substantiation compared to white children (Ards, Myers, Malkis, Sugrue, & Zhou, 2003; Drake, 1996; Eckenrode, Powers, Doris, Munsch, & Bolger, 1988; Rolock & Testa, 2005); and black children were found to be more likely than white children to enter out-of-home care (Hill, 2005; Needell, Brookhart & Lee, 2003). California administrative data show distinctly different rates of placement into foster care for African American and Native American children. As noted in Figure 4, Native American (41.9%) and African American children (41.7%) are most likely to be placed out of the home, followed by whites (32.9%), Hispanics (29.2%) and Asian Americans (25.0%) (Needell et al., 2004).

THEORIES AND RELATED INTERVENTIONS

Although the existence of racial/ethnic disproportionality in child welfare is clear, the reasons for it are not. A number of theories have been developed to explain disproportionality. Regarding disproportionality in the front end of the child welfare system, one theory asserts that bias and inconsistencies in decisions made by the referring community and child welfare agency staff result in disproportionality. A second

FIGURE 3. Referral Incidence in California by Ethnicity

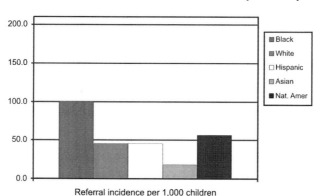

Referral incidence per 1,000 children

FIGURE 4. Cases Investigated, Substantiated, and Placed in California by Ethnicity

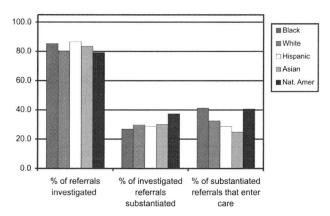

theory suggests that poverty and experiences of oppression in communities of color result in greater stress and higher rates of maltreatment, and thus greater representation in the child welfare system. A third theory focuses on the stressful and sometimes chaotic nature of child welfare agency practice and its relationship to disproportionality. Based upon these theories, a variety of interventions that may affect disproportionality have been developed.

To identify these interventions, we used specific search terms and searched numerous social science and academic databases available through the University of California library. In addition, we searched websites specializing in systematic reviews, as well as research institutes, conference proceedings databases, dissertation databases, and conducted general internet searches. In order to gather information on research that has not been published, inquiries were sent to professional email lists serving professional evaluators and child maltreatment researchers. Since the interventions to address disproportionality in child welfare are so new, they were broadly defined as programs, practices, or strategies. The term "addressing disproportionality" was also broadly defined as those interventions that were directly aimed at reducing disproportionality or those that indirectly addressed disproportionality by improving outcomes for children and families of color.

Bias and Inconsistencies in Decision-Making

The notion that bias and inconsistencies are behind racial/ethnic discrepancies in child welfare is supported by several national studies suggesting that there are no racial/ethnic differences in the occurrence of child maltreatment (Sedlak & Broadhurst, 1996). The National Incidence Studies (NIS) conducted in 1980, 1986 and 1993 are federally funded studies that estimate the number of children who are maltreated in the U.S. The NIS uses two sources of information: 1) child welfare system data and 2) community professionals likely to encounter cases of child maltreatment that may not necessarily be reported to the child welfare system. The NIS is believed to provide more accurate estimates of child maltreatment than estimates derived solely from child welfare system data. All three NIS studies have found child maltreatment to be unrelated to race/ethnicity. In a later study using NIS-3 data, racial/ethnic differences in the incidence of child maltreatment were explored in conjunction with demographic risk factors such as income, number of children in a household, and employment status. After controlling for these risk factors, African American families were found to have less risk of child maltreatment than White families (Sedlak & Schulz 2005a).

And yet, studies have shown increased rates of referral, investigation, substantiation, and placement for children of color, even after controlling for other explanatory variables such as poverty (Ards et al., 2003; Chasnoff, Landress, & Barrett, 1990; Drake, 1996; Needell et al., 2003; Sedlak & Schulz, 2005b; Willis & Wells, 1988; Zellman, 1992). Some argue that disproportionality instead may be due to bias and inconsistency in staff decision-making.

RELATED INTERVENTIONS

Risk assessment tools. The use of risk assessments to guide child welfare decision-making has grown steadily in recent years. The goal is to help predict the risk of future harm in order to provide appropriate services to a family (Hollinshead & Fluke, 2000). There are two major types of risk assessment tools: (1) consensus-based systems, which are based on the consensus of risk assessment judgments made by experts in the field; and (2) actuarial systems, which are based on empirical evidence of factors statistically associated with future maltreatment (Baird & Wagner, 2000).

Many California counties use an actuarial tool called the California Family Risk Assessment (CFRA). Findings from several studies suggest that the CFRA accurately classifies families into risk categories (Baird & Wagner, 2000; Johnson, 2004). Additionally, research indicates that the risk assessments completed by staff using the CFRA are equally valid for white children and families of color (Johnson, 2004). Additionally, in one jurisdiction using an actuarial risk assessment tool developed by the Children's Research Center, disproportionality of African American children existing at early case decision points (referral and substantiation) was significantly less at case opening, the decision point at which workers utilized the CRC risk assessment tool (Baird, 2005). These findings suggest that actuarial risk assessment instruments like the CFRA may contribute to reducing bias in child welfare decision-making and thereby have potential to reduce disproportionality.

Family group conferencing. In cases where maltreatment is substantiated and decisions regarding child placement and safety must be made, family group conferencing (also referred to as Family Group Decision Making) has been adopted as an inclusive, strengths-based approach to improve decision-making. Family group conferencing began in New Zealand as a response to the overrepresentation of Maori children in systems of care and in 1989 the New Zealand government mandated its use in both juvenile justice and child welfare systems (Waites, Macgowan, Pennell, Carlton-LaNey, & Weil, 2004). This intervention is based on the premise that families have the right to be involved with decisions about their children and that family members and others involved in the child's life can help create a better plan for the child (Sundell & Vinnerljung, 2004).

The inclusive nature of family group conferencing may not only improve decision-making but also increase the engagement of families of color. Studies have reported that family group conferences are culturally compatible with culturally diverse groups (Waites et al., 2004) and that the practice may result in a fairly high level of client satisfaction (Sieppert, Hudson, & Unrau, 2000). One study found that after implementing the family group conferencing model, the number of children of color who entered the child welfare system was reduced (Crampton & Jackson, 1999). However, not all research supports the effectiveness of family group conferencing. For example, children in Sweden who received family group conferences (compared to a group receiving traditional child welfare services) actually experienced higher rates of out-of-home placement as well as higher rates of subsequent episodes of substantiated maltreatment based on a three year follow-up study (Sundell & Vinnerljung, 2004).

Improving cultural competence. Some researchers and practitioners note that white, middle class family values tend to be the standard by which culturally diverse parents and children are compared (Miller & Gaston, 2003). As such, children and families exhibiting alternative cultural values or those experiencing circumstances such as poverty or single parenthood may be seen as deviant in the child welfare system (Miller & Gaston, 2003; Pinderhughes, 1989). Green defines cultural competence as the ability to "deliver professional services in a way that is congruent with the behavior and expectations normative for a given community and that are adapted to suit the specific needs of individuals and families from that community" (1999, p. 87). Acknowledging and incorporating cultural responsiveness into the delivery of services may reduce bias in decision-making and improve the effectiveness of child welfare services for children and families of color (Derezotes & Snowden, 1990; McPhatter & Ganaway, 2003; McPhatter, 1997; Miller & Gaston, 2003; Pierce & Pierce, 1996).

One way to approach this task is to increase the diversity of the workforce. A child welfare workforce that is reflective of the ethnicity of the agency's clients may help to improve child welfare outcomes (U.S. Department of Health and Human Services, 2003). Research from psychology suggests that racial/ethnic matching of therapist and client may have some benefits, such as lower rates of treatment drop-out, better attendance, and better therapeutic outcomes (Flaskerud, 1986; Sue, 1998).

A second strategy is to improve the cultural competence of child welfare staff members in order to become more effective in working with culturally diverse clients (Derezotes & Snowden, 1990). Increasing the cultural competence of child welfare staff may reduce disproportionality and improve outcomes for children and families of color by improving decision-making and overall service provision. However, there is little research linking the use of cultural competence training programs to improved outcomes for children and families of color. Outcome evaluations of a program in Washington State aimed at improving the cultural competence of workers are currently underway but are not yet available (McKenna & Trujillo, 2004).

POVERTY AND OPPRESSION OF FAMILIES OF COLOR

The disproportionate representation of children of color in the child welfare system may have another explanation. Risk factors such as poverty, living in impoverished neighborhoods, or single parent status have been shown to be associated with child welfare system involvement

(Coulton, Korbin, Su, & Chow, 1995; Coulton, Korbin & Su, 1999; Hines et al., 2002); African Americans and Hispanics are more likely than Whites to live in impoverished neighborhoods (Jargowsky, 2003). The provision of adequate resources and supports to families of color to prevent maltreatment and removal of children from the home could reduce disproportionality and increase the well-being of vulnerable children and families. However, child welfare resources directed toward prevention represent only a small proportion of all child welfare resources. Moreover, during difficult economic times, prevention programs are often the target of budget cuts (Thomas, Leicht, Hughes, Madigan & Dowell, 2002). Thomas et al. (2002) note that the level of prevention services currently available is inadequate in both secondary and tertiary prevention services. Secondary prevention focuses on providing services to families that have risk factors for child maltreatment, but have not yet been reported to the child welfare system. Tertiary prevention focuses on providing services to families who have already been reported to the child welfare system for maltreatment.

According to this theory, poverty (and other risk factors) combined with a lack of adequate prevention services bring African American children to the attention of the child welfare system in greater numbers than children whose families are not confronting the same stressors. These problems and stressors can contribute to the differences in referral, investigation, substantiation, and placement rates for families of color.

Related Interventions

Differential response. Differential response, also referred to as alternative response or dual response provides child welfare agencies with greater flexibility in responding to reports of child maltreatment. Only reports that involve clear and imminent danger to the child or that involve potential criminal charges are put on the "investigation track." Less serious reports are put on the "assessment track" in which families are offered intensive and culturally appropriate services (Schene, 2001). The non-confrontational and supportive nature of engaging families whose children are not in imminent danger represents a more responsive service strategy for culturally diverse children and families who may be distrustful of the child welfare system. Differential response systems also help to keep out of the system those families whose children are not in imminent danger.

The use of differential response has grown considerably in recent years and these systems have been identified as a strategy to help reduce disproportionality (U.S. DHHS, 2003). Evaluations suggest that differential response systems are effective in producing positive outcomes in certain areas, such as greater satisfaction with services (Institute of Applied Research, 2004), reduction of child maltreatment reports (Loman & Siegel, 2004; Siegel & Loman, 2000), improved child behavior and fewer problems with alcohol, drugs or domestic violence for families who participate in services (Institute of Applied Research, 2004). Related to disproportionality, other studies have found that services appeared to be received equally well by white families and families of color (Institute of Applied Research, 2004).

Out-stationing child welfare workers. One way to establish strong partnerships between the child welfare system and community resources is to locate child welfare staff within family-focused neighborhood-based agencies. Locating child welfare staff within such settings may help to foster a less stigmatized location for public social services to help families feel more comfortable with accessing these services (Daro, 2003). Locating staff within community centers and schools can also provide an opportunity for workers to educate colleagues in other settings about the child welfare system in order to reduce the number of inappropriate referrals coming into the system (U.S. DHHS, 2003). However, there is no direct evidence that out-stationing child welfare workers results in reductions in disproportionality or improved outcomes for children and families of color.

Neighborhood-based ethnic-specific services. These services are designed to respond to the cultural needs of specific ethnic groups by: (1) locating services in ethnic communities, (2) employing bicultural and bilingual staff, and (3) incorporating cultural customs, values and beliefs into agency practices (Sue, 1998). The following evidence suggests that ethnic-specific services may be a useful strategy with culturally diverse families: (a) clients perceive staff from non-ethnic agencies as unfriendly and not understanding of their cultures or their language, (b) clients are unable to trust such agencies, and (c) clients perceive the staff as too busy to provide quality services (Holley, 2003). In another study, clients who participated in ethnic-specific services had lower drop-out rates and stayed in programs longer than those in mainstream services (Sue, 1998).

Leaders of ethnic agencies report several inter-related reasons why community members prefer ethnic-specific agencies; namely, shared cultures and experiences, specific cultural elements within agency programs (dances, stories, food, holidays and cultural history), shared language, and the strong commitment of staff who are also members of the ethnic community (Holley, 2003).

Home visitation services. Although variations exist, most home visitation programs seek to improve parenting and health outcomes of parents and their young children by providing emotional and problem-solving support and concrete assistance. The research suggests that home visitation services are linked to a variety of positive outcomes among children and mothers, including child maltreatment outcomes (Olds, Eckenrode, Henderson, Kitzman, Powers, Cole et al., 1997). In addition, there is evidence to suggest that home visitation services may be effective with families of color. Several studies have found improved outcomes, including greater access to services and a slight improvement in psychological well-being among African American mothers (Kitzman Olds, Henderson, Hanks, Cole, Tatelbaum et al., 1997; Marcenko, Spence, Samost, 1996). There is also evidence to suggest that home visitation programs are better able to retain the involvement of families of color than they are for white families (Daro McCurdy, Falconnier, & Stojanovic, 2003; McGuigan Katzev, & Pratt, 2003).

However, not all research has supported the effectiveness of home visitation programs. In an evaluation of Hawaii's Healthy Start Program, few effects on child maltreatment were found (Duggan, Fuddy, Burrell, Higman, McFarlane, Windham et al., 2004). In addition, an eighteen-month follow-up evaluation focused on the effectiveness of a postnatal home visiting program using nurses, social workers and parent aides for those at risk of child abuse and neglect revealed no significant differences between parents receiving the intervention and those in the control group on measures of parenting stress, parenting competence and quality of the home environment (Fraser, Armstrong, Morris, & Dadds, 2000). Other studies suggest that the positive benefits of home visitation programs may be mediated by other risk factors such as domestic violence. For example, in an analysis of the Nurse Family Partnership Program, results indicated that mothers in the home visitation program who reported more than 28 incidents of domestic violence during a 15-year follow-up period did not experience a reduced likelihood of verified child maltreatment (Eckenrode, Ganzel, Henderson, Smith, Olds, Powers et al., 2000). These results suggest that different risk factors may impact outcomes for home visitation program participants.

Increasing involvement of fathers in child welfare services. Most research suggests that African American families in the child welfare system are primarily headed by mothers (Sedlak & Broadhurst, 1996). In a review of the literature on the involvement of fathers in child welfare services, it was found that caseworkers tend to tailor services to mothers and focus more attention on mothers than on fathers; and that the judicial system, with its preference for keeping children with their primary caretakers, may ignore fathers as a potential placement option (Sonenstein, Malm, & Billing, 2002). Moreover, there are no national standard procedures for establishing paternity, making the identification of non-custodial parents difficult (Sonenstein et al., 2002).

Efforts to increase the involvement of fathers, especially non-custodial fathers, may help stabilize these families so that further child welfare system involvement is unnecessary. In addition, involving fathers expands the potential supports for the mother and child because of the father's kin network. Some practices currently underway include the coordination of child welfare and child support services, involving incarcerated fathers in services, improving fathers' parenting skills, and utilizing non-custodial fathers as placement alternatives when children cannot be placed with their custodial mother (Sonenstein et al., 2002). However, no evaluation data on these programs are yet available.

SYSTEM-RELATED FACTORS

A third "theory" regarding disproportionality in child welfare suggests that system-related factors (e.g., agency infrastructure, organizational culture, resources, and leadership) can influence the delivery of child welfare services and thereby impact on racial/ethnic disproportionality. Research suggests that these system-related factors affect the quality of services delivered and outcomes within child welfare settings (Glisson & Hemmelgarn, 1998; Glisson & James, 2002; Grasso, 1994; Smith & Donovan, 2003; Yoo, 2002). Child welfare organizations with high workloads and staff turnover can be chaotic and crisis-driven environments (Smith & Donovan, 2003; Vinokur-Kaplan & Hartman, 1986). The American Humane Association (2000) reports that workloads in family maintenance programs are approximately three times the optimum recommended workloads; family reunification programs are at approximately twice the recommended optimum workloads; and permanent placement programs are at approximately three times recommended optimum workloads.

These system-related factors affect job satisfaction and the quality of services delivered. In one study investigating the impact of organizational culture within an agency serving children and families indicated that a positive organizational climate (low conflict, high degree of cooperation, role clarity, personalization and low conflict) was related to better service quality and improved client outcomes (Glisson & Hemmelgarn, 1998). Similarly, Yoo (2002) investigated the relationship between child welfare organizational variables and client outcomes and found that employees tended to rate their job satisfaction as low in relationship to heavy workloads and high job stress. They also reported an overall lack of leadership in the organization where feelings of disconnection between workers and management led to an overall chaotic working environment. In the 2003 federal government report on children and families of color in the child welfare system (U.S. Department of Health and Human Services, 2003), participants noted an overall lack of agency resources as a contributing factor to racial/ethnic disproportionality and poor outcomes for children and families of color.

Related Interventions

Leadership and sustained commitment to reducing disproportionality. Strong organizational leadership and a sustained commitment to addressing disproportionality may help bring about the organizational changes needed to better serve children and families of color. Since organizational leaders can set the overall tone of the organization, agency administrators and managers need to be integral to improving services to children and families of color (Mcphatter & Ganaway, 2003). Significant commitments of time and resources are necessary to integrate culturally competent practices and social justice values into agency environments (Chesler, 1994; Hyde, 2004; Mederos & Woldeguiorguis, 2003). Although studies focusing on the links between leadership and a sustained commitment to reduce disproportionality in the child welfare system are not available, a recent inquiry into factors related to closing the racial/ethnic educational achievement gap among Bay Area schools in California suggests that strong leadership and sustained commitment are critical factors for schools that have successfully improved educational outcomes for children of color (Symonds, 2003). Evaluations in the child welfare system are currently underway but are not yet available (Ramsey County Community Human Services Department, 2004).

Organizational re-structuring through vertical case management. Most child welfare agencies use a traditional hierarchical organizational structure in which specific tasks within the organization are allocated to various units. As a case comes into the system, one worker screens the case, another investigates, a different worker facilitates family reunification or family preservation services, and yet another worker facilitates permanency planning services. This service model can hinder the ability of workers to form the types of collaborative relationships with clients necessary for culturally competent practices. In contrast, the vertical case management model assigns the same worker to oversee all phases of the family's involvement with the child welfare system. In agencies that have implemented this model as a way to reduce disproportionality, workers have reported it to be particularly effective for culturally diverse families (U.S. Department of Health and Human Services, 2003).

Collaborations with racial/ethnic communities. Improved collaborations between the child welfare system and racial/ethnic communities may also help improve outcomes for children and families of color and reduce disproportionality. Such collaborations involve concerted outreach efforts to diverse communities, an area that is largely neglected in child welfare practice (Woodroffe & Spencer, 2003). Improved collaboration and communication can be mutually beneficial; agencies can gain information on how to tailor services to communities of color and these communities can learn about the role of the child welfare system (U.S. Department of Health and Human Services, 2003). In human service agencies that have successfully integrated multicultural and social justice values into their organizations, outreach activities to client populations were the key aspects of successful implementation (Hyde, 2003). Research on the impact of these efforts on reducing disproportionality is underway (Ramsey County Community Human Services Department, 2004). Figure 5 summarizes each of the three theories and the interventions related to them.

Considering the Nature of Available Evidence

The available evidence regarding the effectiveness of these interventions is limited. Few studies attempted to determine whether interventions affected disproportionality rates. Most studies assessed whether some child welfare case process was improved by the intervention or whether the intervention worked well for children and families of color.

None of the interventions had evidence suggesting that they reduced disproportionality in child welfare front-end processes. However, there was evidence that three of the interventions improved the following as-

FIGURE 5. Summary of Interventions by Theory

Theory #1: BIAS	*Theory #2:* POVERTY	*Theory #3:* SYSTEMS
Actuarial Risk Assessment	Differential Response	Leadership
Family Group Conferencing	Out-Stationing Social Workers	Vertical Case Management
Improving Cultural Competence	Ethnic-Specific Services	Community Collaborations
	Home Visiting	
	Involving Fathers	

pects of child welfare case processes related to disproportionality: (1) actuarial risk assessment tools appear to be more accurate at predicting the likelihood of maltreatment recurrence than clinical judgment or consensus-based risk assessment instruments, thereby reducing the chance of bias; (2) family group decision-making may result in reductions in the number of children of color entering foster care; and (3) differential response models may result in a decrease in child maltreatment reports, improvement in child behavior, and reductions in substance abuse and domestic violence problems.

The two interventions that appear to work well with children and families of color were: (1) ethnic-specific agencies, which had lower drop-out rates and longer participation time frames with families of color than did non-ethnic specific agencies; and (2) home visiting programs, which documented positive outcomes for African American mothers and increased retention for families of color over white families. The evidence for differential response suggests that clients of color were satisfied with the intervention. However, for many interventions there was no empirical research available regarding whether they reduced disproportionality, improved child welfare case processes related to disproportionality were especially effective with families of color or were well received by families of color. In some cases relevant research was pending. It is important to note that this categorization of interventions should not be interpreted as an evaluative assessment of their efficacy, especially since the evidence available for each intervention varies in its focus and quality. And finally, the effectiveness of any interventions depends upon the quality of its implementation.

IMPLICATIONS

Implications for Practice

Another model explaining disproportionality in child welfare proposes that there are multiple causes; African American families *are* at greater risk of child maltreatment, *and* problems with agency decision-making (along with other factors) contribute to the problem (Barth, 2005). If this is the case, attempts to achieve sustained reductions in racial/ethnic disproportionality may benefit from the implementation of a variety of interventions related to several of the theories noted. For example, the Family-to-Family Initiative of the Annie E. Casey Foundation seeks to improve a variety of child welfare outcomes (e.g., reducing length of stay, re-entry to care, and placement moves.) An important new goal of this initiative is to reduce racial/ethnic disparities in outcomes. The Family-to-Family initiative utilizes several of the interventions described in this report, including collaborations with racial/ethnic communities, family group conferencing within the context of group decision-making, and leadership through sustained commitment in the form of self-evaluation teams that use data to focus and track agency efforts (Annie E. Casey Foundation, n.d.).

A second Casey initiative in the juvenile justice arena focuses on the disparities in detention rates by ethnicity. For example, the Santa Cruz County Probation Department utilized several interventions described in this report as part of that initiative: (1) agency administrative leaders made the goal of reducing disproportionality a primary organizational objective (leadership); (2) data at each key decision point was mapped and trends tracked quarterly (sustained commitment); (3) objective criteria for decisions made at each point were developed, aiming for a quantifiable set of risk factors (actuarial risk assessment); (4) cultural competence and staff diversity was enhanced (cultural competence training); (5) barriers to family involvement in case processes were eliminated; (6) alternatives to formal case handling and incarceration were developed (differential response); and (7) a full continuum of treatment, supervision and placement options was developed. Subsequently, Santa Cruz experienced an almost 20% reduction in the proportion of Latino/Hispanic youth in detention from 1998-2000, from 66% to 46%, in a community in which 33% of the youth population is Latino (Cox & Bell, 2001; Hoyt, Schiraldi, Smith, & Ziedenber, n.d.).

Linking together interventions that target a particular area is another way to maximize agency resources. For example, if most of the disproportionality in the front end of an agency's system was from referrals, the agency might target that decision point, using several interventions drawn from the different theories. For example, based upon the theory that greater poverty and stresses experienced by parents of color result in a higher maltreatment rate, the agency could make use of home-visiting services to aid poor parents with supports and services to relieve some of that stress. To address a lack of cultural sensitivity or awareness possibly behind the disproportionality of referrals from schools and hospitals, an agency could provide cultural competence training for staff in those institutions. Based on the theory that system factors contribute to disproportionality, collaborations with neighborhood communities could be used to improve relationships between agencies and communities in order to inform referring parties about community resources that might be of use to struggling families.

Implications for Research

Much work remains to be done in terms of understanding the causes of racial/ethnic disproportionality at the front end of the child welfare system as well as identifying the most effective interventions. Much of the research on disproportionality documents the disproportionate representation of various racial/ethnic groups throughout the service system as well as the differences in permanency outcomes, while relatively little investigates or tests theoretical explanations of disproportionality. While there is increasing attention to this area (see Derezotes, Poertner & Testa, 2005), more study is required before the field can be confident that causal factors underlying disproportionality are fully understood.

Evaluating the effectiveness of interventions intended to decrease racial/ethnic disproportionality in the child welfare system will benefit from collaborations between researchers and public agencies. Such studies need to explicitly articulate the theoretical foundation for the use of each intervention as well as the logic linking program inputs with anticipated outcomes. The best tests of the effectiveness of particular interventions would involve true experiments where clients are randomly assigned to an intervention so that any differences in decision-making practices and/or overall disproportionality rates could be ascribed to the intervention. Given the complex nature of both interventions and the effects of race and ethnicity, studies need to disentangle any differential effects that exist between the intervention, the environment in which it is implemented, and different racial/ethnic groups.

CONCLUSION

The preponderance of evidence in the literature indicates that cases involving children of color are referred, investigated, substantiated and placed out of the home at higher rates than cases involving white children. Bias and inconsistencies in decision-making may play a role, as may poverty and oppression in communities of color combined with the limited availability of prevention services. And agencies that fail to develop strong leadership, sustained commitment, and a work environment that facilitates high quality services provided by culturally competent staff may exacerbate disproportionality.

Although the child welfare community has been aware of racial/ethnic disproportionality for many years, there is a critical need for more research on interventions designed to reduce disproportionality. While no specific intervention has been shown to be effective in decreasing disproportionality in child welfare, this review of the literature should be a useful starting point for agencies to address the issue of racial/ethnic disproportionality at the front end of the child welfare system.

REFERENCES

Annie E. Casey Foundation (n.d.) Family to family tools for rebuilding foster care: Outcomes, goals and strategies.

Ards, S. D., Myers, S. L., Malkis, A., Sugrue, E., & Zhou, L.(2003). Racial disproportionality in reported and substantiated child abuse and neglect: An examination of systematic bias. *Children and Youth Services Review, 25*(5/6), 375-392.

Baird, C. & Wagner, D. (2000). The relative validity of actuarial- and consensus-based risk assessment systems. *Children and Youth Services Review, 22*(11/12), 839-871.

Baird, C. (2005). The effect of risk assessments and their relationship to maltreatment recurrence across races. In D.M. Derezotes, J. Poertner, & M.F.Testa (Eds.), *Race matters in child welfare: The overrepresentation of African American children in the system (pp. 131-146).* Washington D.C.: CWLA.

Barth, R.P. (2005). Child welfare and race: Models of disproportionality. In D.M. Derezotes, J. Poertner, & M.F. Testa (Eds.), *Race matters in child welfare: The overrepresentation of African American children in the system (pp. 25-46).* Washington DC: CWLA.

Chasnoff, I. J., Landress, H.J. & Barrett, M. E. (1990). The prevalence of illicit drug or alcohol use during pregnancies and discrepancies in mandatory reporting in Pinellas County, Florida. *The New England Journal of Medicine, 322,* 1202-1206.

Chesler, M. A. (1994). Strategies for multicultural organizational development. *The Diversity Factor,* 12-18.

Coulton, C. J., Korbin, J., Su, M., & Chow, J. (1995). Community level factors and child maltreatment rates. *Child Development, 66,* 1262-1276.

Coulton, C. J., Korbin, J. E. & Su, M. (1999). Neighborhoods and child maltreatment: A multi-level study. *Child Abuse and Neglect, 239*(11), 1019-1040.

Courtney, M. E., Barth, R. P., Berrick, J. D., Brooks, D., Needell, B., & Park, L. (1996). Race and child welfare services: Past research and future directions. *Child Welfare, 75*(2), 99-137.

Cox, J.A.& Bell, J. (2001). Addressing disproportionate representation of youth of color in the juvenile justice system. *Journal of the Center for Families, Children and the Courts,* v(3), 31-42.

Crampton, D. & Jackson, W. L. (1999). Beyond justice: Using family group decision making to address the over-representation of children of color in the child welfare system. *American Humane Association Family Group Decision Making Roundtable Proceedings.*

Daro, D., McCurdy, K., Falconnier, L., & Stojanovic, D. (2003). Sustaining new parents in home visitation services: Key participant and program factors. *Child Abuse and Neglect, 27*(10), 1101-1125.

Derezotes, D.M. & Poertner, J. (2005). Factors contributing to the overrepresentation of African American children in the child welfare system. In D.M. Derezotes, J. Poertner, & M.F. Testa (Eds.), *Race matters in child welfare: The overrepresentation of African American children in the system (pp. 131-146).* Washington D.C.: CWLA.

Derezotes, D.M., Poertner, J., & Testa, M.F. (2005). *Race matters in child welfare: The overrepresentation of African American children in the system.* Washington DC: CWLA.

Derezotes, D. S., & Snowden, L. R. (1990). Cultural factors in the intervention of child maltreatment. *Child and Adolescent Social Work Journal, 7*(2), 161-175.

Drake, B. (1996). Predictors of preventive services provision among unsubstantiated cases. *Child Maltreatment, 1*(2), 168-175.

Eckenrode, J., Powers, J., Doris, J., Munsch, J., & Bolger, N. (1988). Substantiation of child abuse and neglect reports. *Journal of Consulting and Clinical Psychology, 56*(1), 9-16.

Flaskerud, J. H. (1986). The effects of culture-compatible intervention on the utilization of mental health services to minority clients. *Community Mental Health Journal, 22*(2), 127-141.

Fluke, J. D., Yuan, Y. T., Hedderson, J., & Curtis, P. A. (2003). Disproportionate representation of race and ethnicity in child maltreatment: Investigation and victimization. *Children and Youth Services Review, 25*(5/6), 359-373.

Glisson, C. & Hemmelgarn, A. (1998). The effects of organizational climate and interorganizational coordination on the quality and outcomes of children's service systems. *Child Abuse and Neglect, 22*(5), 401-421.

Glisson, C. & James, L. R. (2002). The cross-level effects of culture and climate in human services teams. *Journal of Organizational Behavior, 23,* 767-794.

Grasso, A. J. (1994). Management style, job satisfaction, and service effectiveness. *Administration in Social Work, 18*(4), 89-105.

Green, J. W. (1999). *Cultural awareness in the human services: A multi-ethnic approach.* Boston: Allyn and Bacon.

Hill, R.B. (2005). The role of race in foster care placements. In D.M. Derezotes, J. Poertner, & M.F. Testa (Eds.), *Race matters in child welfare: The overrepresentation of African American children in the system (pp. 187-200)*. Washington D.C.: CWLA.

Hines, A. M., Lee, P. A., Drabble, L., Snowden, L. R., & Lemon, K. (2002). *An Evaluation of Factors Related to the Disproportionate Representation of Children of Color in Santa Clara County's Child Welfare System: Phase 2 Final Report.* Online, retrieved October 21, 2004 from: http://www2.sjsu.edu/depts/SocialWork/cwrt/

Hines, A. M., Lemon, K., Wyatt, P., & Merdinger, J.(2004). Factors related to the disproportionate involvement of children of color in the child welfare system: A review and emerging themes. *Children and Youth Services Review, 26*(6), 507-527.

Holley, L. C. (2003). The influence of ethnic awareness on ethnic agencies. *Administration in Social Work, 27*(3), 47-63.

Hollinshead, D. & J. Fluke (2000). What Works in Safety and Risk Assessment for CPS. *What Works in Child Welfare.* M. P. Kluger, G. Alexander & P. Curtis, A. Washington, DC, CWLA Press: 370.

Hoyt, E.H., Schiraldi, V., Smith, B.V. & Ziedenberg, J. (n.d.). *Pathways to juvenile detention reform: Reducing racial disparities in juvenile detention.* Baltimore, MD: The Annie E. Casey Foundation.

Hyde, C. A. (2003). Multicultural organizational development in nonprofit human services agencies: Views from the field. *Journal of Community Practice, 11*(1), 39-59.

Hyde, C. A. (2004). Multicultural organizational development in human service agencies: Challenges and solutions. *Social Work, 49*(1), 7-16.

Institute of Applied Research (2004). *Minnesota alternative response evaluation: Select interim evaluation findings.* Online, retrieved October 27, 2004 from: http://www.iarstl.org

Jargowsky, P. (2003). *Stunning progress, hidden problems: The dramatic decline of concentrated poverty in the 1990s.* Washington, DC: Brookings Institution.

Johnson, W. (2004). *Effectiveness of California's Child Welfare Structured Decision-Making (SDM) model: A prospective study of the validity of the California Family Risk Assessment.* Alameda County Social Services Agency.

Jones, L. (1998). The social and family correlates of successful reunification of children in foster care. *Children and Youth Services Review, 20*(4), 305-323.

Kemp, S. P. & Bodonyi, J. M. (2002). Beyond termination: Length of stay and predictors of permanency for legally free children. *Child Welfare, 81*(1), 59-86.

Kitzman, H., Olds, D.L., Henderson, C. R., Hanks, C., Cole, R., Tatelbaum, R., McConnochie, K. M., Sidora, K., Luckey, D. W., Shaver, D., Engelhardt, K., James, D., & Barnard, K. (1997). Effects of prenatal and infancy home visitation by nurses on pregnancy outcomes, childhood injuries, and repeated childbearing: A randomized controlled trial. *Journal of the American Medical Association, 278*(8), 644-652.

Loman, L. A., & Siegel, G. L. (2004). *Differential response in Missouri after five years.* Online, retrieved December 12, 2004 from: http://www.iarstl.org

Marcenko, M. O., Spence, M. & Samost, L. (1996). Outcomes of a home visitation trial for pregnant and postpartum women at-risk for child placement. *Children and Youth Services Review, 18*(3), 243-259.

McGuigan, W. M., Katzev, A. R. & Pratt, C. C. (2003). Multi-level determinants of retention in a home-visiting child abuse prevention program. *Child Abuse and Neglect, 27*(4), 363-380.

McKenna, M & Trujillo, I. (2004). *Frontline Connections quality improvement center: Project report.* Northwest Institute for Children and Families: University of Washington.

McPhatter, A. R. & Ganaway, T. L. (2003). Beyond the rhetoric: Strategies for implementing culturally effective practice with children, families, and communities. *Child Welfare, 82*(2), 103-124.

McPhatter, A. R. (1997). Cultural competence in child welfare: What is it? How do we achieve it? What happens without it? *Child Welfare, 76*(1), 255-278.

Mederos, F. & Woldeguiorguis, I. (2003). Beyond cultural competence: What child protection managers need to know and do. *Child Welfare, 82*(2), 125-142.

Miller, O. A. & Gaston, R. J. (2003). A model of culture-centered child welfare practice. *Child Welfare, 82*(2), 235-249.

Needell, B., Brookhart, M. A. & Lee, S. (2003). Black children and foster care placement in California. *Children and Youth Services Review, 25*(5/6), 393-408.

Needell, B., Webster, D., Cuccaro-Alamin, S., Armijo, M., Lee, S., Lery, B., Shaw, T., Dawson, W., Piccus, W., Magruder, J., & Kim, H. (2004). *Child Welfare Services Reports for California.* Retrieved October 21, 2004, from University of California at Berkeley Center for Social Services Research Website. URL: < http://cssr.berkeley.edu/CWSCMSreports/>.

Olds, D.L., Eckenrode, J., Henderson, C. R., Kitzman, H., Powers, J., Cole, R., Sidora, K., Morris, P., Pettitt, L. M., & Luckey, D. (1997). Long-term effects of home visitation on maternal life course and child abuse neglect: 15-year follow-up of a randomized trial. *Journal of the American Medical Association, 278*(8), 637-643.

Pierce, R. L. & Pierce, L. H. (1996). Moving toward cultural competence in the child welfare system. *Children and Youth Services Review, 18*(8), 713-731.

Pinderhuges, E. (1989). *Understanding race, ethnicity, and power: The key to efficacy in clinical practice.* New York: Free Press.

Rolock, N. & Testa, M.F. (2005). Indicated child abuse and neglect reports: Is the investigation process racially biased? In D.M. Derezotes, J. Poertner, & M.F.Testa (Eds.), *Race matters in child welfare: The overrepresentation of African American children in the system (pp. 119-130).* Washington D.C.: CWLA.

Schene, P. (2001). Meeting Each Family's Needs: Using Differential Response in Reports of Child Abuse and Neglect, Examples of Differential Response in Several States, Making Differential Response Work: Lessons Learned. *Best Practice/Next Practice, (Differential Response in Child Welfare),* 1-24.

Sedlak, A. J. & Broadhurst, D. D. (1996). *Third National Incidence Study of Child Abuse and Neglect.* Washington, DC: U.S. Department of Health and Human Services, National Center on Child Abuse and Neglect.

Sedlak, A. J. & Schulz, D. (2005a). *Race differences in risk of maltreatment in the general child population.* In D.M. Derezotes, J. Poertner, & M.F. Testa (Eds.), *Race matters in child welfare: The overrepresentation of African American children in the system (pp. 47-62).* Washington DC: CWLA.

Sedlak, A. J. & Schulz, D. (2005b). *Race differences in child protective investigations of abused and neglected children.* In D.M. Derezotes, J. Poertner, & M.F. Testa (Eds.), *Race matters in child welfare: The overrepresentation of African American children in the system (pp. 97-118).* Washington DC: CWLA.

Sieppert, J. D., Hudson, J. & Unrau, Y. (2000). Family Group Conferencing in Child Welfare: Lessons from a Demonstration Project. *Families in Society: The Journal of Contemporary Human Services, 81*(4), 382-391.

Smith, B. D. & Donovan, S. E. F. (2003). Child welfare practice in organizational & institutional context. *Social Services Review, 77*(4), 541-563.

Sonenstein, F., Malm, K. & Billing, A. (2002). *Study of fathers' involvement in permanency planning and child welfare casework.* Online, retrieved April 17, 2003 from: http://aspe.hhs.gov

Sue, S. (1998). In search of cultural competence in psychotherapy and counseling. *American Psychology, 53*(4), 440-448.

Sundell, K. & Vinnerljung, B. (2004). Outcomes of Family Group Conferencing in Sweden: A 3-year follow-up. *Child Abuse and Neglect, 28*(3), 267-287.

Symonds, K. W. (2003). *After the test: How schools are using data to close the achievement gap.* SF: Bay Area School Reform Collaborative.

Waites, C., Macgowan, M. J., Pennell, J., Carlton-LaNey, I., & Weil, M. (2004). Increasing the Cultural Responsiveness of Family Group Conferencing. *Social Work, 49*(2), 291-300.

Wells, S. J., Fluke, J. D. & Brown, C. H. (1995). The decision to investigate: Child protection practice in 12 local agencies. *Children and Youth Services Review, 17*(4), 523-546.

Wells, K., & Guo, S. (1999). Reunification and reenty of foster children. *Children and Youth Services Review, 21*(4), 273-294.

Willis, C. L. & Wells, R. H. (1988). The police and child abuse: An analysis of police decisions to report illegal behavior. *Criminology, 26*(4), 695-716.

U.S. Department of Health and Human Services (2003). *Children of color in the child welfare system: Perspectives from the child welfare community.* Washington, DC: Author.

Vinokur-Kaplan, D. & Hartman, A. (1986). A national profile of child welfare workers and supervisors. *Child Welfare, 65*(4), 323-335.

Yoo, J. (2002). The relationship between organizational variables and client outcomes: A case study in child welfare. *Administration in Social Work, 26*(2), 39-61.

Zellman, G. (1992). The impact of case characteristics on child abuse reporting decisions. *Child Abuse and Neglect, 16*, 57-74.

Zuravin, S., & DePanfilis, D. (1999). Predictors of child protective service intake decisions: Case closure, referral to continuing services, or foster care placement. In P.A. Curtis, G. Dale, Jr., & J.C. Kendall (Eds.). *The foster care crisis* (pp. 63-83). Lincoln, NE: University of Nebraska.

Risk and Safety Assessment in Child Welfare: Instrument Comparisons

Amy D'Andrade, PhD
Michael J. Austin, PhD
Amy Benton, MSW

SUMMARY. The assessment of risk is a critical part of child welfare agency practice. This review of the research literature on different instruments for assessing risk and safety in child welfare focuses on instrument reliability, validity, outcomes, and use with children and families of color. The findings suggest that the current actuarial instruments have stronger predictive validity than consensus-based instruments. This review was limited by the variability in definitions and measures across studies, the relatively small number of studies examining risk assessment instruments, and the lack of studies on case decision points other than the initial investigation.

KEYWORDS. Risk assessment, safety assessment, child welfare, actuarial instruments, consensus-based instruments

INTRODUCTION

Before child welfare agencies intervene with families, they are generally required to identify maltreatment or the risk of maltreatment. As a

Amy D'Andrade is Research Director, Michael J. Austin is Professor, and Amy Benton is Doctoral Research Assistant; all are affiliated with Bay Area Social Services Consortium, School of Social Welfare, University of California, Berkeley.

result, the assessment of risk is a critical part of child welfare agency practice (Wald & Woolverton, 1990). Most states in the US formalize the process of assessing risk by using some type of structured decision-making process or tool. Risk assessment instruments generally include broad categories of areas related to abuse and neglect, behavioral descriptions, procedures to determine levels of risk, and standardized forms to record this information (Rycus & Hughes, 2003). After describing current approaches to risk and safety assessment and related issues, this review of the research literature describes instruments for risk assessment in terms of their reliability, predictive validity, outcomes, and use with children and families of color. The review concludes with implications for practice and research.

THE PURPOSE OF RISK ASSESSMENT IN CHILD WELFARE

One goal of risk assessment is to focus limited resources on the children who are at the greatest risk of maltreatment. Given the limited resources of social services agencies, risk assessment serves as a strategy for targeting scarce resources and services toward those who have the greatest need (Camasso & Jagannathan, 2000; Leschied, Chiodo, Whitehead, Hurley & Marshall, 2003; Rycus & Hughes, 2003; Wald & Woolverton, 1990). A second purpose of a structured risk assessment process is to facilitate an accurate, less biased decision-making process for determining which cases should receive services (Rycus & Hughes, 2003).

Researchers from a variety of academic fields, particularly psychology, have studied human decision-making and identified a number of common errors people tend to make in their predictions and decisions. For example, researchers have found that people tend to disregard information regarding the base-rate of a phenomenon in a population (such as child abuse or neglect) when attempting to predict or diagnose the presence of the phenomenon in a specific situation (such as a child abuse investigation) (Kahneman & Tversky, 1982). In addition, people tend to be overconfident of their ability to predict an event (Kahneman & Tversky, 1982), and to have difficulty weighing factors related to a decision (Grove & Meehl, 1996). Part of the difficulty for decision-makers may relate to the availability of too much information, some of which is likely unrelated to the outcomes and may thereby increase the chance that irrelevant information is used in the decision (Dawes, 1994).

Several studies focus on decision-making within the field of the child welfare. In a study by Schuerman, Rossi & Budde (1999), case vignettes were presented to social workers, expert practitioners and academics in the field. In considering the same vignette, workers made different choices from one another in deciding whether or not a child should be removed from the home. While this variability was less when cases were of very low or very high risk, "...similar cases in the midrange of severity of family problems are treated quite differently by different experts and workers" (Schuerman et al., 1999, p.609). In a second study, researchers conducted a content analysis of 45 "public inquiries" completed in England on two types of cases: cases of child deaths by parental actions, and sexual abuse cases in which the actions of professionals were suspected of being overzealous. The formal inquiries identified three general types of errors made by child welfare workers. First, "the most striking and persistent criticism was that professionals were slow to revise their judgments . . . (adherence to) the current risk assessment of a family had a major influence on responses to new evidence" (Munro, 1999, p. 748). Secondly, professionals were skeptical of new information when it conflicted with their initial view of a family, yet uncritical of new information when it supported their initial view. And third, evidence from some sources was more highly valued (e.g., doctor's statements regarding abuse and social worker's witnessing of injury) than other sources (neighbors, concerns of the public) (Munro, 1999). These findings suggest that child welfare workers are prone to the same difficulties in decision-making as those in other fields and that valid risk assessment processes are needed to aid social workers in decision-making.

DIFFERENT APPROACHES TO RISK ASSESSMENT

Currently, there are two major approaches to risk assessment in child welfare decision-making: a consensus-based model, and an actuarial model. Both involve a list of family or case characteristics believed to be associated with risk of maltreatment (a risk assessment "instrument"). However, the two approaches differ in the processes used to identify factors for inclusion in the instrument and how the instruments are utilized in practice.

Consensus-based instruments emphasize a comprehensive assessment of risk based upon various theories of child maltreatment, the research literature on maltreatment, and/or the opinions of with expert

practitioners (English, 1999). Items on one instrument are often combined with items from another instrument, creating hybrid instruments
that vary according to the needs or beliefs of the user. Sometimes factors are assessed numerically and families categorized by their total
score, while other instruments simply describe areas that are to be assessed by the worker without necessarily providing direction in terms of
that assessment. Either way, the worker considers the area identified
and codes it high, moderate or low risk based upon his or her judgment.
Consensus-based instruments tend to use the same instrument to predict
all forms of maltreatment (English, 1999).

In contrast, actuarial instruments are developed using statistical procedures that identify and weigh factors that predict future maltreatment
(Rycus & Hughes, 2003). Often the statistical analysis is done in the
state or county in which the instrument is applied. Factors identified as
predictive of maltreatment are incorporated into a checklist. Social
workers score each factor, scores are summed into overall risk scores
for each type of maltreatment, and families are categorized into low,
moderate or high-risk groups. Actuarial instruments tend to use fewer
factors than do consensus-based instruments and generally use different
factors to predict the likelihood of physical abuse and of neglect.

There is some debate regarding the best approach to risk assessment
in the field of child welfare. A consensus-based approach to risk assessment utilizes the underlying theoretical assumption that the causes of
child maltreatment are multi-dimensional and complex, and therefore
utilizes many related domains (English & Graham, 2000). These instruments can also help structure a worker's process of information gathering for clinical assessments of risk (English, 1999), and provide
documentation of the reasoning underlying their decision-making
(Doueck, English, DePanfalis & Moote, 1993; English, 1999). Some argue that the more comprehensive approach of consensus-based instruments provides better information for casework decisions (Nasuti &
Pecora, 1993).

However, consensus-based models are criticized in the research literature for the following reasons: (1) poor conceptualization (according
to Rycus and Hughes, "measures are often poorly defined, nebulous and
ambiguous, overly global, illogical, and very subjective" (2003, p. 13));
(2) inconsistency in the type and number of variables included (Rycus
& Hughes, 2003); (3) use of the same variables to predict physical
abuse, neglect, and sexual abuse, even though contributing factors are
often different for these types of maltreatment (Rycus & Hughes,
2003); and (4) reliance upon characteristics associated with maltreat-

ment (rather than recurrence of maltreatment) (Wald & Woolverton, 1990) or upon characteristics for which there is no research support (McDonald & Marks, 1991).

Actuarial instruments help practitioners focus their risk assessments on a small set of case characteristics that have demonstrated a strong statistical relationship to future maltreatment (Ereth, Johnson & Wagner, 2003). In a meta-analysis of over 100 studies of various health and behaviorally oriented predictions that compared actuarial methods to clinical judgment, about 95% of the studies found actuarial processes to be equal to or superior to clinical judgment (Grove & Meehl, 1996). According to proponents, even a small set of factors generally does a better job predicting outcomes than does simply the use of clinical judgment (Dawes, 1979).

Critics of actuarial instruments assert that these instruments do not facilitate the clinical judgment of skilled practitioners. In addition, since the basis for including a factor on an actuarial instrument is its statistical association with a poor outcome (generally recurrence of maltreatment), factors may not appear to be causally related to the outcome. This perceived lack of a logical, theoretical connection between the items may lead to discounting the value of an actuarial instrument and objections to its use (Schwalbe, 2004).

It is not clear which approach to assessing risk is more commonly used. There is no national database regarding risk assessment approaches used by states (Lyons, Doueck & Wodarski, 1996). As of 1996, Lyons et al. (1996) reported that 15 states used the Illinois CANTS 17B instrument or some derivation of it, 4 used the CARF system, and 4 used WARM or some derivation, all consensus-based instruments. However, an increasing number of states are using an actuarial instrument as part of a "Structured Decision Making (SDM)" case management system developed by the Children's Research Center (CRC, n.d.).

USE ACROSS THE LIFE OF A CASE

Since a family's risk may change over time, it is important that risk be periodically reassessed (Munro, 2004). For example, few states have explicit guidelines for making screening decisions, and fewer still have formal instruments to guide this decision (Downing, Wells, & Fluke, 1990). The percentage of referrals that are screened out varies dramatically by state, from 5% in New Jersey to 78% in Vermont, yet states with higher investigation rates were just as likely to substantiate a referral as states with lower investigation rates (Tumlin & Geen, 2000). In addition, caseworkers have difficulty revising their assessments of families once they have been made (Munro, 1999). Therefore, a structured instrument could help workers attend to critical factors that would indicate changes in risk across the life of a case. However, using the same instrument to assess risk at different case points may be unwise (Wald & Woolverton, 1990). Factors that predict maltreatment at one point, such as at investigation and prior to services, may not be the same as those that predict subsequent maltreatment at another time point, such as at reunification after service provision. For example, one study examining two time points (within 24 hours of the initial investigation of a case and within 5 days of a case opening for in-home services) found that factors that predicted maltreatment recurrence at each time point were not always the same (Fuller, Wells & Cotton, 2001).

Unfortunately, there is very little research regarding the reliability or validity of instruments used at case time points other than the initial investigation (Rycus & Hughes, 2003; Zuravin, Orme & Hegar, 1995). For some relevant outcomes, validity is difficult to assess. For example, the safety assessment focuses on assessing imminent or current risk to a child and is usually concerned with maltreatment "...of a moderate to severe nature" (Fuller et al., 2001). While the likelihood of subsequent maltreatment within sixty days is fairly rare, the likelihood of subsequent maltreatment occurring within several days is even more so. When events are rare, it is very difficult to accurately predict them (Johnson, 2004; Munro & Rumgay, 2000).

IMPORTANT QUALITIES OF A RISK ASSESSMENT INSTRUMENT

When considering the value of any risk assessment approach, two psychometric qualities are of particular importance; namely, *predictive validity* which refers to the accuracy of the instrument in predicting a particular outcome and *inter-rater reliability* which involves the degree to which the use of an instrument leads to consistent worker decisions for similar cases (Rycus & Hughes, 2003). In child welfare, most studies focus on whether or not risk assessment instruments accurately predict the occurrence of subsequent maltreatment.

Most diagnostic or predictive instruments will produce some errors; that is, using the instrument, some cases will be identified as 'high risk' even though they are truly low risk (resulting in false positives) and some cases will be identified as low risk although they are truly high risk (resulting in false negatives). In child welfare, these classification errors are important because false negatives can be dangerous to the child and false positives can result in poor targeting of agency resources (Camasso & Jagannathan, 2000).

Some researchers assess the validity of an instrument in terms of the degree to which false negatives or false positives are minimized (Lyons et al., 1996). However, when considering a rare phenomenon like subsequent maltreatment, a low false negative and false positive rate can be achieved by simply predicting the event never happens (Baird, Ereth & Wagner, 1999; Dawes, 1994). Such a strategy, of course, is not useful for protecting children and/or providing services to families in need. An alternative strategy for assessing the validity of a prognostic instrument is to classify individuals into risk categories so that an individual can be categorized in terms of a low, moderate, or high risk of some adverse event. In medicine, this framework provides important information for a patient and doctor to make decisions about the most appropriate preventive approach to take (Altman & Royston, 2000; Baird & Wagner, 2000). Proponents of this approach to classification assert that it provides important information for case decisions and should be the basis for determining the validity of a risk assessment instrument, even if it produces more false results than does predicting that the event never happens (Baird, Ereth & Wagner, 1999; Rycus & Hughes, 2003).

Some have argued other forms of validity are also important to consider in risk assessment instruments. English & Graham (2000) assert that convergent validity, which involves the degree to which a measure corresponds to other measures of the same or similar constructs, is also relevant. In addition to considering the validity of the instruments overall, it is also important to consider the validity of the measures and/or outcomes assessed by an instrument. For example, there is some question regarding the appropriate indicator to use for maltreatment recurrence. If *substantiated maltreatment* is used, it could underestimate the future occurrence of maltreatment, especially if it is not detected (English & Graham, 2000). If *subsequent referral* is used, it could overestimate occurrence because some referrals will be unfounded. If substantiation decisions are themselves biased, using them as the basis for assessing the validity of a risk assessment instrument would be inappropriate (Morton, 1999). Some researchers believe that the severity of the maltreatment should be incorporated into the criterion (Morton & Salovitz, n.d.). Another critique of both consensus-based and actuarial risk assessment instruments is that they focus almost exclusively on the interpersonal factors of parents and rarely upon neighborhood, community or societal factors that may be associated with maltreatment (Galasso, 2001).

Inter-rater reliability refers to the degree to which an instrument results in similar decisions on similar cases when those cases are assessed by different workers (Rycus & Hughes, 2003; Schuerman et al., 1999). Assessing reliability also involves challenges. The goal is to determine whether multiple users of the same instrument would reach the same decision for the same situation. However, the practice environment of one person cannot be replicated for another person in order to determine if he or she would make the same decision. Two alternative strategies have been used to assess inter-rater reliability: (1) different workers read the same case file and their assessments or predictions of risk are compared, and (2) different workers read a hypothetical case vignette and their assessments or predictions of risk are compared. Both of these strategies are problematic for different reasons. A vignette is consistent, but artificial and limited in terms of the information that is provided to the decision-maker. Case files are complex and reflect the "real world" but could be missing critical information that was present in the real world situation (Baird, Ereth & Wagner, 1999). In addition, the statistical estimate used to assess reliability can be problematic; there could be a high correlation between two scores, even if the two coders have consistently different scores (Baird, Ereth & Wagner, 1999).

Child welfare agencies have an expectation that "risk assessment will have some effect on services provided" (Fluke, Wells, England, Walsh, English, Johnson, Gamble & Woods, 1993, p. 118). Therefore, another way to evaluate risk assessment strategies is to consider whether they have improved safety and risk decisions, facilitated services for high risk children, and thus improved outcomes (assuming services are effective). For example, one might expect to see fewer recurrences of maltreatment after implementation of a risk assessment instrument, as high risk cases would be targeted for services. Similarly, if workers were doing a better job assessing risk and safety in reunification decisions, one would expect to see a reduction in foster re-entry rates and/or maltreatment after reunification. In addition, some studies assess the use of various instruments with children and families of color because it is important to determine whether a particular instrument is equally valid for different racial/ethnic groups (Baird & Wagner, 2000; Baird, Ereth & Wagner, 1999; English, Marshall, Brummell & Orme, 1995; Johnson, 2004, 2005; Loman & Siegel, 2004).

Comparing the performance of various instruments is difficult because not all instruments have been assessed for their reliability, validity, or effects. Comparisons are further complicated by the variety of events used by different researchers to measure maltreatment recurrence. For example, many researchers use substantiated maltreatment (subsequent to the initial investigation) as the criterion against which to measure predictive validity. Others use subsequent referral, or a measure of the chronicity of subsequent referrals or substantiation, or placement of the child outside the home. Furthermore, the observation time frame varies (30 days, 60 days, 6 months, or 12 months or longer). Finally, different strategies are employed to assess the both reliability and validity and different kinds of statistics are used to estimate them.

Review of Studies

This review considered studies examining risk assessment instruments for reliability and validity, as well as studies examining the effects of the implementation of a risk assessment system on child and case outcomes and the effects for families of various different racial/ethnic groups. Specific search terms were used to search the social science and academic databases available through the University of California library, Websites specializing in systematic reviews, and publications of research institutes. Studies were excluded if they did not assess a particular identified instrument of risk assessment appropriate for use in a CPS investigation situation, or in the case of predictive validity studies, if the outcome assessed did not relate to maltreatment recurrence or case re-referral.

The search process identified studies examining the following seven instruments of risk and safety assessment: (1) the Washington Risk Assessment Matrix (WRAM), (2) the California Family Assessment Factor Analysis (CFAFA, the "Fresno" instrument), (3) the Child At Risk Field System (CARF), (4) the Child Emergency Response Assessment Protocol (CERAP), (5) the actuarial Risk Assessment instruments developed by the Children's Research Center, (6) the Risk Assessment Model of Child Protection from Ontario, and (7) the Utah Risk Assessment Scale. Findings from available studies related to predictive validity, convergent validity, inter-rater reliability, outcomes after implementation, and racial/ethnic group differences are summarized here.

WRAM

The WRAM was developed by Washington State social service agency in 1986 as a consensus-based instrument. Its contents are continuously updated based on new research evidence. Used at the initial investigation, the instrument currently includes 37 items based on seven major domains: (1) child characteristics, (2) severity of abuse/neglect, (3) chronicity of abuse/neglect, (4) caretaker characteristics, (5) caretaker/child relationship, (6) socio-economic factors, and (7) perpetrator access. To use the instrument, child welfare workers assess and rate the level of risk that they perceive for each item on a five point scale. Based on these ratings, families are categorized into risk levels. The instrument assesses risk of maltreatment in general rather than considering the risks for each kind of abuse (e.g., neglect, abuse, sexual abuse, etc.).

In tests of predictive validity, performance of the WRAM was mixed. One study of 1400 cases from four sites across the country found that while rates of subsequent investigation were higher for moderate or high risk families than for low risk families, rates of substantiated maltreatment for families in low, moderate or high risk groups were not significantly different (Baird & Wagner, 2000). When a slightly different outcome was used (the number of subsequent substantiated reports received by a family within two years), the same difficulty in accurately classifying families emerged (Baird & Wagner, 2000).

Another study of WRAM using different analytic techniques and outcomes produced similar findings. In this study of ten child welfare agency offices in New Jersey (n = 239), Camasso and Jagannathan (1995) adapted five of the seven major domains of the instrument into scales to measure the domains, and two domains were assessed individually. When these variables were entered into a regression model designed to predict subsequent maltreatment, the variables that measured the severity of abuse were found to be *negatively* correlated with maltreatment (i.e., the more severe the abuse the less likely the parent to maltreat again). The variables measuring child characteristics, caretaker characteristics, the parent-child relationship, and socio-economic status were not associated with subsequent maltreatment, while the variable measuring child behavior problems was positively associated with subsequent maltreatment. The model had poor predictive power overall, explaining approximately 6% of the variability in the outcome. In addition, based on a plot of the sensitivity and specificity of the instrument overall, authors concluded that the performance of the instrument ". . . . might be characterized as generally poor" (Camasso & Jagannathan, 1995).

In a different study of the WRAM in the state of Washington (n = 12,329), cases coded "low or no risk" were less likely to have a subsequent referral within 18 months than were cases coded as moderate and high risk. The cases coded as moderate risk, however, were not less likely to be re-referred than were high risk cases. Eleven items from the instrument were positively associated with re-referral, and eight items with recurrence of substantiated maltreatment. This study also showed that the average risk ratings of re-referred cases did not differ significantly from risk ratings of cases not re-referred (English, Marshall, Brummel & Orme, 1999).

Another study by English and Graham (2000) considered the convergent validity of the WRAM. In this study (n = 261), the instrument items were used as scales and correlated with other scales or items from well-known measures of the same constructs. A strong correlation would suggest the WRAM item did a good job of measuring that area. Alternative measures of constructs were available for only nine of the 37 items on the WRAM. Of these, items assessing child development and behavior problems were not associated with measures of similar constructs. Four of the 5 items related to the caregiver were found to be associated with measures of similar constructs, but the item related to stress and social support was not associated with related measures (English & Graham, 2000). As a result, the findings are mixed; some items do appear to have a degree of convergent validity, while others do not.

Two studies were identified that assessed the inter-rater reliability of the instrument. In the first study, four raters were asked to rate the same 80 cases using the instrument. All four workers classified families in the same way ess than 14% of the time, and three out of four workers did so just over half the time. Because some portion of these agreements could be due to chance, a statistical correction was done which produces a "kappa" score. Kappa varies from -1 to + 1; a kappa of 0 would mean the performance of the instrument was no better than chance. According to the authors of the study, a kappa in the range of .5 to .6 is generally considered acceptable. The score for the WRAM was 0.18 (Baird, Wagner, Healy & Johnson, 1999).

No studies were found that considered the effects of implementation of the WRAM on case outcomes. Several studies have considered the use of the WRAM with different racial/ethnic groups. One study of 8785 cases in Washington state found that African American and Native American families were more likely to be assigned to the highest risk level than their numbers in the referral population would suggest; Asian American families were under-assigned to the highest risk level

(English et al., 1995). However, it should also be noted that in a subsequent multivariate analysis of 12,329 cases in the same state, Native American families were in fact more likely to be re-referred, and Asian families less likely to be re-referred (English et al., 1999). Another study of 1400 cases in four sites found that approximately equal percentages for African American and White families were classified into each risk level by the WRAM (Baird & Wagner, 2000).

CFAFA (The "Fresno Model")

This consensus-based instrument, the CFAFA (California Family Assessment Factor Analysis) or the "Fresno Model," is derived from an instrument originally developed by the state of Illinois (the Child Abuse and Neglect Tracking System or CANTS 17B). The instrument is no longer used in Illinois, but has been used most recently in California. The instrument can be used throughout the life of a case. The CFAFA has 23 items that fit within five theoretical domains: (1) precipitating incident, (2) child assessment, (3) caregiver assessment, (4) family assessment, and (5) family-agency interaction. All types of maltreatment are considered together. A social worker rates each item as low, moderate or high risk and sums the number of items coded at each risk level in order to determine the overall level of risk.

In tests of predictive validity, the CFAFA did not perform well. While in a study of 1400 cases rates of subsequent investigation were higher for moderate or high risk families than for low risk families, rates of substantiated maltreatment for low, moderate or high risk families were not significantly different (Baird & Wagner, 2000). This was also true when the number of subsequent substantiated reports received by a family within two years was used as the outcome instead of the presence of any subsequent substantiated report (Baird & Wagner, 2000).

Another study examined the Illinois CANTS 17B that is the foundation of the CFAFA. When four items from this instrument were used as variables in a multivariate model predicting subsequent maltreatment (n = 239), none were associated with the outcome and the model had poor predictive power overall (explaining only 1% of the variability in the outcome). In addition, when authors plotted the sensitivity and specificity of the instrument, they concluded that "performance. . . . might be characterized as generally poor" (Camasso & Jagannathan, 1995).

One study attempted to determine the inter-rater reliability of the instrument. Four raters were asked to rate the same 80 cases using the instrument. Just over 16% of the time, all four workers classified families into the same risk groups; about 45% of the time, three out of four workers did so. The kappa for the CFAFA was 0.184 (Baird, Wagner, Healy & Johnson, 1999).

No studies were found that considered the effects of implementation of the CFAFA on case outcomes of the CFAFA. One study of 1400 cases considered use of the CFAFA with different racial/ethnic groups. In this study, the CFAFA classified approximately equal percentages of African American and White families into each risk level (Baird & Wagner, 2000).

CARF

The CARF (Child At Risk Field System) was one of the first risk assessment instruments to focus on safety as distinct from risk and was developed by ACTION for Child Protection. This consensus-based instrument can be used throughout the life of a case. It includes fourteen items within the following five domains: (1) child; (2) parent; (3) family; (4) maltreatment; and (5) intervention. Four "qualifiers" are also to be considered: (1) duration of a negative influence; (2) pervasiveness of a negative influence; (3) acknowledgement by parents of a negative influence; and (4) control of the negative influence. All types of maltreatment are considered together. Each item or qualifier is rated on a four point scale; the average of the 14 items plus the average of the four qualifiers is summed and divided by 2 to arrive at a final risk score. The family is then categorized into no risk, low risk, moderate risk, significant risk, or high risk groups.

The performance of CARF on tests of predictive validity was mixed. In one study of 207 cases in New York state, families assigned to the highest risk group were more likely to have a subsequent referral than families assigned the lowest risk group, though the relationship only "approached" statistical significance. Particular items were not found to be associated with subsequent maltreatment (Doueck, Levine & Bronson, 1993).

One study (Kolko, 1998) assessed the convergent validity of CARF (n = 90). The child welfare worker ratings of the "parent risk field" and the "family risk field" were not found to be associated with any of eight clinical measures of related constructs against which they were each tested. The child welfare worker ratings of the "child risk field" was found to be associated with one clinical measure of parent-reported "child to parent violence." However, the rating of the child risk field was also found to be negatively associated with the level of child PTSD (Post Traumatic Stress Disorder) which was the opposite direction than expected and no relationship was found between the ratings and five other clinical measures of related constructs (Kolko, 1998).

Only one study that assessed the inter-rater reliability of CARF was found. In this study (Fluke et al., 1993), 25-50 workers from several counties in Pennsylvania were asked to read case vignettes and assess the level of risk using the risk assessment instrument. The scores of all pairs of coders of a case vignette were correlated and those correlations averaged. Alpha coefficients for the CARF instrument overall risk scores for three different vignettes varied widely, ranging between .067 to .952 (Fluke et al., 1993).

In a study comparing substantiation rates before and after implementation of CARF in one New York county (n = 207), no differences were found. When maltreatment type was considered separately, physical neglect was found to be somewhat more likely to be substantiated before CARF was implemented than after it was implemented. No difference in "before and after" substantiation rates were found for physical maltreatment, sexual maltreatment, medical neglect, emotional maltreatment, or educational neglect (Doueck, Levine & Bronson, 1993).

No studies were found that considered the use of CARF with different racial/ethnic groups.

CERAP

A consensus-based instrument, the CERAP (Child Emergency Response Assessment Protocol) was developed as a "safety assessment" by Illinois Department of Child and Family Services, the American Humane Association, the University of Illinois, and experts in the field. All types of maltreatment are considered together. The instrument includes fourteen items where and can be used throughout the life of the case. The child welfare worker notes the presence or absence of each item; if any of the items are present, the worker decides whether the child is "safe" or "unsafe." If the worker decides the child is unsafe, a safety plan is developed. The training for using the instrument includes a rigorous testing and certification process.

One study attempted to assess the predictive validity of the CERAP. Since the CERAP focuses on safety assessment, the outcome used was subsequent substantiated maltreatment within 60 days. The use of the CERAP was assessed at two different points in time in the case; namely, initial investigation (n = 380) and within five days of case opening (n = 350). At initial investigation, neither overall safety assessment nor number of safety factors identified were associated with subsequent maltreatment within 60 days, either in bi-variate or multivariate tests that controlled for CERAP completion, prior reports, total number care-giver problems, and service receipt (Fuller, Wells & Cotton, 2001). Within five days of opening the case, both the safety assessment and the number of safety factors identified were found to be associated with subsequent maltreatment within 60 days in bi-variate tests, but these relationships did not remain in multivariate tests once other factors had been controlled for. Completion of the instrument, regardless of safety rating, was negatively associated with subsequent maltreatment (Fuller et al., 2001).

In considering changes in the 60 day maltreatment recurrence rates after implementation of CERAP compared to the year before implementation in one state, a series of studies found a reduction in the maltreatment recurrence rates that has been maintained for six years following implementation (Garnier & Nieto, 2002; Nieto & Garnier, 2001). Several alternative explanations for the reductions (increased use of out of home placement, another policy, nationwide trend) were considered and ruled out in a follow-up study (Fluke, Edwards, Bussey, Wells & Johnson, 2001).

No studies were found that considered the inter-rater reliability of the CERAP, or the use of the CERAP with different racial/ethnic groups.

CRC ACTUARIAL INSTRUMENTS FOR RISK ASSESSMENT

Slightly different versions of this actuarial risk assessment instrument have been developed by the Children's Research Center (CRC) for various jurisdictions. These instruments are based upon the statistical association of variables with substantiated maltreatment injury, foster care placement, and reinvestigation within two years in each location. The instrument is used at the initial investigation and includes two subscales of ten items each; one subscale assesses risk of neglect and the other risk of physical or sexual abuse. Each item is scored with a 0, 1, or 2 as indicated on the instrument and each subscale is summed. Based on the highest subscale score, a family is classified into a low, moderate, high, or very high risk category. In most jurisdictions, workers can override the risk classification and increase the risk rating by one level.

A number of studies have assessed the predictive validity of the CRC risk assessment instruments and found that the instruments are able to distinguish between low, medium and high levels of risk of subsequent maltreatment. Families categorized as high risk by the instrument have a distinctly higher rate of subsequent maltreatment than do families categorized as moderate risk. Similarly, moderate risk families have a distinctly higher rate of subsequent maltreatment than do families categorized as low risk. This was found to be true for subsequent maltreatment within 6 months (Johnson, 2004), 18 months (Baird & Wagner, 2000), and 2 years (Johnson, 2004; Loman & Siegel, 2004), and for the total number of subsequent substantiated reports received by a family at 18 months (Baird & Wagner, 2000) and 24 months (Loman & Siegel, 2004). Additionally, in a multivariate study, families coded as higher risk showed a stronger association with subsequent maltreatment (controlling for ethnicity, county size, service receipt, and safety finding) than did families coded as moderate or low risk (Johnson, 2004).

The CRC risk assessment instruments performed fairly well in reliability studies. In one study (Baird, Wagner, Healy & Johnson, 1999), four raters were asked to rate the same 80 cases using the instrument. Over half of the time, all four workers classified families in the same way; 85% of the time, three out of four workers did so. The kappa score for the CRC Risk Assessment instrument was .562 (Baird, Wagner, Healy & Johnson, 1999). In a second study that involved coding case vignettes, most workers scored the subscales within 4 points of one another (scores ranged from 0-20). Somewhat lower consistency was realized when scores were combined for an overall risk score.

No study was found that assessed the use of the CRC risk assessment instrument with respect to outcomes. One study (Wagner, Hull & Luttrell, 1995) assessed outcomes in one state following the implementation of an *array* of CRC instruments that included the actuarial risk assessment. Compared to a demographically matched set of counties that were not implementing the array of instruments, counties implementing the CRC array had: (1) lower rates of re-referral or substantiation for cases closed without services, (2) families received more services, particularly if they were high risk, and (3) and referral rates, substantiation rates, removal rates, and injuries were lower (Wagner, Hull & Luttrell, 1995).

The findings from studies that assess the use of the instruments with different racial/ethnic groups are mixed. Some studies found that the instrument classifies approximately equal percentages of all ethnic groups into each risk level (Baird & Wagner, 2000; Baird, Ereth & Wagner, 1999; Johnson, 2004), that rates of recurrence for different risk categories are consistent across ethnic groups (Baird, Ereth & Wagner, 1999), and that the association of scores with subsequent maltreatment does not differ by ethnic group (Johnson, 2005; Johnson, 2004). However, studies have also found that white families were somewhat more likely to be coded higher on more items than families of color (Johnson, 2005; Johnson, 2004); African American families scored slightly higher on neglect scale, and white families scored slightly higher on physical abuse/sexual abuse scale (Baird, Ereth & Wagner, 1999), Southeast Asian and Hispanic families in Minnesota were slightly more likely to be coded as low risk than other ethnic groups, and Native American families were slightly more likely to be coded High and Intensive Risk (differences were greatest on the neglect scale) (Loman & Siegel, 2004). Additionally, in the Minnesota study, when predictive validity was considered separately by ethnic group, distinctions between maltreatment rates of risk groups were smaller for Native American families due to the high referral rate in the Low Risk group (Loman & Siegel, 2004).

Risk Assessment Model of Child Protection (Ontario)

Based upon scales originally developed by Magura and Moses (1986), this consensus-based instrument was modified by a research team from the University of Toronto in consultation with the Ontario Association of Children's Aid Societies. Twenty-two items within five domains (caregiver, child, family, intervention, and abuse/neglect) are assessed by means of a 4-point Likert-type scale scoring system. The child welfare worker determines a total overall assessment of risk (low to high) and the cumulative risk score (the total of the ratings from the five domains). The instrument is used to decide whether or not a child should be removed and placed into foster care. All types of maltreatment are considered together. No studies were found that assessed predictive validity (using outcomes of subsequent referral or maltreatment), outcomes, or racial/ethnic differences of the Ontario Risk Assessment Model.

One study (Lescheid et al., 2003) was found that assessed the inter-rater reliability of the Ontario Risk Assessment Model. A reliability score of $r = .92$ is reported for the cumulative risk score, and of $r = .96$ for the overall risk (Lescheid et al., 2003). However, it is not clear how many coders were used in the reliability assessment, how many cases were assessed for reliability, or by what means reliability was determined.

Utah Risk Assessment Scales

The Utah Risk Assessment Scales are based upon Family Risk Scales and Child Well-Being Scales originally developed by Magura and Moses (1986) along with additional scale items developed by members of the Utah Department of Social Services and the Utah Child Welfare Training Project. These additions reflected the practice experience of the staff members involved in the development of the instrument (Nasuti, 1998). This consensus-based Likert-type instrument is composed of 32 items within five domains: parent, child, family, maltreatment, and intervention. The instrument was designed for all types of maltreatment and can be used by child welfare intake and investigative workers. No studies were found that considered the predictive validity, outcomes, or racial/ethnic differences for the Utah Risk Assessment Scales.

One study (Nasuti, 1998; Nasuti & Pecora, 1993) assessed the inter-rater reliability of the Utah Risk Assessment Scales. To assess inter-rater reliability, eight vignettes were developed describing cases of varying severity. Child welfare workers, supervisors and child welfare experts were asked to review each case vignette and provide a risk rating using the Utah Risk Assessment Scales. These risk scores were then correlated to determine reliability scores. Pearson's r coefficients ranged from .568 to .855 for the eight vignettes, each of which was assessed by 22 to 28 raters. A "Spearman-Brown prophecy formula" was applied to these scores to provide a "stepped-up" reliability estimate that was perceived to provide a more accurate estimate of inter-rater reliability. Stepped-up estimates were all above .970 (Nasuti, 1998; Nasuti & Pecora, 1993).

DISCUSSION AND IMPLICATIONS

Overall, the available research suggests that the CRC risk assessment instruments appear to have greater predictive validity than the available consensus-based instruments. This may be related to their development via the statistical identification of the strongest predictors of a particular outcome in that state or county. Unless the sample used to develop that model was different from the typical population referred to child welfare agencies in that jurisdiction (or there were major changes in the local context or population demographics), it would be reasonable to assume that those variables in the model would continue to be predictive of outcomes experienced by subsequent cohorts. The processes for identifying factors for consensus-based instruments may simply be less accurate at identifying the strongest predictors of maltreatment.

Convergent validity was not formally assessed for the CRC risk assessment instruments, and the performance of consensus-based instruments in this area was generally poor. These instruments may be unreliable and/or include measures that do not adequately reflect underlying concepts. It is difficult to draw conclusions across studies on inter-rater reliability. Only one study compared several instruments at the same time and found that the consensus-based instruments performed less effectively than the CRC actuarial instruments. Other studies of a consensus-based instrument have found variable or high inter-rater reliability. Higher inter-rater reliability might be expected from actuarial instruments because items in these instruments are more often objective while items in consensus-based instruments are more often subjective and less precise. For example, in a question related to prior CPS history using the consensus-based WRAM, the child welfare worker is required to determine whether past incidents were 'isolated' or 'intermittent,' and whether there is evidence of 'minor' abuse and neglect or 'moderate' abuse and neglect. In comparison, the actuarial CRC instrument asks 'whether or not' there was a prior injury to a child from abuse or neglect, or 'whether or not' there was a prior investigation. Generally, well-defined, objective, and clearly articulated measures are more likely to be reliable because differences of opinion about the meaning or coding of factors are minimized (Rycus & Hughes, 2003). In support of this conclusion, English & Graham (2000) noted that in a study of the CRC actuarial instrument (Wood, 1997), objective items on the instrument, such as the age of a child, had higher reliability than subjective items, such as "was child inadequately supervised?" In addition, some consensus-based instruments often require coders to use their judgment regarding the level or risk related to an area. That is, rather than asking workers "whether or not" maltreatment previously occurred, a consensus-based instrument asks workers to assign a level of risk to the broad area of previous maltreatment. Because different workers could perceive or define risk differently, different levels of risk could be assigned to similar situations.

In terms of outcomes, studies of the CERAP and the CRC instruments suggested that implementation resulted in improved outcomes. These instruments may be improving the accuracy of worker assessments of risk, resulting in fewer high risk children being left at home to be re-abused. The findings regarding the use of the instruments with different racial/ethnic groups are mixed.

It is important to note that the available research is limited. For any particular instrument, there were only a few studies available and sometimes only a single study was found. Therefore, conclusions about the risk assessment instruments should be considered preliminary and in need of further study.

IMPLICATIONS FOR PRACTICE

The debate about the best approach to assessing risk and safety may be related to a lack of clarity regarding the purposes of "risk assessment." Distinctions between *risk assessment* and *family assessment* can be somewhat unclear (Lyons et al., 1996), and a number of researchers have argued that they have often been confused (Rycus & Hughes, 2003; Wald & Woolverton, 1990). "While risk assessment is designed to accurately estimate the likelihood of future incidents of maltreatment, the purpose of family assessment is to identify and explore, in considerable depth, the unique complex of developmental and ecological factors in each family and their environment that may contribute to or mitigate maltreatment" (Rycus & Hughes, 2003, p. 11). Some researchers assert that risk assessment and family assessment are separate and distinct, and that neither activity is served by attempting to use a single instrument to do them both, or even by attempting to do them at the same time (Rycus & Hughes, 2003; Wald & Woolverton, 1990).

If the goal of an assessment is to *predict the likelihood of the recurrence of maltreatment* in order to provide services to the families at greatest risk, this is clearly a risk assessment. The research evidence suggests that the actuarial instrument will produce a more accurate and reliable prediction than the consensus-based instruments. On the other hand, if the goal of an assessment activity is to *gain a comprehensive understanding of the service needs of a family or individual,* a family needs assessment instrument incorporates more items and thus provides more information. However, consensus-based instruments did not have high convergent validity, suggesting they may not accurately measure the relevant characteristics and thus would not necessarily be helpful in family assessments.

Finally, most research on risk assessment acknowledges that the use of any kind of risk assessment instrument, actuarial or consensus-based, requires good clinical skills (Doueck et al., 1993; Johnson, 2004). For example, the CRC actuarial instrument contains numerous items that require clinical judgment to score, and allow for a clinical over-ride based on family characteristics or dynamics that are likely to affect risk but are not included on the actuarial instrument. As Ereth et al. have noted, ". . . A caseworker can sense things that an actuarial instrument would ignore or could not employ . . . Many characteristics of human subjects simply cannot be quantified empirically and actuarial models cannot easily account for rare events" (2003, p. 3). Therefore, clinical judgment can never be eliminated from any risk assessment process. In fact, many researchers in child welfare stress that the instruments for risk and safety assessment should be understood as decision aids to enhance or expand upon clinical judgment, rather than as a competing approach (Ereth et al., 2003; Fuller et al., 2001; Munro, 1999). As Munro observed, ". . . Errors can be reduced if people are aware of them and strive consciously to avoid them. The challenge is to devise aids to reasoning that recognize the central role of intuition and do not seek to ignore or parallel it but, by using our understanding of its known weakness, offer ways of testing and augmenting it" (1999, p. 756).

IMPLICATIONS FOR RESEARCH

Most of the available research on risk and safety assessment instruments is limited to five well-known instruments: the WRAM, CERAP, CARF, CFAFA (the "Fresno" instrument), and the CRC actuarial instrument. Clearly, further research in the area of risk assessment is needed. One next step in this area might be an on-going survey of the utilization of risk assessment instruments across all the states, as currently there is no process by which such information is gathered, updated and made available to the practice and research community. As a result, it is not clear how many jurisdictions use actuarial instruments, consensus-based instruments, or none at all, nor which instruments are used. In addition, much of the research on various instruments has been conducted by researchers who are associated with the development of those instruments. While this research is of high quality and has been published in respected peer-reviewed publications, studies conducted by independent researchers are also needed.

It is also important to note that current research focuses primarily on one decision point in the case; namely, the initial investigation. There is growing interest in utilizing instruments that can assist child welfare workers in making decisions at other points in the life of a case. Therefore, there is a clear need for the development of research-based instruments that can be validated for other decision points such as placement and reunification.

While predictive validity studies are needed for any instrument that attempts to assess the likelihood of future maltreatment, some researchers have suggested that other relevant outcomes besides recurrence need to be considered, such as severity of abuse (Wald & Woolverton, 1990). On-going validity and reliability studies are necessary so that the instruments can be continually refined and improved over time. Many researchers have also suggested that the effects of services provision need to be taken into consideration (English & Aubin, 1990; Milner, 1994; Nasuti, 1998). Wald and Woolverton assert that a risk assessment instrument is "truly useful only if it identifies the likelihood of re-abuse *given specific interventions*" (1990, p. 491). Since the provision of services may reduce risk, predictions of future abuse and neglect that fail to take services into account may possibly overestimate risk. For example, the lack of consideration of child-caregiver interactions (Morton, 2004b) or neighborhood factors in current instruments need to be taken into account in future research. Lastly, more research should consider the quality and nature of the implementation process, especially worker acceptance or resistance to the use of risk assessment instruments (English & Aubin, 1990).

CONCLUSION

This review of the available research literature on instruments of risk and safety assessment in child welfare suggests that CRC actuarial instruments have stronger predictive validity than available consensus-based instruments. This structured review was limited by: (1) the lack of studies on decision points other than initial investigation, (2) the variability in definitions and measures across studies, and (3) the relatively small number of studies examining risk assessment instruments. Nonetheless, the findings should be useful to practitioners and researchers evaluating the various approaches to risk and safety assessment in child welfare.

REFERENCES

Albers, M. & Roditti, M. (2004). *Management values and decision-making instruments: Nuts and bolts of risk assessment in California.* Bay Area Academy, Berkeley, CA.

Altman, D.G. & Royston, P.R. (2000). What do we mean by validating a prognostic model? *Statistics in Medicine,* 19, 453-473.

American Federation of State County and Municipal Employees (1999). *Liability and child welfare workers.* Available online at: http://www.afscne.org/publications/child/*cww99205.htm.*

Baird, C., Ereth J. & Wagner, D. (1999). *Research-based risk assessment: Adding equity to CPS decision-making.* Madison, WI: Children's Research Center.

Baird, C. & Wagner, D. (2000). The relative validity of actuarial and consensus-based risk assessment systems. *Children and Youth Services Review, 22*(11-12), 839-871.

Baird, C. Wagner, D. Healy, T. & Johnson, K. (1999). Risk assessment in child protective services: Consensus and actuarial instrument reliability. *Child Welfare, 78*(6), 723-748.

Camasso, M. J. & Jagannathan, R. (2000). Instrumenting the reliability and predictive validity of risk assessment in child protective services. *Children and Youth Services Review, 22*(11/12), 873-896.

Camasso, M. J. & Jagannathan, R. (1995). Prediction accuracy of the Washington and Illinois risk assessment instruments: An application of receiver operating characteristic curve analysis. *Social Work Research, 19*(3), 174-183.

Children's Research Center (n.d.). SDM: Structured decisions made in child welfare. Retrieved August 15, 2005 from www.nccd-crc.org/crc/c_sdm_about.html.

Child Welfare Services Stakeholders Group (2003). *CWS Redesign: The future of California's child welfare services–final report.* State of California Health and Human Services Agency, Department of Social Services.

Cicchinelli, L. (1990). Risk assessment: Expectations, benefits and realities. *Fourth National Roundtable on CPS Risk Assessment.* San Francisco, CA: American Public Welfare Association.

Costello, T. (1995). Why is it so hard to implement risk assessment? *Ninth National Roundtable on CPS Risk Assessment.* San Francisco, CA: American Public Welfare Association.

Curran, T. F. (1995). Legal issues in the use of CPS risk assessment instruments. *From the APSAC Advisor, 8*(4), 1-4.

Davidson, H. (1991). Risk assessment and the law: Unsettled issues. *Fifth National Roundtable on CPS Risk Assessment.* San Francisco, CA: American Public Welfare Association.

Dawes, R. M. (1979). The robust beauty of improper linear models in decision-making. *American Psychologist, 34,* 571-582.

Dawes, R. M. (1994). *House of cards: Psychology and psychotherapy built on myth.* New York, NY: The Free Press.

DePanfilis, D. (1996). Implementing child mistreatment risk assessment systems: Lessons from theory. *Administration in Social Work, 20*(2), 41-59.

Doueck, H. J., English, D. J., DePanfalis, D. & Moote, G. T. (1993). Decision-making in child protective services: A comparison of selected risk assessment systems. *Child Welfare, 72*(5), 441-452.

Doueck, H. J., Levine, M. & Bronson, D. E. (1993). Risk assessment in child welfare services: An evaluation of the Child at Risk Field System. *Journal of Interpersonal Violence, 8*(4), 446-467.

Downing J. D. Wells S. J. & Fluke J. (1990). Gatekeeping in child protective services: A survey of screening policies. *Child Welfare, 69* (4), 357-369.

English, D. J. (1999). Evaluation and risk assessment of child neglect in public child protection services. In H.Dubowitz, (Ed.), *Neglected children: Research, practice, and policy* (pp. 191-210). Thousand Oaks, CA: Sage Publications, Inc.

English, D. & Aubin, S. W. (1990). Outcomes for screened-out and low-risk cases within a child protective services risk assessment system. *Fourth National Roundtable on CPS Risk Assessment* (pp. 41-58). San Francisco, CA: American Humane Association.

English, D. J. & Graham, J. C. (2000). An examination of relationship between children's protective services social worker assessment of risk and independent LONGSCAn measures of risk constructs. *Children and Youth Services Review, 22*(11-12), 897-933.

English, D. J., Marshall, D., Brummel, S. & Orme, M. (1995). A preliminary examination of similarities and differences I the assessment of risk for different ethnic groups. *Ninth National Roundtable on CPS Risk Assessment,* pp. 195-218. San Fransisco, CA: American Human Association.

English, D. J., Marshall, D., Brummel, S. & Orme, M. (1999). Characteristics of repeated referrals to child protective services in Washington state. *Child Maltreatment* 4(4), 297-307.

Ereth, J., Johnson, K. & Wagner, D. (2003). *New Mexico Children, Youth and Families Department Foster Provider Risk Assessment Study.* Madison, WI: Children's Research Center.

Fluke, J., Edwards, M., Bussey, M., Wells, S. & Johnson, W. (2001). Reducing recurrence in child protective services: Impact of a targeted safety protocol. *Child Maltreatment, 6*(3), 207-218.

Fluke, J., Wells, S., England, P., Walsh, W., English, D., Gamble, T. & Woods, L. (1993). Evaluation of the Pennsylvania approach to risk assessment. *Seventh National Roundtable on CPS Risk Assessment* (pp. 116-170). San Francisco, CA: American Humane Association.

Fuller, T. L., Wells, S. J. & Cotton, E. E. (2001). Predictors of maltreatment recurrence at two milestones in the life of a case. *Children and Youth Services Review, 23*(1), 49-78.

Galasso, L. B. (2001). *Toward the prevention of child maltreatment through risk assessment:* Evaluation of an ecological, prospective instrument of risk for child abuse potential. Dissertation, Michigan State University Department of Psychology.

Garnier, P. & Nieto, M. (2002). *Illinois Child Endangerment Risk Assessment Protocol evaluation: Impact on short-term recurrence rates–year six + .* Children and Family Research Center, University of Illinois at Urbana-Champaign.

Grove, W. M. & Meehl, P. E. (1996). Comparative efficiency of informal (subjective, impressionistic) and formal (mechanical, algorithmic) prediction procedures: The clinical-statistical controversy. *Psychology, Public Policy, and Law,2*(2), 293-323.

Hollinshead D. & Fluke J. (2000). What works in safety and risk assessment for child protective services. In M. Kluger G. Alexander and P. Curtis (Eds.), *What Works in Child Welfare* (pp. 67-74). Washington D.C.: CWLA Press.

Johnson, W. (2004). *Effectiveness of California's child welfare Structured Decision-making Instrument (SDM): A prospective study of the validity of the California Risk Assessment.* Unpublished report.

Johnson, W. (2005). Effects of a research-based risk assessment on racial/ethnic disproportionality in service prevision decisions. In D. Derezotes, J. Poertner & M. F. Testa (Eds.), *Race Matters in Child Welfare: The Overrepresentation of African American Children in the System.* Washington, D.C.: CWLA.

Kahneman, D. & Tversky, A. (1982). On the psychology of prediction. in D. Kahneman, P. Slovic & A. Tversky (Eds.), *Judgment under Uncertainty: Heuristics and Biases* (pp. 50-98). New York, NY: Cambridge University Press.

Kanani, K., Regehr, C. & Bernstein, M.M. (2002). Liability considerations in child welfare: Lessons from Canada. *Child Abuse and Neglect, 26,* 1029-1043.

Kolko, D. J. (1998). CPS operations and risk assessment in child abuse cases receiving services: Initial findings from the Pittsburgh service delivery study. *Child Maltreatment,* 3(3), 262-275.

Leschied, A. W., Choido, D., Whitehead, P. C., Hurley, D., & Marshall, L. (2003). The empirical basis of risk assessment in child welfare: The accuracy of risk assessment and clinical judgment. *Child Welfare, 82*(5), 527-540.

Loman L. A. & Siegel G. L. (2004). *An evaluation of the Minnesota SDM Family Risk Assessment.* St. Louis, MO: Institute for Applied Research. Available from: http://www.iarstl.org.

Lyle, C. G. & Graham, E. (2000). Looks can be deceiving: Using a risk assessment instrument to evaluate the outcomes of child protection services. *Children and Youth Services Review, 22*(11/12), 935-949.

Lyons, P., Doueck, H. J. & Wodarski, J. S. (1996). Risk assessment for child protective services: A review of the empirical literature on instrument performance. *Social Work Research, 20*(3), 143-155.

McDonald, T.P. & Marks, J. (1991). A review of risk factors assessed in child protective services. *Social Services Review,* 65, 112-132.

Milner, J. S. (1994). Assessing physical child abuse risk: The Child Abuse Potential Inventory. *Clinical Psychology Review, 14*(6), 547-583.

Morton, T.D. (1999). The increasing colorization of America's child welfare system: The overrepresentation of African American children. *Policy & Practice,* 57(4), 23-30.

Morton, T. D. (April, 2004a). Where assessment fails. *Commentary.* Duluth, GA: Child Welfare Institute.

Morton, T. D. (Sept, 2004b) *Caretaker and child interactions in child maltreatment.* Duluth, GA: Child Welfare Institute.

Morton, T. D. & Salovitz, B. (n.d.) *Evolving a theoretical instrument of child safety in maltreating families.* Unpublished manuscript.

Munro, E. (1999). Common errors of reasoning in child protection work. *Child Abuse and Neglect, 23*(8), 745-758.

Munro, E. (2004). A simpler way to understand the results of risk assessment instruments. *Children and Youth Services Review, 26*(9), 873-883.

Munro, E. & Rumgay, J. (2000). Role of risk assessment in reducing homicides by people with mental illness. *British Journal of Psychiatry,* 176, 116-120.

Nasuti, J. P. (1998). Risk assessment in child protective services: Challenges in measuring child well-being. *Journal of Family Social Work, 3*(1), 55-70.

Nasuti, J. P & Pecora, P. J. (1993). Risk assessment scales in child protection: A test of the internal consistency and interrater reliability of one stateside system. *Social Work Research and Abstracts, 29*(2), 28-33.

Nieto, M. & Garneir, P. (2001). *Illinois Child Endangerment Risk Assessment Protocol evaluation: Impact on short-term recurrence rates–year five.* Children and Family Research Center, University of Illinois at Urbana-Champaign.

Nohejl C. Doueck H. J. & Levine M. (1992). Risk assessment implementation and legal liability in CPS practice. *Law & Policy,* 14(2 & 3),185-203.

Repetosky C. & Bailey D. (1988). The risk "fit": Integrating risk assessment with case management and practice decisions in child protection and child welfare services. *Second National Roundtable on CPS Risk Assessment.* San Francisco, CA: American Public Welfare Association.

Rycus, J. S. & Hughes, R. C. (2003). *Issues in risk assessment in child protective services: Policy white paper.* Columbus, OGH: North American Resource Center for Child Welfare, Center for Child Welfare Policy.

Scheurman, J., Rossi, P. H. & Budde, S. (1999). Decisions on placement and family preservation. *Evaluation Review, 23*(6), 599-618.

Schwalbe, C. (2004). Re-visioning risk assessment for human service decision making. *Children and Youth Services Review, 26*(6), 561-576.

Sheets, D. (1992). How Texas Got S.M.A.R.T.: A description of the rapid application design and development process used by Texas to design and implement a statewide risk assessment system. *Sixth National Roundtable on CPS Risk Assessment.* San Francisco, CA: American Public Welfare Association.

Squadrito, E., Neuenfeldt, D., & Fluke, J. (1994). Findings of Rhode Island's two-year research and development efforts. *Eighth National Roundtable on CPS Risk Assessment.* San Francisco, CA: American Public Welfare Association.

Thompson L., Brown J. & Pecora P. J. (1989). Implementation of risk assessment systems: Training and quality assurance issues. *Third National Roundtable on CPS Risk Assessment.* San Francisco, CA: American Public Welfare Association.

Tumlin, K. C. & Geen, R. (2000). The decision to investigate: understanding state child welfare screening policies and practices. *No.A-38 in New Federalism Issues and Options for States, Series A.* Washington, D.C.: The Urban Institute.

Wagner, D., Hull, S. & Luttrell, J. (1995). Structured decision making in Michigan. *Ninth National Roundtable on CPS Risk Assessment,* pp. 167-191. San Francisco, CA: American Humane Association.

Wald, M.S. & Woolverton, M. (1990). Risk assessment: The emperor's new clothes? *Child Welfare, 69*(6), 483-511.

Wood, J.M. (1997). Risk predictors for re-abuse or re-neglect in a predominantly Hispanic population. *Child Abuse and Neglect,* 21(4), 379-389.

Zuravin, S. J., Orme, J. G. & Hegar, R. L. (1995). Disposition of child physical abuse reports: Review of the literature and test of a predictive instrument. *Children and Youth Services Review 17*(4), 547-566.

Family Assessment in Child Welfare Services: Instrument Comparisons

Michelle A. Johnson, PhD
Susan Stone, PhD
Christine Lou, MSW
Catherine M. Vu, MPA, MSW
Jennifer Ling, BA
Paola Mizrahi, BA
Michael J. Austin, PhD

SUMMARY. Family assessment instruments can enhance the clinical judgment of child welfare practitioners by structuring decision-making processes and demonstrating the linkages between assessment, service provision, and child and family outcomes. This article describes the concept of family assessment in the child welfare context and provides an overview of the theoretical and disciplinary influences in the family assessment field. Based on a structured review of 85 instruments, the article discusses 21 that appear to the be the most valid and reliable for evaluating four federally-defined domains of family assessment: (1) patterns of social interaction, (2) parenting practices, (3) background and

Michelle A. Johnson is Doctoral Research Assistant, Susan Stone is Assistant Professor, Christine Lou is Doctoral Research Assistant, Catherine M. Vu is Doctoral Research Assistant, Jennifer Ling is Master's Research Assistant, Paola Mizrahi is Research Assistant, and Michael J. Austin is BASSC Staff Director; all are affiliated with University of California, Berkeley, School of Social Welfare.

history of the parents or caregivers, and (4) problems in access to basic necessities such as income, employment, and adequate housing. Key measurement criteria as well as practical considerations in the selection and implementation of family assessment instrumentation in child welfare are discussed.

KEYWORDS. Family assessment, child welfare, instruments, parenting practices, social interaction, basic needs, comprehensive measures

INTRODUCTION

For child welfare services to be relevant and effective, workers must systematically gather information and continuously evaluate the needs of children and their caregivers as well as the ability of family members to use their strengths to address their problems. Several kinds of assessments are conducted with children and families that come to the attention of child welfare services, such as risk and safety assessments that are used to guide and structure initial decision-making and predict future harm. However, the states' performance on the federal Child and Family Services Reviews, in both outcomes and systemic factors, suggests that it is not often clear how caseworkers gain a full understanding of family strengths, needs, and resources or how this information is incorporated into ongoing service planning and decision-making (HHS, 2006). Family assessment instruments hold promise for enhancing clinical judgment by structuring decision-making processes and demonstrating the linkages between assessment, service provision, and child and family outcomes.

Risk and Safety Assessment in Child Welfare: Instrument Comparisons (2005),[1] described approaches to assessing risk and summarized research findings regarding the validity and reliability of existing instruments. The primary focus of this article is to evaluate the family assessment literature and provide recommendations for promising instruments that may be useful in structuring the family assessment process. We first describe the concept of family assessment in the child welfare context, followed by an overview of the theoretical and disciplinary influences in the family assessment field and key measurement criteria. Next, we present practical considerations in the selection of a family assessment instrument for use in child welfare. The framework and methods of the review are then presented, followed by major findings and implications for practice.

FAMILY ASSESSMENT IN CHILD WELFARE

Comprehensive family assessment has been defined as the process of identifying, gathering and weighing information to understand the significant factors affecting a child's safety, permanency, and well-being, parental protective capacities, and the family's ability to assure the safety of their children. The Children's Bureau of the U.S. Department of Health and Human Services recently released guidelines for comprehensive family assessment to provide an initial framework to facilitate the development of best practices (HHS, 2006). The guidelines identify key points in the life of a case for comprehensive family assessment, beginning with the initial contact with the family and continuing through several decision making stages, including placement, reunification, termination of parental rights, and case closure. Other assessment points include decisions related to changes in the service plan or case goal, independent living decisions, formal progress reviews, and anytime new information triggers the need for additional assessment. However, existing guidelines for family assessment in child welfare services typically do not recommend particular tools or instruments for monitoring the complex and often challenging circumstances that bring families to the attention of child welfare services (HHS, 2006; DePanfilis & Salus, 2003).

Previous literature on family assessment instruments for use in child welfare includes descriptions of instruments (Pecora, Fraser, Nelson, McCroskey, & Meezan, 1995; Berry, Cash, & Mathiesen, 2003) and guides for developing comprehensive assessment strategies as part of community-based child welfare services reform (Day, Robison, & Sheikh, 1998). This structured literature review builds on these efforts by identifying the most valid and reliable instruments that address the following four federally-defined domains of family assessment: (1) patterns of social interaction, including the nature of contact and involvement with others, and the presence or absence of social support networks and relationships; (2) parenting practices, including methods of discipline, patterns of supervision, understanding of child development and/or of the emotional needs of children; (3) background and history of the parents or caregivers, including the history of abuse and neglect; and (4) problems in access to basic necessities such as income, employment, adequate housing, child care, transportation, and other needed services and supports (HHS, 2006). Several additional behaviors and conditions have been associated with child maltreatment, such as domestic violence, mental illness, poor physical health, disabilities, and alcohol and drug use. Ideally, a comprehensive family assessment instrument will address these conditions and indicate whether a need for more specialized assessment exists. An objective of this review was to identify measures that addressed these behaviors and conditions as part of a comprehensive family assessment strategy. However, the review of specialized instruments for these conditions and various disabilities was outside the scope of this review. A structured review on the assessment of children and youth in the child welfare system is the focus of a separate review.

FAMILY ASSESSMENT AND MEASUREMENT CRITERIA

Interest in family relationships began expanding in research and clinical practice with the advent of systems of child protection in the 1970s; however, only in recent years have significant efforts been made to develop family assessment instruments specifically for the child welfare practice setting. Three related sets of literatures, stemming from academic psychology during the 1970s and 1980s and medicine during the 1980s and 1990s, inform the general topic of family assessment (Boss, Doherty, LaRossa, Schumm, & Steinmetz, 1993). Rooted in family systems theory and family therapy research, a first literature seeks to capture overall family functioning, focusing on the family as a primary unit of analysis. Typically, three general within-family dimensions are assessed including overall structural and organizational patterns, communication processes, and affective qualities and cohesiveness. For example, the McMaster Model (Epstein, Bishop, & Levin, 1978), the Circumplex Model (Olson, 2000), and the Beavers Systems Model (Beavers & Hampson, 2000) represent assessment models in this tradition.

Informed by developmental psychology, a second literature includes research on the assessment of parenting. This literature identifies relevant components of parenting and typically relates them to child developmental and functional outcomes. In short, it focuses on the caregiver-child dyad as the key unit of attention. Conceptual and empirical work in this area highlights the following five parenting factors that are particularly salient for assessment: (1) parent beliefs about the child, (2) perceived efficacy in the parenting role, (3) parenting style, (4) parent-child relational qualities, and (5) parenting skills and behaviors. Finally, the stress and coping literature, as well as related literatures on risk and resilience, informs family assessment (see Hill, 1949). For example, McCubbin and McCubbin (1987) provide a model of family stressors (normative or unexpected; acute or chronic) and the extent to which families manage the stressor without negative effects on the family system. Research identifies two protective factors, including the internal and external social support resources of families as well as how the family perceives the stressor (i.e., the extent to which the family views the stressor as manageable). In short, this work places attention on social supports and family appraisal processes as a way to understand and assess family functioning.

These major theoretical and disciplinary influences have given rise to several practical issues when considering the appropriateness of a family assessment measure and method. While there are many approaches, family assessment methods typically fall into three categories: client self-report, observation, and interviews. Each of these methods has its advantages and disadvantages. A key distinction is the degree to which the method is formalized. Formal methods, such as self-report questionnaires, tend to have procedures that are clearly outlined to facilitate consistently repeated administrations. By contrast, informal methods such as interviews may be less clear in their specification and more variable in terms of administration.

Family assessment measures also vary in terms of the perspective obtained. Typically, child welfare practitioners will consider the perspectives of multiple individuals during the family assessment process, including "insider" reports from family members and children as well as "outsider" reports from school personnel, extended family members, and others that may be involved with the case. Integration of the assessment of multiple reporters with insider and outsider perspectives is reflected in the "multisystem-multimethod" (MS-MM) approach (Cromwell & Peterson, 1983).

Self-report questionnaires provide a unique insider view of family life as well as reliable methods, simplified administration and scoring, and a measurable link between an individual's perceptions or attitudes and behaviors. Given these advantages, they are by far the most commonly used method in research as well as in practice. Observation rating scales provide another cost-effective method of generating outsider information regarding family interaction patterns that can also be evaluated for reliability and validity. However, rating scales can also be limited in their usefulness by the competence of the rater and the psychometric quality of the scale. Raters must have a clear understanding of the concepts that are measured and the behaviors that represent the concepts in practice. They must also possess adequate knowledge of different populations in order to place observed behavior on a continuum, a concern that adequate training and clinical supervision can begin to address. However, as with self-report measures, evidence of the validity and reliability of an observational rating scale is critical in the instrument selection process, particularly with regard to specific stages of assessment.

Family assessment includes several sequential functions, including (1) screening and general disposition, which typically occur at intake; (2) definition of the problem, which may include diagnostic assessments (or quantification of problem severity) that occur during intake and investigation procedures; (3) planning, selecting, and matching services with identified problems; and (4) monitoring progress and evaluating service outcomes (Hawkins, 1979). Validity and reliability are the primary psychometric issues when selecting family assessment measures. Briefly, validity is the degree to which the instrument measures what it intends to measure (e.g., family functioning or perceptions of family life) whereas reliability is a measure of consistency. In other words, a high level of reliability indicates confidence in the fact that similar results will be obtained if similar procedures are used and if the results are assessed in the same manner time after time. As Figure 1 suggests, there are many types of validity and reliability to consider for each stage of assessment when selecting a family assessment instrument. Appendix A provides more details about these measurement criteria.

CONSIDERATIONS FOR SELECTING
FAMILY ASSESSMENT INSTRUMENTS
FOR USE IN CHILD WELFARE

There are many clinical and measurement criteria for evaluating the adequacy of a family assessment method and they vary depending upon the function for which they are developed and used. In the child welfare setting, the choice of method will also be governed by the following practical considerations (adapted from Johnson & Wells, 2000):

1. Will the instrument be used for initial assessment only or for the monitoring of progress? If it is the latter, is the instrument sensitive to

clinical change? Many instruments are designed to detect the existence of a given condition, not to measure improvement in a child or family's functioning over time. Only instruments sensitive enough to detect client change can reliably measure it, a distinction that may not be apparent to many users. Since child welfare decisions are often made when there appears to be a "lack of progress" on the part of a client, assessment instruments need to be very sensitive to measuring change.

2. What domains of family assessment are assessed? Family assessment instruments cover a wide array of factors, from tangible outcomes such as the cleanliness of the home environment, to less tangible factors such as self-esteem. Before selecting measures, such as parental functioning, parental behavioral health, or quality of the home environment, it is important for agencies and programs to clearly identify the goals and desired outcomes of services for children and families.

3. How long does it take to administer the instrument? Child welfare workers generally have limited time to spend with clients. Therefore, the time needed to administer an assessment instrument needs to be brief. Managers will also want to consider the time it takes to train workers to use the instrument and the length of time required to interpret the results.

4. What is the developmental stage or age focus with respect to the instrument? The broad range of ages of parents and children served by the child welfare system will require agencies to select multiple instruments in most cases.

5. Is it useful with the intended target group of clients? For example, if an agency works primarily with Latino clients, knowing that a particular instrument has been tested with Latino individuals will be a defining factor in selection. As most instruments have been normed with white English speaking individuals in research settings, serious consideration needs to be given to the appropriateness of using instruments in practice that are not culturally validated. Managers will also need to consider how the instrument is administered. If a client completes the form, it is important to consider the reading level of the instrument and the languages available.

6. What are the advantages and disadvantages of using this instrument? Certain clinical instruments have the advantage of assessing a range of child or family functioning. Other instruments are useful in that they can be used along with other tools as part of a "package." Any time an instrument can provide information on multiple outcomes, managers are able to conserve resources. Several instruments may only tap one aspect of family functioning, or are useful only with a particular popula-

tion. For example, some instruments may be written for a higher reading level than would be sensible for use with an agency's client population. Managers and administrators also need to consider the costs of purchasing copyrighted materials or reproducing other instruments.

7. What does the instrument tell a practitioner, administrator, or policy maker? Decisions about instruments should be guided by a clear idea of what information is needed, how it will be used, and who will be using it.

8. Is psychometric data available? Again, reliability and validity indices establish the credibility of instruments. Without this information, various alternative explanations for the findings (e.g., examiner bias, chance, and effects of maturation) cannot be ruled out, which seriously restricts the usefulness of findings.

Given measurement criteria and practical considerations, the goal of this review is to identify instruments that (a) comprehensively address the major domains of family assessment, (b) are valid and reliable for

FIGURE 1. Stages of Assessment, Criteria for Evaluation, and Child Welfare Services (CWS) Decision Making (adapted from Carlson, 1989)

CWS Decision-Making Stage	Assessment Stage	Clinical Criteria	Measurement Criteria
Intake	Screening	Detects the nature of a problem; provides guidance as to further assessment; cost-effective	Adequacy determined by predictive validity
Investigation	Diagnosis	Confirms hypotheses regarding family functioning; quantifies or measures the severity of dysfunction; determines the primary locus of the problem; provides standardized measures and validated clinical cutoff scores	Adequacy determined by discriminative and differential predictive validity
Case Planning	Service Planning	Specifies objectives for change; analyzes factors that produce and maintain problematic behavior; identifies family strengths and resources; determines both intervention sequence and level of change adequate for treatment termination; may require multimethod assessment approach if multiple goals cannot be systematically measured using a single method	Adequacy determined by content validity and inter-rater reliability regarding specific behavioral patterns relevant to the problem
Continuing Services/Placement and Reunification Decisions	Monitoring Progress/ Evaluation	Focuses on the behavior to be changed; amenable to a repeated-measures; generalizable beyond the treatment setting; sensitive to change; easily administered	Unresponsive to spurious influences such as retesting effects and instrument decay

the appropriate stage of assessment, and (c) are practical for use in child welfare settings.

METHODS

Search Strategy

This review used pre-determined search terms and search sources to identify research literature within a given topic. This method of searching can reduce the potential for bias in the selection of materials. Using specified search terms, we searched numerous social science and academic databases available through the University of California library. In addition, we conducted overall internet searches and also searched the websites of research institutes and organizations specializing in systematic reviews, conference proceedings databases, dissertation databases, internet databases. In order to gather information on research that has not been published, inquiries were sent to national child welfare resource centers, federal agencies such as the Children's Bureau, and child welfare researchers (see Appendix B for a description of the search strategy). The references in reviews and primary studies were scanned to identify additional articles. The references reviewed were limited to those printed in the English language.

Evaluation Methods

The instruments that were obtained through the structured search strategy were evaluated with regard to their appropriateness for child welfare settings based on seven criteria: (1) their relationship to the family assessment domains identified and their comprehensiveness in relation to these domains; (2) the appropriateness of the assessment methods employed; (3) the number of stages of assessment addressed, with emphasis on the appropriateness for use at multiple points in the life of the case; (4) the populations with which instruments were normed; (5) ease of administration, in terms of time, instructions, scoring, and clarity of interpretation; (6) other advantages and disadvantages related to use in the child welfare setting, such as the reading level required of clients or prior use by caseworkers; and (7) psychometric properties. The psychometric properties of the instruments were rated on a four point scale, from those having the least psychometric information available to those having psychometric information available for all of the stages of assessment that the instrument addressed.

A ten percent sample of the instrument evaluations was reviewed by an independent reviewer to establish the inter-rater reliability of the evaluation process. Two discrepancies were found with regard to the comprehensiveness of the family assessment domains that an instrument addressed and in one case, with regard to the stage of assessment that the instrument addressed. These differences were reconciled with the introduction of additional sub-criteria for evaluation.

MAJOR FINDINGS

Overview

Eighty five (n = 85) instruments pertaining to family assessment were evaluated (see Appendix C). Of these, the majority typically addressed one to two domains of family assessment, such as patterns of social interaction and parenting practices (see Figure 2). The majority of the instruments relied on self-report methods and/or observational rating scales (80%). A smaller number of instruments included structured interviews (15%) and methods relying on structured tasks such as games (4%).

In terms of measurement criteria, half of the instruments (50%) had some type of information available about their reliability and/or validity. In twenty-two cases (26%), psychometric information was available for (1) some stages of assessment but not all, or (2) for specific stages but overarching psychometric properties of the instrument had yet to be established (such as content validity or test-retest reliability). Ten instruments had information available for all stages of the assessment addressed (12%), while another ten provided little to no psychometric information (12%).

As mentioned, seven criteria were used to evaluate the 85 instruments with regard to their appropriateness for child welfare settings. Seven instruments appeared to be the most comprehensive and appropriate for use in the child welfare setting. These are presented first, followed by instruments that appear to be promising for specialized purposes within specific domains. For example, the specialized assessments of patterns of social interaction presented (n = 4) might be made to better target referrals for mental health services or family therapy. Similarly, the assessments of parenting practices identified (n = 5)

FIGURE 2. Instruments/Models Addressing Family Assessment Domains (n = 85)[2]

Family Assessment Domains	Number of Instruments Addressing Domain
Patterns of Social Interaction (the nature of contact and involvement with others, the presence or absence of social support networks and relationships)	58
Parenting Practices (methods of discipline, patterns of supervision, understanding of child development and/or of emotional needs of children)	43
Background and History of Caregivers (including the history of abuse and neglect)	20
Problems in Access to Basic Necessities (such as income, employment, adequate housing, child care, transportation and needed services and supports)	23
Other Behaviors and Conditions (domestic violence, mental illness, physical health, physical, intellectual, and cognitive disabilities, alcohol and drug use)	18

might be made to refer clients to the most appropriate parenting program. Community-based providers of mental health services and parenting programs might also use these specialized instruments to assess family strengths and needs, develop service plans, and monitor and report on progress. Promising instruments for the specialized assessment of background characteristics (n = 3) and basic needs (n = 2) are also discussed.

Comprehensive Measures of Family Assessment

As noted in Figure 3, the seven family assessment instruments that are the most comprehensive and appear the most promising for child welfare practice include three instruments that have been developed specifically for use in child welfare settings: (1) the North Carolina Family Assessment Scale (NCFAS) and two modified versions of the NCFAS, (2) the NCFAS for Reunification (NCFAS-R) and (3) the Strengths and Stressors Tracking Device (SSTD). Four additional instruments include (4) the Family Assessment Form (FAF), (5) the Family Assessment Checklist (FAC), (6) the Ackerman-Schoendorf Scales for Parent Evaluation of Custody (ASPECT), and (7) the Darlington Family Assessment System (DFAS). Each instrument is discussed briefly. Figure 4 presents the various stages of assessment that each instrument is designed to address.

North Carolina Family Assessment Scale (NCFAS) and Related Instruments. The NCFAS (Reed-Ashcraft, Kirk, & Fraser, 2001) was developed in the mid-1990s to allow caseworkers working in intensive family preservation services (IFPS) caseworkers to assess family func-

FIGURE 3. Promising Measures of Comprehensive Family Assessment for Child Welfare by Assessment Domain

Instruments	Family Assessment Domains				
	Patterns of Social Interaction	Parenting Practices	Background of Caregivers	Basic Needs	Other Behaviors and Conditions
North Carolina Family Assessment Scale (NCFAS)	X	X	X	X	X
NCFAS-Reunification (NCFAS-R)	X	X		X	X
Strengths and Stressors Tracking Device (SSTD)	X	X	X	X	X
Family Assessment Form (FAF)	X	X		X	
Family Assessment Checklist (FAC)		X	X	X	X
Ackerman-Schoendorf Scales for Parent Evaluation of Custody (ASPECT)	X	X	X	X	X
Darlington Family Assessment System (DFAS)	X	X	X		X

X = assesses family functioning in this domain

tioning at the time of intake and again at case closure. The 39-item instrument was designed to assist caseworkers in case planning, monitoring of progress, and measuring outcomes. The NCFAS provides ratings of family functioning on a six-point scale ranging from "clear strengths" to "serious problems" in the following five domains: (1) environment, (2) parental capabilities, (3) family interactions, (4) family safety, and (5) child well-being. Internal consistency and construct validity have been established for early versions as well as the most recent version of the NCFAS (Version 2.0; Reed-Ashcraft et al., 2001, Kirk et al., in press) and the instrument is able to detect changes in functioning over time. The instrument also appears to have some degree of predictive validity in relation to placement prevention; however, the authors caution that the relatively weak capability of the intake ratings to predict placement at closure or thereafter suggest that the NCFAS should not be used as a device to screen out families from service at the time of intake (Kirk et al., in press). Additional research with sufficiently large samples is necessary to establish predictive validity for outcomes of interest.

The NCFAS for Reunification (NCFAS-R), a collaborative effort between the National Family Preservation Network the University of North Carolina at Chapel Hill, is an assessment instrument used to assist caseworkers using intensive family preservation service strategies to successfully reunify families where children have been removed from the home due to substantiated abuse and or neglect, juvenile delinquency, or the receipt of mental health services in a "closed" treatment setting (Reed-Ashcraft et al., 2001). The scale provides family functioning assessment ratings on seven domains relevant to reunification: (1) environment, (2) parental capabilities, (3) family interactions, (4) family safety, (5) child well-being, (6) caregiver/child ambivalence, and (7) readiness for reunification. Like the NCFAS, change scores for the NCFAS-R illustrate the amount of measurable change that is achieved during the service period from intake ratings through closure ratings. Internal consistency and concurrent validity in relation to the success or failure of reunification cases have been established for this measure.

The Strengths and Stressors Tracking Device (SSTD) is another modification of the NCFAS that assesses the strengths and needs of families at intake to help guide case planning and evaluate the effectiveness of treatment. The SSTD is shorter than the NCFAS in its two-page form but includes an additional 16 items (for a total of 55 items). The SSTD can be completed by caseworkers in less than 30 minutes. Like the NCFAS, family strengths and stressors are rated on a Likert type scale, with -2 indicating a serious stressor to $+2$ indicating a clear strength. Unlike the NCFAS, psychometric information for the SSTD is somewhat limited. In a small validation study in a single agency, the SSTD demonstrated high internal consistency in all domains, distinguished between physical abuse and neglect cases at intake, and appeared to be sensitive to specific changes made by families during the treatment period (Berry, Cash, & Mathiesen, 2003). However, further use and validation are needed to establish content and criterion related validity, including predictive validity, as well as test-retest reliability.

Family Assessment Form (FAF). The FAF is a practice-based instrument that was developed by workers at the Children's Bureau of Los Angeles, a nonprofit child welfare agency, to help practitioners improve the assessment of families receiving home-based services. It includes 102 items that relate to the following five factors: (1) living conditions, (2) financial conditions, (3) interactions between adult caregivers and between caregivers and children, (4) support available to the family, and (5) developmental stimulation available to children. The FAF is completed at assessment and termination along with a two-page termination review. A comparison of initial and termination scores provides data on changes during the service period so workers and families can evaluate progress and plan for the future. Content validity for the FAF was developed through a committee and reliability testing has yielded positive results for its internal consistency and inter-rater reliability (McCroskey & Nelson, 1989; McCroskey, Nishimoto, & Subramanian, 1991; Children's Bureau of Southern California, 1997). However, its consistency in repeated administrations and its ability to distinguish between groups and predict outcomes of interest is unclear.

Family Assessment Checklist (FAC). The FAC is a comprehensive assessment of family problems and strengths that was developed for use in an urban, home-based child welfare program to assist workers in establishing goals, planning services, and monitoring changes. The FAC addresses seven major areas: (1) financial status, (2) condition of the home environment, (3) developmental level of the client, (4) the developmental level of the child(ren), (5) parenting skills, (6) nutrition knowledge and practice, and (7) physical and mental health of family members. The FAC is sensitive to changes in family functioning over the course of home-based services. It appears to be economic in terms of personnel demands and time expenditure given that it can be completed by caseworkers based upon observations made in the routine course of service. In a single study, the FAC appeared to have high inter-rater reliability and convergent validity (Cabral & Marie, 1984). However, like the FAF, its consistency in repeated administrations and its ability to distinguish between groups and predict outcomes of interest is unclear.

Ackerman-Schoendorf Scales for Parent Evaluation of Custody (ASPECT). The ASPECT was designed to assist mental health professionals in making child custody recommendations by assessing characteristics of parents and parent-child interactions that are related to effective parenting. The scales include 56 items and represent a system that combines the results of psychological testing, interviews, and observations of each parent and child to provide data regarding the suitability of the parent for custody. While the scales are comprehensive in relation to the family assessment domains, obtaining the data needed for the ASPECT involves considerable time and entails several assessment steps. Nonetheless, the scale has adequate internal consistency and inter-rater reliability and correctly predicted the final disposition of court orders regarding custody in approximately 75% of cases. However, it is important to note that these scales were developed and tested primarily with predominantly white, married and well-educated parents; therefore, the generalizability of the scale to child welfare populations is unknown (Heinze & Grisso, 1996; Touliatos, Perlmutter, & Holden, 2001).

Darlington Family Assessment System (DFAS). The DFAS is a multisystem-multimethod assessment that consists of three components: (1) the Darlington Family Interview Schedule (DFIS), a structured family interview with an integrated rating scale called the Darlington Family Rating Scale, (DFRS), (2) a battery of self-report questionnaires, including the Social Support Index, Goldberg's General Health Questionnaire, the Eyberg Child Behavior Inventory, the Marital Satisfaction Index, and the McMaster Family Assessment Device, and (3) a task with an associated behavior coding system. DFAS measures twelve problem dimensions using four major perspectives: (1) child-centered (including physical health, development, emotional behavior, relationships, and conduct), (2) parent-centered (including physical health, psychological health, marital partnership, parenting history, and social supports), (3) parent-child interactions, including care, and control, and (4) the whole family/total system perspective (closeness and distance, power hierarchies, emotional atmosphere and rules, and family development). The DFIS requires approximately 1 1/2 hour to complete the interview, twenty minutes for clients to complete the self-report questionnaire battery, and fifteen minutes for completion of the task activity. The DFIS has been developed and tested with psychiatric and healthy populations and may be helpful to novice and non-specialty practitioners as a training device. Experienced practitioners may use DFIS to organize clinical observations and inferences and the DFRS can assist practitioners with summarizing clinical observations and treatment planning. The DFIS enhances understanding of both objective and subjective views of family problems, is useful as an integrated package of tools, and appears promising in guiding therapeutic strategies. While it has relatively good inter-rater reliability, concurrent and content validity, and is sensitive to clinical change, the DFIS has not been used with child welfare populations (Wilkinson, 2000; Wilkinson, & Stratton, 1991).

In summary, of the seven most promising assessment instruments, the NCFAS the NCFAS-R appear to be the most relevant for use in child welfare settings due to its strengths-based orientation and extensive testing with child welfare populations, despite some of its psychometric limitations. The Darlington Family Assessment System (DFAS) also appears promising given its multi-system, multi-method approach, which mirrors the family assessment process in child welfare by using multiple methods to gain multiple perspectives in a case. It has excellent psychometric properties and is comprehensive nature. However, more research is needed to establish its validity with child welfare

FIGURE 4. Promising Measures of Comprehensive Family Assessment for Child Welfare

Instruments	Child Welfare Decision/Stage of Assessment			
	Intake/ Screening	Investigation/ Diagnosis	Case Planning	Continuing Services, Placement & Reunification/ Monitoring & Evaluation
North Carolina Family Assessment Scale (NCFAS)		X	X	X
NCFAS for Reunification (NCFAS-R)			X	X
Strengths and Stressors Tracking Device (SSTD)		X	X	X
Family Assessment Form (FAF)		X	X	X
Family Assessment Checklist (FAC)		X	X	X
Ackerman-Schoendorf Scales for Parent Evaluation of Custody (ASPECT)	X		X	
Darlington Family Assessment System (DFAS)	X	X	X	X

X = child welfare decision/stage of assessment for which instrument is used

populations and to evaluate its feasibility due to lengthy administration time.

Patterns of Social Interaction and Support

We identified four measures for specialized assessment for use at multiple points in the life of the case that focus on patterns of social interaction (including the nature of contact and involvement with others, and the presence or absence of social support networks and relationships at multiple points in the life of the case). As noted in Figure 5, these instruments include the McMaster Model, the Assessment of Strategies in Families-Effectiveness (ASF-E), the Circumplex Model, and the Family Assessment Measure III.

McMaster Model. The McMaster Model relies on multiple instruments to assess six dimensions of functioning: (1) problem solving, (2) roles, (3) communication, (4) affective responsiveness, (5) affective involvement, and (6) behavior control. The three complementary instruments include: the Family Assessment Device (FAD), a 60-item self-report questionnaire; the McMaster Clinical Rating Scale (MCRS), an observational rating used by clinician or other observer; and the McMaster Structured Interview of Family Functioning (McSiff), which provides a series of structured questions on each of the six domains. The MCRS and the FAD provide a single score for each of the six dimen-

FIGURE 5. Promising Measures of Social Interaction

Instrument	Child Welfare Decision/Stage of Assessment			
	Intake/ Screening	Investigation/ Diagnosis	Case Planning	Continuing Services, Placement & Reunification/ Monitoring & Evaluation
McMaster Model	X	X	X	X
Assessment of Strategies in Families-Effectiveness (ASF-E)	X	X		X
Circumplex Model		X	X	X
Family Assessment Measure III		X		X

X = child welfare decision/stage of assessment for which instrument is used

sions, and the McSiff is used to obtain a reliable clinical rating on the MCRS. The clinical utility and psychometric validity and reliability of the McMaster instruments have been documented in several studies (Epstein et al., 2003; Miller et al., 2000). The FAD is easy to administer and cost effective, has predictive validity for several clinically relevant outcomes, can differentiate between clinical and non-clinical families and is available in at least sixteen languages (Epstein et al., 2003; Miller et al., 2000). The Chinese and Spanish versions of the FAD appear to possess good psychometric properties (Shek, 2001; Shek, 2002; Walrath et al., 2004). While the instruments presently lack normative data on child welfare populations, they may provide early identification of families who may benefit from therapy despite reluctance to seek services (Akister & Stevenson-Hinde, 1991; Miller et al., 2000).

Assessment of Strategies in Families-Effectiveness (ASF-E). The ASF-E is a brief, 20-item screening instrument to determine the perceived need for therapy and to determine progress as a result of family therapy in clinical settings. The ASF-E measures congruence and family health on four dimensions of family behavior patterns and strategies; namely, stability, growth, control, and connectedness/spirituality. High internal consistency and validity have been established for the ASF-E in the U.S. and the measure has been tested with populations internationally (Friedemann, Astedt-Kurki, & Paavilainen, 2003).

Circumplex Model. The Circumplex battery of instruments integrates three dimensions of family functioning (communication, cohesion, and flexibility) and is designed for use in clinical assessment, treatment planning, and family intervention research. The Circumplex Model includes the Family Adaptability and Cohesion Scale (FACES), a self-report questionnaire that has gone through multiple revisions over the past 20 years to improve the reliability and validity of the instrument. The latest version, the FACES IV, has been found to be reliable and valid for clinical use (Olson & Gorall, 2003). Additional Circumplex measures include the Clinical Rating Scale (CRS) for rating couples and family systems based on clinical interviews or observations; the Family Communication Scale, which focuses on the exchange of factual and emotional information; the Family Satisfaction Scale to determine the family's satisfaction with their functioning; the Family Strengths Scale, which focuses on family characteristics and dynamics that enable families to demonstrate resilience and deal with family problems; and the Family Stress Scale, which taps into levels of stress currently being experienced by family members within their family system (Olson, 2000; Olson & Gorall, 2003). While the CRS has been validated, it is unclear whether self-report questionnaires other than the FACES IV have established validity and reliability.

Family Assessment Measure III. The FAM III is a set of self-report questionnaires that measure family strengths and weaknesses in the seven constructs related to: (1) task accomplishment, (2) role performance, (3) communication, (4) affective expression, (5) affective involvement, (6) control, and (7) values and norms. While the concepts are similar to those measured in the McMaster Model, the FAM III is unique in assessing family strengths and weaknesses from perspectives on three scales: the family as a system (general scale), various dyadic relationships (dyadics scale), and individual family members (self-rating scale). The collection of data from all three perspectives facilitates the analysis of family processes from multiple system levels. The FAM III consists of 94 items and can be completed by family members at least 10-12 years of age. Numerous studies attest to the clinical utility of the FAM III, including its ability to differentiate between clinical and non-clinical families and it predictive validity in relation to children's problems. The FAM III has demonstrated sensitivity to change in treatment, has been developed and tested with clinical and non-clinical families, and has twenty years of research to support its efficacy (Skinner et al., 2000).

In summary, research has found the FACES, the FAM III, and the FAD to be highly correlated, to suggest that these three instruments may be interchangeable (Olson, 2000; Beavers & Hampson, 2000). Although the Circumplex instruments appears best at providing a multisystem-multimethod assessment of the family, the McMaster instruments provide the clearest link with a therapeutic model of intervention (Carlson, 2003). McMaster instruments also have demonstrated superior sensitivity in identifying families with clinical needs and greater correspondence between clinical rating scales and family member self-report inventories when compared to the Circumplex instruments (Drumm & Fitzgerald, 2002). More studies comparing the treatment utility of the various instruments are needed, especially with respect to child welfare populations.

Parenting Practices

In addition to the seven comprehensive measures of family assessment and the four specialized measures of patterns of family social interaction, five measures were identified as promising for the specialized assessment of parenting practices among families that have come to the attention of the child welfare system: (1) the Adult-Adolescent Parenting Inventory (AAPI); (2) the Child Abuse Potential Inventory (CAPI); (3) the Parental Empathy Measure (PEM); (4) the Parenting Stress Index (PSI); (5) and the Beavers Model of Family Assessment (see Figure 6).

Adult-Adolescent Parenting Inventory (AAPI). The AAPI is designed to identify high-risk parenting activities and behaviors that are known to be attributable to child abuse and neglect, and may also be used to assess patterns of family social interaction. It is a self-report inventory consisting of forty five-point Likert scale items, and can be administered at multiple points over the course of a child welfare case for the purposes of screening, diagnosis, and monitoring progress and clinical change over time. Advantages of this instrument include a brief administration time of approximately twenty minutes and suitability for parents with a fifth-grade reading level or above. Additionally, the AAPI can be read orally to non-readers and a Spanish version is available for Spanish-reading parents. Over twenty years of research have provided considerable evidence of the psychometric strength of this instrument, including high internal consistency and significant diagnostic and discriminatory validity in discerning non-abusive parents and known abusive parents (Bavolek & Keene, 2001).

Child Abuse Potential Inventory (CAPI). The CAPI is also designed to identify parents who are most likely to be at risk for child abuse by assessing problematic parenting practices and social interaction, and was developed as a tool specifically for child protective services workers in their investigations of reported child abuse cases. While the CAPI was originally designed as a preliminary screening tool to discriminate between abusive and non-abusive parents, treatment/intervention programs have successfully used the CAPI at pre- and post-treatment to assess progress and clinical change (Milner, 1994). It is a self-administered 160-item questionnaire that assesses six primary clinical factors: (1) distress, (2) rigidity, (3) unhappiness, (4) problems with child and self, (5) problems with family, and (6) problems with others. Additionally, the instrument includes three validity subscales that help mitigate potential self-report bias. Other advantages of the CAPI include a brief administration time of approximately twenty minutes and a third-grade reading level requirement that permits its suitability for use with parents with limited literacy proficiency. Similarly to the AAPI, the CAPI has undergone substantial psychometric evaluations and has demonstrated significant discriminative validity, high internal consistency and test-retest reliabilities (Heinze & Grisso, 1996).

Parental Empathy Measure (PEM). The PEM is a promising instrument for screening for abusive or neglecting parenting behaviors/practices. It is a semi-structured interview with open-ended questions assessing parental attention to signals, attributes, emotional/behavioral responses to, and perceptions of their children. In addition to these parenting practices and behaviors, the PEM includes items addressing past involvement with child protective services. One of the strongest features of this instrument is the comprehensiveness of its psychometric evaluation; reliability and validity tests indicate that the PEM has good sensitivity for identifying abusive parents, good inter-rater reliability, high internal consistency, and high construct reliability when measured against the CAPI. Furthermore, the PEM also includes a measure of social desirability that was found to be effective in detecting biased responses. However, the PEM lacks the advantage of administrative brevity exhibited by the previous measures; for example, the PEM contains open-ended items and general administration time cannot be estimated because it depends on specific case characteristics (Kilpatrick, 2005).

Parenting Stress Index (PSI). The PSI also screens for abusive or neglecting parenting behaviors/practices, and assesses social interaction

FIGURE 6. Promising Measures of Parenting Practices

Instrument	Child Welfare Decision/Stage of Assessment			
	Intake/ Screening	Investigation/ Diagnosis	Case Planning	Continuing Services, Placement & Reunification/ Monitoring & Evaluation
Adult-Adolescent Parenting Inventory	X	X		X
Child Abuse Potential Inventory (CAPI)	X			X
Parenting Stress Inventory (PSI)	X			
Parental Empathy Measure (PEM)	X			
Beavers Model of Family Assessment	X	X	X	X

X = child welfare decision/stage of assessment for which instrument is used characteristics that may affect the quality of family functioning. The current version of the PSI contains 101 self-report items assessing the parenting domain (competence, social isolation, attachment to child, health, role restriction, depression, spouse) and the child domain (distractibility, adaptability, parent reinforcement, demandingness, mood, acceptability). An optional nineteen-item life stress scale is also provided (Terry, 1991a). The advantages include a brief administration time of 20-25 minutes for the full instrument (recommended for a more comprehensive assessment), and a 36-item short form is also available for situations requiring more rapid assessment. Additionally, the PSI is available in eight languages permitting its use with non-English reading populations. Psychometric evaluations have demonstrated high internal consistency, high correlations with instruments measuring the same construct, and relatively good test-retest reliabilities (Terry, 1991b). However, evaluators caution that low ratings on the PSI do not necessarily indicate the absence of problems, in part due to the lack of validity measures that address potential social desirability bias (Touliatos et al., 2001).

Beavers Model of Family Assessment. The Beavers Model of Family Assessment consists of three instruments that assess parenting practices using a combination of self-report and observational methods: (1) the Beavers Self-Report Family Inventory (SRFI) which measures self-reported parenting practices and competence; and (2) the Beavers Interactional Style Scale (BISS) and the Beavers Interactional Competence Scale (BICS), which are both scored using observer ratings of parenting style and competence based on a ten minute observation of a semi-structured episode of family interaction (Beavers & Hampson, 2000). The Beavers instruments may be administered throughout the course of a child welfare case, and consequently, assist with multiple stages of assessment, including screening, diagnosis, treatment planning, and monitoring progress/follow-up. The SFRI is a 36-item Likert-format questionnaire that may be completed by family members eleven years of age or older, and is brief and easy to score (McCubbin, McCubbin, Thompson, & Huang, 1989). Psychometric evidence of its reliability and validity is substantial; studies demonstrate a 91% correct classification of clinical versus non-clinical cases, high test-retest reliability, high internal consistency, and concurrent validity (Halvorsen, 1991). The BICS also has demonstrated strong reliability and validity; studies indicate that this instrument has a 65% sensitivity rate for clinical families, a 90% specificity rate for non-clinical families, high inter-rater reliability, high overall test-retest reliability, and high construct validity (Carlson, 2003). Psychometric evidence of the reliability/validity of the BISS is still in progress; however, one study suggests that it has limited descriptive and discriminative power in comparison to the other two Beavers measures (Drumm, Carr, & Fitzgerald, 2000). Although some studies have administered and evaluated these instruments separately, the developers of the Beavers model indicate that a more comprehensive family assessment would be facilitated by the conjunctive use of all three instruments (Beavers & Hampson, 2000).

BACKGROUND CHARACTERISTICS

Three measures were identified as possible candidates for the assessment of family background characteristics related to a history of child abuse and neglect; namely, the Family Systems Stressors Strength Inventory (FSSSI), the Hispanic Stress Inventory (HIS), and the Ontario Child Neglect Index (CNI). While these measures have been designed for clinical use, more psychometric evaluation is needed to determine their validity and reliability.

Family Systems Stressors Strength Inventory. The FSSSI is a 53-item self administered questionnaire that is designed to identify the perceptions of family members regarding general and specific family stressors and strengths. When used as a clinical tool, the instrument can provide direction for intervention planning and has the advantage of assessing family strengths as well as difficulties. Content validity was assessed through inter-rater agreement for conceptual fit and for clarity of items. However, as previously mentioned, very little psychometric data are available for this instrument and reliability of this instrument is unknown (Touliatos et al., 2001).

Hispanic Stress Inventory. The HIS is designed as a culturally appropriate tool for assessing stressors within Hispanic families, including marital stress, family stress, occupational stress, economic stress, discrimination stress, and acculturation stress. Two versions of the instrument are available, a 73-item self-report questionnaire designed for use with immigrant families and a 59-item self-report questionnaire adapted for US-born family members. A key advantage of the HIS is its culture-specific application for diagnosing and planning interventions for Hispanic families, and its subscales have been found to have high internal consistency and high test-retest reliabilities (Cervantes, Padilla, & De Snyder, 1991). Additional psychometric tests should be conducted in order to further substantiate its reliability and validity (Touliatos et al., 2001).

Ontario Child Neglect Index (CNI). The Ontario CNI is a brief 6-item caseworker-rated instrument, which is designed to identify the type and severity of neglect that children experience from their primary caretakers. In addition to evaluating history of physical abuse, sexual harm and criminal activity, the CNI can also be used to identify problematic areas in basic needs provision, including nutrition, clothing and hygiene, physical care, mental health care, and developmental/educational care. The brevity of the instrument helps facilitate an immediate screening and diagnostic impression of the family, however, may also pose a potential limitation through loss of accuracy, comprehensiveness, and susceptibility to bias (Touliatos et al., 2001). The CNI has demonstrated a high level of consistency in repeated administrations and high inter-rater reliability (Trócme, 1996).

ASSESSING BASIC NEEDS

Few measures have been developed for the sole purpose of assessing a family's basic needs. As previously mentioned, the Ontario Child Neglect Index includes items that screen for potential deficiencies in basic needs provision; however, it does not provide a thorough assessment of this domain. The Home Observation for the Measurement of Environment (HOME) is a perhaps the most comprehensive and widely used measure that assesses the family's capacity to fulfill basic needs, in addition to assessing patterns of social interaction and parenting practices. The HOME may be used clinically for screening and intervention planning purposes. Several versions of the HOME that are tailored to age-specific populations are available, including versions suitable for assessing families with infants/toddlers (age 0-3 years), children in early childhood (age 3-6 years), children in middle childhood (age 6-10 years), and early adolescents (age 10-15 years). Although different versions of the measure vary in number of items, ranging from 45-60 items, all versions employ observation and semi-structured interviewing methods to obtain evaluation scores for the family and can be administered in about one hour. The HOME has been used in a number of studies with minority and special needs populations, and versions adapted for these populations are also available (Caldwell & Bradley, 2003). Psychometric properties of the HOME include high inter-rater reliability and high internal reliability (Elardo & Bradley, 1981).

The Family Economic Strain Scale (FES) is another measure that is potentially promising for the assessment of basic needs fulfillment for families in the child welfare system. It is a 13-item self-administered questionnaire that is designed to evaluate the financial difficulties of single and two-parent families (Hilton & Devall, 1997). Preliminary reliability tests have demonstrated high internal consistency for the measure, however additional psychometric evaluations should be conducted to ensure its reliability and validity (Touliatos et al., 2001).

IMPLICATIONS FOR PRACTICE

Rather than replacing clinical judgment, psychometrically validated family assessment instruments can enhance the family assessment process by structuring the collection of information and ensuring that relevant categories of family assessment are evaluated. Practitioners can use the results of these assessments to appropriately refer clients to services and to demonstrate the linkages between assessment, referrals, service provision, and child and family outcomes to supervisors, the courts, and other professionals working on the case, and to monitor client progress over time. At the programmatic level, assessment results can be aggregated and analyzed to assess overall program performance and to identify service areas in need of improvement.

ADDITIONAL PSYCHOMETRIC TESTING

The large number of measures related to patterns of social interaction and parenting practices suggest that the family assessment field has been rapidly expanding based on theoretically diverse but overlapping research traditions (including family systems theory, family therapy research, the literature on risk and resilience and the assessment of parenting). Significant effort has been made to bridge these research traditions to produce comprehensive family assessment instruments that meet the needs of child welfare practitioners. These efforts, which have been made incrementally by a small number of researchers over the past fifteen years, are reflected in the introduction and refinement of measures such as the Family Assessment Form and the North Carolina Family Assessment Scale (NCFAS). In the case of new instruments, it can take several years to establish their structural components and validate them (Skinner, 1987). However, establishing additional psychometric information for existing measures that appear appropriate for child welfare services represents a task that agencies can manage through pilot testing and smaller scale studies by way of university-agency partnerships, inter-agency research consortiums, or independent contracting.

KEY ADMINISTRATIVE SUPPORTS

In addition to carefully reviewing the measurement criteria and the practical implications for use of a family assessment instrument in child welfare, it is important for managers to assess the agency resources that may be necessary to successfully integrate family assessment. Comprehensive family assessment is a process rather than the simple completion of a tool; therefore, once decisions are made regarding the selection of instruments, consideration will need to be given to how the agency will build or modify the existing infrastructure to support it. The family assessment process includes at least nine components: (1) the evaluation of information; (2) interviewing; (3) obtaining and integrating information from more specialized assessments; (4) identifying family strengths and needs; (5) decision-making; (6) documenting and maintaining records; (7) linking assessments to service plans; (8) evaluating outcomes; and (9) disseminating information to other providers, as needed (HHS, 2006). Figure 7 outlines four areas of administrative support (adapted from HHS, 2006).

For example, policy needs to reflect the institutional support for the family assessment process, the parameters and expectations of the family assessment process, and the needed staffing support. A comprehensive family assessment process incorporates information collected through other assessments, such as safety, risk, and child assessments. Policies also need to address how these multiple assessments are conducted in day-to-day practice and how this information will be incorporated into the development of service plans that address the major factors that affect safety, permanency, and child well-being over time. Given that the engagement and building of worker-client rapport are of central importance in gathering information from families regarding their needs and strengths, organizational and administrative supports are necessary for implementing family assessment techniques. These include allocating staff time for assessment, formal training, clinical supervision, and mentoring in areas such as completing comprehensive assessments in a culturally sensitive manner, engaging families in a

FIGURE 7. Administrative Supports for Family Assessment

Administrative Support	Description
Policies	Policies that require family assessment processes; incorporate workload requirements into staffing needs and time frames; define its characteristics and its overarching framework, distinguish it from risk and safety assessment, and clarify relationships between multiple assessments
Training, Clinical Supervision, and Mentoring	Training, supervision and mentoring on the family assessment process and its relationship to other types of assessment; training on engagement; interviewing skills; interpretation of specialized assessments; information integration and decision-making; documentation; linkage of assessment information to service planning; coordination of information with other service providers; timing of re-assessment; outcomes evaluation
Systems of Accountability and Evaluation	Systems that assure that the family assessment process takes place and guidelines are followed; assessing how results are used in service plans; evaluating whether service needs are addressed and how case progress is tied to the assessment; establishing a system whereby the entire process of assessment, service planning, service delivery, progress reviews, key decisions, and program outcomes are documented and evaluated
Contracting	Requirements such as purchase of service contract provisions for family assessment that are consonant with child welfare family assessment processes; clarification of reporting requirements and policies and processes of information sharing; examination of cross-training opportunities

change process, and reaching the appropriate conclusions about the meaning of the information gathered.

Systems of accountability, such as quality assurance programs, represent a key support for building the infrastructure that links assessment information to service plans. To illustrate, Figure 8 demonstrates one approach to quality assurance that is currently in place at a local community-based agency that provides differential response services. After the agency receives the child welfare referral, a new worker and a Master's level mentor meet with the family, make their observations, and then jointly complete the NCFAS afterwards during a case conference to establish inter-rater reliability. Results of the NCFAS are then used to develop the service plan, which guides the provision of services. Case notes are used to continuously update the case and to document decisions. The NCFAS is conducted at multiple points during the case to monitor progress and to evaluate the outcomes of service at case closure. The quality assurance component of the process is enhanced through a peer review process using accreditation standards for child welfare developed by the Council on Accreditation. This process is used to monitor and evaluate the linkage of assessment information, service plan specifications, case notes, and service outcomes.

FIGURE 8. Quality Assurance Steps in Family Assessment

Step 1:	Step 2:	Step 3:	Step 4:	Step 5:	Step 6:
Evaluation of Child Welfare Referral	Joint NCFAS Assessment (Worker & Master's Level Mentor)	Development of Service Plan, Service Provision and Linkage	Linkage of Case Notes to Service Plan	Repeat NCFAS to Monitor Progress and Evaluate Outcomes of Service at Case Closure	Council on Accreditation Peer Review Process

Quality assurance programs represent an important administrative support for monitoring and evaluating the implementation and outcomes of the family assessment process and can also be used to identify needs for changes in policies, training, clinical supervision, and mentoring. While child welfare agencies have the ultimate responsibility for the case plan, increasingly, community-based organizations are often the contracted providers of services. Therefore, systems of accountability naturally extend to services that are provided through other agencies. In relation to family assessment, contract provisions and memoranda of understanding represent the mechanisms through which family assessment processes and information sharing can be coordinated and clarified.

NOTES

1. Available at http://cssr.berkeley.edu/bassc/projects_practice.asp
2. Numbers do not add to 85 given that instruments address multiple domains

REFERENCES

Akister, J., & Stevenson-Hinde, J. (1991). Identifying families at risk: Exploring the potential of the McMaster Family Assessment Device. *Journal of Family Therapy, 13*(4), 411-421.

Bavolek, S. J., & Keene, R. G. (2001). *Adult-Adolescent Parenting Inventory AAPI-2: Administration and Development Handbook.* Park City, UT: Family Development Resources, Inc.

Beavers, R., & Hampson, R. B. (2000). The Beavers System Model of Family Functioning. *Journal of Family Therapy, 22*(2), 128-143.

Berry, M., Cash, S. J., & Mathiesen, S. G. (2003). Validation of the strengths and stressors tracking device with a child welfare population. *Child Welfare, 82*(3), 293-318.

Boss, P., Doherty, W., LaRossa, R., Schumm, W., & Steinmetz, S. (Ed.). (1993). *Sourcebook of Family Theories and Methods.* New York: Plenum Press.

Cabral, R. J., & Strang, M. (1984). Measuring child care: An examination of three assessment measures. *Journal of Social Service Research, 7*(2), 65-77.

Caldwell, B. M., & Bradley, R. H. (2003). *HOME Inventory Administration Manual.* Little Rock, AR: Print Design, Inc.

Carlson, C. I. (1989). Criteria for family assessment in research and intervention contexts. *Journal of Family Psychology, 3*(2), 158-176.

Carlson, C. I. (2003). Assessing the family context. In C. R. Reynolds, & R. W. Kamphaus (Eds.), *Handbook of Psychological and Educational Assessment of Children: Intelligence, Aptitude, and Achievement* (2nd ed., pp. 473-492). New York: Guilford Press.

Cervantes, R. C., Padilla, A. M., & de Snyder, N. S. (1991). The Hispanic Stress Inventory: A culturally relevant approach to psychosocial assessment. *Psychological Assessment, 3*(3), 438-447.

Cromwell, R. E., & Peterson, G. W. (1983). Multisystem-Multimethod Family Assessment in Clinical Contexts. *Family Process, 22*(2), 147-163.

Day, P., Robison, S., & Sheikh, L. (1998). *Ours to Keep: A Guide for Building a Community Assessment Strategy for Child Protection.* Washington, DC: CWLA Press.

DePanfilis, D., & Salus, M. K. (2003). *Child Protective Services: A Guide for Caseworkers.* Rockville, MD: U.S. Department of Health & Human Services.

Drumm, M., Carr, A., & Fitzgerald, M. (2000). The Beavers, McMaster and Circumplex clinical rating scales: A study of their sensitivity, specificity and discriminant validity. *Journal of Family Therapy, 22*(2), 225-258.

Elardo, R., & Bradley, R. (1981). The Home Observation for Measurement of the Environment: A review of research. *Developmental Review, 1*, 113-145.

Epstein, N. B., Bishop, D. S., & Levin, S. (1978). The McMaster model of family functioning. *Journal of Marriage and Family Counseling, 40*, 585-593.

Epstein, N. B., Ryan, C. E., Bishop, D. S., Miller, I. W., & Keitner, G. I. (2003). The McMaster Model: A view of healthy family functioning. In F. Walsh (Ed.), *Normal Family Processes: Growing Diversity and Complexity* (3rd ed., pp. 581-607). New York: Guilford Press.

Friedemann, M., Åstedt-Kurki, P., & Paavilainen, E. (2003). Development of a Family Assessment Instrument for Transcultural Use. *Journal of Transcultural Nursing, 14*(2), 90-99.

Halvorsen, J. G. (1991). Self-Report Family Assessment Instruments: An Evaluative Review. *Family Practice Research Journal, 11*(1), 21-53.

Hawkins, R. P. (1979). The functions of assessment: Implications for selection and development of devices for assessing repertoires in clinical, educational, and other settings. *Journal of Applied Behavior Analysis, 12*, 501-516.

Heinze, M. C., & Grisso, T. (1996). Review of instruments assessing parenting competencies used in child custody evaluations. *Behavioral Sciences and the Law, 14*, 293-313.

Hill, R. (1949). *Families under Stress.* Westport, CT: Greenwood Press.

Hilton, J. M., & Devall, E. L. (1997). The Family Economic Strain Scale: Development and evaluation of the instrument with single and two-parent families. *Journal of Family Economics Issues, 18*(3), 247-271.

Johnson, M. A., & Wells, S. J. (2000). *Measuring Success in Child Welfare, National Study of Outcome Measurement in Public Child Welfare Services: Results and Recommendations*. Urbana, IL: Children and Family Research Center, School of Social Work, University of Illinois at Urbana-Champaign.

Kilpatrick, K. L. (2005). The Parental Empathy Measure: A New Approach to Assessing Child Maltreatment Risk. *American Journal of Orthopsychiatry, 75*(4), 608-620.

Kirk, R. S., Kim, M. M., & Griffith, D. P. (2005). Advances in the reliability and validity of the North Carolina Family Assessment Scale. *Journal of Human Behavior in the Social Environment*.

McCroskey, J., & Nelson, J. (1989). Practice-based research in a family-support program: The Family Connection project example. *Child Welfare, 68*(6), 573-587.

McCroskey, J., Nishimoto, R., & Subramanian, K. (1991). Assessment in family support programs: Initial reliability and validity testing of the family assessment form. *Child Welfare, 70*(1), 19-33.

McCubbin, M. A., & McCubbin, H. I. (1987). Family stress theory and assessment: The T-double ABCX model of family adjustment and adaptation. In H. I. McCubbin, & A. I. Thompson (Eds.), *Family Assessment Inventories for Research and Practice* (pp. 1-32). Madison, WI: University of Wisconsin-Madison.

McCubbin, H. I., McCubbin, M. A., Thompson, A. I., & Huang, S. (1989). Family assessment and self-report instruments in family medicine research. In C. Ramsey (Ed.), *Family Systems in Medicine* (pp. 181-214). New York: Guilford Press.

Miller, I. W., Ryan, C. E., Keitner, G. I., Bishop, D. S., & Epstein, N. B. (2000). The McMaster Approach to Families: Theory, assessment, treatment and research. *Journal of Family Therapy, 22*(2), 168-189.

Milner, J. (1994). Assessing physical child abuse risk: The Child Abuse Potential Inventory. *Clinical Psychology Review, 14*(6), 547-583.

Olson, D. H. (2000). Circumplex Model of Marital and Family Systems. *Journal of Family Therapy, 22*(2), 144-167.

Olson, D. H., & Gorall, D. M. (2003). Circumplex Model of Marital and Family Systems. In F. Walsh (Ed.), *Normal family processes: Growing diversity and complexity* (3rd ed., pp. 514-548). New York: Guilford Press.

Pecora, P. J., Fraser, M. W., Nelson, K. E., McCroskey, J., & Meezan, W. (1995). *Evaluating Family-Based Services*. New York: Aldine de Gruyter.

Pedhazur, E. J., & Schmelkin, L. P. (1991). *Measurement, Design, & Analysis*. Hillsdale, NJ: Lawrence Erlbaum Associates.

Perlmutter, B. F., & Czar, G. (2001). Developing, interpreting, and using family assessment techniques. In J. Touliatos, B. F. Perlmutter, & G. W. Holden (Eds.), *Handbook of Family Measurement Techniques*. Thousand Oaks, CA: Sage Publications, Inc.

Reed-Ashcraft, K., Kirk, R. S., & Fraser, M. W. (2001). The reliability and validity of the North Carolina Family Assessment Scale. *Research on Social Work Practice, 11*(4), 503-520.

Shek, D. T. L. (2001). The general functioning scale of the Family Assessment Device: Does it work with Chinese adolescents? *Journal of Clinical Psychology, 57*(2), 1503-1516.

Shek, D. T. L. (2002). Assessment of family functioning in Chinese adolescents: The Chinese version of the Family Assessment Device. *Research on Social Work Practice, 12*(4), 502-524.

Skinner, H. A. (1987). Self-report: Instruments for family assessment. In J. Theodore (Ed.), *Family Interaction and Psychopathology: Theories, Methods, and Findings* (pp. 427-452). New York: Plenum Press.

Skinner, H., Steinhauser, P., & Sitarenios, G. (2000). Family Assessment Measure (FAM) and Process Model of Family Functioning. *Journal of Family Therapy, 22*(2), 190-210.

Terry, D. J. (1991). Predictors of subjective stress in a sample of new parents. *Australian Journal of Psychology, 43*(1), 29-36.

Terry, D. J. (1991). Stress, coping and adaptation to new parenthood. *Journal of Social and Personal Relationships, 8*, 527-547.

Touliatos, J., Perlmutter, B., & Holden, G. (2001). *Handbook of Family Measurement Techniques: Abstracts* (Vol. 2). Thousand Oaks, CA: Sage Publications.

Trocme, N. (1996). Development and preliminary evaluation of the Ontario Child Neglect Index. *Child Maltreatment, 1*(2), 145-155.

U.S. Department of Health and Human Services. (2006). *Comprehensive Family Assessment Guidelines for Child Welfare*. Washington, DC: Administration for Children and Families Children's Bureau.

Walrath, C., Franco, E., Liao, Q., & Holden, W. (2004). Measures of child emotional and behavioral strengths and family functioning: A preliminary report on the reliability and validity of their Spanish translations. *Journal of Psychoeducational Assessment, 22*, 209-219.

Wilkinson, I. (2000). The Darlington Family Assessment System: Clinical guidelines for practitioners. *Journal of Family Therapy, 22*(2), 211-224.

Wilkinson, I., & Stratton, P. (1991). The reliability and validity of a system for family assessment. *Journal of Family Therapy, 13*(1), 73-94.

APPENDIX A

Measurement Criteria (Perlmutter & Czar, 2001; Pedhazur & Schmelkin, 1991)

Measurement Criteria	Definitions
VALIDITY	A valid instrument measures what it claims to measure. Major types of validity include content-related validity, criterion-related validity, and construct-related validity.
Content-Related Validity	A well-constructed instrument can be considered to adequately represent a specified area of knowledge as well as avoid the effects of unrelated variables. Judges that render opinions about the suitability of items in an instrument commonly assess content validity. There is no accepted standard of agreement established for retaining an item, however, better scales tend to elicit greater agreement among judges.
Criterion-Related Validity	Relates to predicting an individual's performance against a score on an existing instrument or a future outcome. Two methods for establishing criterion-related validity include concurrent and predictive strategies. *Concurrent validity.* Using this method, tests are administered to individuals for whom criterion data are already available for accurate indicators of the construct under study (e.g., an existing measure of family functioning). Correlations between scores or ratings on the new instrument and those obtained on the existing instrument are then established. *Predictive validity.* Denotes an instrument's ability to predict future outcomes or status from scores on an instrument. *Differential predictive validity* refers to an instrument's ability to predict these outcomes for different groups (e.g., abusive vs. non-abusive families).
Construct-Related Validity	Relates to the degree to which an instrument successfully measures a theoretical concept. Two methods, convergent and divergent validity, establish the construct-related validity of a test. *Convergent-Divergent Validity.* When different measures of a concept yield similar results they converge; demonstrating convergent validity typically involves correlating two existing measures or correlating a new measure with an existing measure. When concepts can be empirically differentiated from other concepts they diverge; therefore, measures of different constructs will possess low linear correlations.
RELIABILITY	Reliability is an index of the degree to which individual differences in scoring reflect actual differences in the characteristic under consideration versus chance errors. There are four types of reliability: test-retest, alternate form, inter-rater, and internal consistency.
Test-Retest Reliability	Refers to the degree to which generalizations can be made about test scores from one administration to the next. Established by correlating results of baseline and subsequent administrations. Higher test-retest coefficients generally mean that scores are less susceptible to random changes in the condition of test takers or the testing environment
Alternate-Form	When equivalent forms of a test are administered to the same person on two occasions, the reliability coefficient is the correlation between scores obtained on the two tests. The higher the scores, the more likely it is that the different test forms are measuring the same characteristics.
Inter-rater Reliability	Relates to the extent to which two or more people arrive at the same result when observing and/or rating the same event. It is most frequently reported for observational techniques when events are recorded or ratings of behaviors are made.
Internal Consistency	Cronbach's alpha is the measure of internal consistency by which we infer that items within a scale or subscale measure the same construct. Alpha rises when the average inter-item correlation between items increases. It also increases with increased numbers of items, so long as the quality of those items remains high. Therefore, when considering the value of alpha for a given instrument or subscale, both the reported alpha and the number of items must be considered.

APPENDIX B
BASSC Search Protocol

Search Terms

1) assessment of families
2) family assessment
3) family assessment and child welfare
4) family assessment and clinical
5) family assessment and device
6) family assessment and evaluation
7) family assessment and guide
8) family assessment and intervention
9) family assessment and measure
10) family assessment and measurement
11) family assessment and mental health
12) family assessment and model
13) family assessment and research
14) family assessment and scale
15) family assessment and school
16) family assessment and service
17) family assessment and social services
18) family assessment and therapy
19) family assessment and treatment
20) family functioning assessment
21) family strengths assessment

Databases
Academic databases for books and articles
Pathfinder or Melvyl
ArticleFirst
ERIC
Expanded Academic ASAP
Family and Society Studies Worldwide
PAIS International
PsychInfo
Social Science Citation Index
Social Services Abstracts
Social Work Abstracts
Sociological Abstracts

Systematic Reviews
Campbell Collaboration–C2-Spectre & C2-Ripe
Children and Family Research Center
Cochrane Library
ESRC Evidence Network
NHS Centre for Reviews & Dissemination
Social Care Institute for Excellence

Research Institutes
Brookings Institute
Manpower Demonstration Research Corporation
Mathematica Policy Research, Inc.
Urban Institute
RAND
GAO
National Academy of Sciences

Chapin Hall
CASRC (San Diego)

Conference Proceedings
PapersFirst (UCB Database)
Proceedings (UCB Database)

Dissertation Abstracts
DigitalDissertations (UCB database)

Professional Evaluation Listserves
EVALTALK
GOVTEVAL
ChildMaltreatmentListserve

Internet
Google
Dogpile

George Warren Brown School of Social Work at Washington University in St. Louis, Center for Mental Health Services Research : http://gwbweb.wustl.edu/cmhsr/measure/category.html

Administration for Children and Families, DHHS, Resources for Measuring Services & Outcome in Head Start Programs Serving Infants & Toddle rs:
http://www.acf.hhs.gov/programs/opre/ehs/perf_measures/reports/resources_measuring/res_meas_toc.html

Violence Institute of New Jersey at UMDNJ:
http://www.umdnj.edu/vinjweb/research_projects/instrument_inventory/instrument_inventory.html

http://www.lib.berkeley.edu/SOCW/socw_instruments.html

APPENDIX C
Instruments Evaluated

Abusive Behavior Inventory
Adult-Adolescent Parenting Inventory
Attitudes toward Wife Abuse Scale
Brother-Sister Questionnaire
Child Abuse Potential Inventory
Circumplex Model (FACES IV)
Culturagrams
Family Adaptation Model
Family Assessment Checklist
Family Assessment Measure III
Family Concept Assessment Method (FCAM)
Family Distress Index
Family Emotional Involvement and Criticism Scale (FEICS)
Family Evaluation Form (FEF)
Family Functioning Questionnaire
Family Hardiness Index
Family Interaction Q-Sort
Family Strengths Inventory
Family Systems Stressor Strength Inventory
Global Coding Scheme
Hispanic Stress Inventory
Interparental Conflict Scale
Inventory of Battering Experiences
Kempe Family Stress Inventory

Maternal Characteristics Scale
MMPI Family Scale
North Carolina Family Assessment Scale (NCFAS)
Ontario Child Neglect Index
Parent Child Relationship Inventory
Parental Stress Scale
Parenting Stress Index
Physical Abuse and Psychological Abuse
Revised Conflict Tactics Scales (CFTS-2/RCTS)
Severity of Violence Scales
Social Environment Inventory
Strengths and Stressors Tracking Device (SSTD)
Structural Family Interaction Scale (SFIS)
Structured Clinical Interview (SCI)

Ackerman-Schoendorf Scales for Parent Evaluation of Custody
Assessment of Strategies in Families-Effectiveness (ASF-E)
Beavers Model
Child Abuse Blame Scale- Physical Abuse
Childhood Level of Living Scale
Colorado Family Assessment
Darlington Family Assessment System (DFAS)
Family APGAR
Family Assessment Form
Family Behavioral Snapshot
Family Daily Hassles Inventory
Family Economic Strain
Family Environment Scale

Family Functioning Index (FFI)
Family Functioning Style Scale
Family Impact Questionnaire
Family Profile II
Family Strengths Scale
Global Assessment of Relational Functioning (GARF)
Global Family Interaction Scales (FIS-II)
Home Observation for Measurement of the Environment
Interpersonal Support Evaluation List (ISEL)
Inventory of Socially Supportive Behaviors
Life Stressors and Social Resources Inventory–Adult & Youth Forms
McMaster Model (Family Assessment Device)
Mother's Activity Checklist
North Carolina Family Assessment Scale for Reunification (NCFAS-R)
Parent Child Conflict Tactics Scale
Parental Empathy Measure (PEM)
Parent-Child Relationship Scale (PCRS, subset of CAPA)
Parenting Stress Inventory
Propensity for Abusiveness Scale
Scale of Neglectful Parenting

Simulated Family Activity Measure (SIMFAM)
Standardized Clinical Family Interview
Stress Index for Parents of Adolescents

Structural Family Systems Rating Scale (SFSR)
Yale Guide to Family Assessment

Assessing Child and Youth Well-Being: Implications for Child Welfare Practice

Christine Lou, MSW
Elizabeth K. Anthony, PhD
Susan Stone, PhD
Catherine M. Vu, MPA, MSW
Michael J. Austin, PhD

SUMMARY. The measurement of child well-being has become increasingly important in child welfare practice in the past ten years with the federal emphasis on measuring positive outcomes for children and families. Practical and methodological barriers to evaluating well-being exist alongside positive developments in the field. This article reviews the research literature related to child and youth well-being, providing a context for the discussion of measurement issues in child welfare settings. Based on a structured review of the literature, the article discusses instruments that appear to be most appropriate for use in a child welfare setting. Instruments are presented within stages of development, including (1) Infancy and Early Childhood, (2) Middle Childhood, and (3) Adolescence. Implications for the design and use of child well-being

---

Christine Lou is Doctoral Research Assistant, Elizabeth K. Anthony is BASSC Research Director, Susan Stone is Research Consultant, Catherine M. Vu is Doctoral Research Assistant, and Michael J. Austin is Staff Director; all are affiliated with Bay Area Social Services Consortium, School of Social Welfare, University of California, Berkeley.

instruments in child welfare practice are discussed.

KEYWORDS. Assessment, child, youth, well-being, strengths-based assessment, instruments

Current guidelines for family assessment from the Children's Bureau of the U. S. Department of Health and Human Services (HHS, 2006) recommend the use of a comprehensive assessment of individual children and youth to guide service planning and delivery. A key component of the assessment process is the concept of child well-being and its systematic measurement. Although the Children's Bureau has consistently included child well-being as one of its three primary goals for child welfare services, the goals of safety and of permanency have traditionally been the principal indicators of program success and, accordingly, represent the most concretely defined and measurable outcomes in child welfare policy and practice (Altshuler & Gleeson, 1999). However, with the passage of the Adoption and Safe Families Act of 1997 (AFSA), well-being has moved to the forefront of child welfare reform, policy development, and program evaluation (Wulczyn, Barth, Yuan, Harden, & Landsberk, 2005). The AFSA explicitly and legislatively mandates that the outcome of child well-being be actively pursued and regularly assessed. These two directives of assessment and outcome indicate the need for identifying and for developing standard assessment tools for use with children and youth by child welfare workers in order to develop and monitor service plans that are rooted in the concept of child well-being.

Child and youth assessments are related to both risk and family assessment, namely constructs of risk for deleterious child/youth outcomes and family functioning for identifying problematic behaviors and ecological difficulties. Two structured reviews included in this special issue, *Risk and Safety Assessment in Child Welfare: Instrument Comparisons* and *Family Assessment in Child Welfare Services: Instrument Comparisons*, address the array of valid and reliable instruments. However, the purpose of this review is to utilize the strengths-based and well-being perspectives to identify valid and reliable assessment tools for use in child welfare practice.

The introduction to this structured review of the literature is divided into three sections. The first section provides an overview of the need for assessing child and youth well-being in child welfare, the existing and potential uses of such assessments, and the challenges related to utilization. The second section highlights the concept of well-being and how it was used to develop the criteria for inclusion/exclusion of reviewed measures and assess existing guidelines for the evaluation of measures. The third section is a brief description of the framework and methodology of the review. The remainder of the report includes major findings and implications for practice.

NEED FOR CHILD AND YOUTH WELL-BEING ASSESSMENT IN CHILD WELFARE

The impetus for assessing child and youth well-being in child welfare is the convergence of conceptual changes, policy directives, and practical concerns that have surfaced in recent years. In response to the shortcomings of the deficit- and pathology-based model that has guided social work policy and practice in the past, the field has undergone a paradigm shift towards incorporating strengths-based practice and policy in order to "discover and embellish, explore and exploit client's strengths and resources in the service of assisting them to achieve their goals" (Saleebey, 2006, p. 1). Influenced by these broad changes, the field of child welfare has increasingly adopted the terms "positive youth development," "youth assets," and "resilience and protective factors" as a part of the lexicon for daily practice (Damon, 2004; Park, 2004). Beyond rhetoric, the child development and child welfare fields have realized that the process of incorporating strengths, assets, and abilities in the assessments of children and youth provides a more complete and accurate picture than those that focus on risks alone and can help identify pathways for successful development (Gilgun, Klein, & Pranis, 2000).

However, as these terms and goals have gained currency in the child welfare field, so have the demands for evaluation of service efficacy and goal attainment. The ASFA indicates that "The child welfare system must focus on results and accountability. The law makes it clear that it is no longer enough to ensure that procedural safeguards are met. It is critical that child welfare services lead to *positive* [italics added] results" (HHS, 1998). Moreover, the federal guidelines for comprehensive family assessment issued by the Children's Bureau make explicit the need to identify individual and family strengths and protective factors that are "relevant and dynamically involved in offsetting the risks related to abuse/neglect" (HHS, 2006). Thus, the child welfare system and its workers are not only charged with the responsibility of ensuring basic safety levels for children and youth, but also must conduct ongoing standardized assessments of children and youth from a strengths-perspective and provide evidence that children and youth demonstrate positive outcomes and well-being as a result of service delivery.

Finally, several research studies have indicated that children and youth that come to the attention or care of the child welfare system demonstrate significantly lower levels of well-being than any other subpopulation of children and youth in the United States (Leslie, Gordon, Ganger, & Gist, 2002; Zimmer & Panko, 2006). Many of these disparities in well-being have been documented by the National Survey of Child and Adolescent Well-Being (NSCAW), a study sponsored by the U.S. Department of Health and Human Services (1997-2007) that examines the characteristics of children and families who come in contact with the child welfare system. Their findings include the following: 53% of all children aged 3 to 24 months whose families were investigated for maltreatment are classified as high risk for developmental delay or neurological impairment, 38% of all children in the study are classified as having "fewer" social skills than the general population, 30% of all children in the study have low or moderately low scores for daily living skills, substantially lower than the general population and, all children in the study were at least five times more likely than the normative sample to have problem behaviors and poor psychosocial functioning (HHS, 2001). While these findings still focus on deficits, they highlight the critical need for comprehensive assessments of children and youth in the child welfare system that also feature strengths and well-being (Leslie et al., 2003). Moreover, the identification of protective factors and the promotion of positive child and youth development can be used to offset deleterious outcomes for such high-risk populations.

Based on these deficit and strengths perspectives, the uses of a comprehensive assessment of child and youth well-being in child welfare can include the following:

1. To ensure normal development and functioning based on observable characteristics, self- and caregiver-reports, and other sources of information (including school records and other care agencies);
2. To identify child/youth strengths in order to inform service/treatment planning, to reduce identified risks, to monitor the course of service, and to provide outcome scores;

3. To obtain a quick "snapshot" of the child or youth's general status in order to make referral to specialty care; and
4. To inform policy and program development and evaluation at a county- or state-wide level based on population surveys.

CHALLENGES TO CHILD AND YOUTH WELL-BEING ASSESSMENTS IN CHILD WELFARE

The concepts, operationalization, and measurement of "well-being" present numerous challenges. One of the major challenges relates to assessment instruments that emphasize deficits, often developed by researchers in medicine, psychiatry, education, and clinical psychology. The tools are often designed to identify physical illness, psychiatric diagnosis or maladaptive child/youth behaviors, educational and intellectual abilities, or personality characteristics. Further, there is no consensus on the definitions, domains, indicators, and measures of child well-being amongst or within these professions (Altshuler & Gleeson, 1999; Wulczyn et al., 2005). To further complicate matters, assessment procedures have historically ignored the context in which the child resides; research now supports the notion that the well-being of a child is not simply the product of the child's internal characteristics but rather the interaction between the child and the environment. As a result, child assessment needs to be multidimensional, including a multisystems perspective that addresses family and community influences (Ungar, 2004).

In addition to instrumentation issues, child welfare workers face additional challenges in the form of federal guidelines and outcome criteria for "well-being" with no accompanying valid and reliable performance indicators. There are no specific measures in the Child and Family Services Review process that monitors state child welfare programs (Wulczyn et al., 2005). Consequently, not only is the concept of well-being not clearly defined by the literature, but also the outcome of well-being is not clearly defined in mandated performance indicators.

In addition to this lack of clarity, child welfare workers are expected to assess the multiple dimensions of each child within the constraints of limited time and resources. For example, the categories for comprehensive child assessment recommended by the federal guidelines include the following: (1) physical and motor skills, (2) intellectual ability and cognitive functioning, (3) academic achievement, (4) emotional and social functioning, (5) vulnerability/ability to communicate or protect themselves, (6) developmental needs, and (7) readiness of youth to move toward independence. In addition to these aspects, the categories of youth assessment include: (1) readiness to live interdependently, (2) ability to care for one's own physical and mental health needs, (3) self-advocacy skills, (4) future plans for academic achievement, (5) life skills achievement, (6) employment/career development, and (7) quality of personal and community connections. Given this wide range of categories it is unclear which aspects of assessment would be most helpful to a child welfare worker, especially since the majority of well-validated and psychometrically sound instruments do not focus on well-being.

CONCEPTUAL FRAMEWORK

While there are multiple approaches to understanding child well-being, this structured review of the literature draws primarily upon the fields of child development, child psychology, and child health and is organized by developmental stages related to certain aptitudes and tasks. Given our emphasis on strengths, competencies, and positive adaptation, the risk and resilience literature informs our conceptualization of well-being. In contrast to the "fixed" indicators of healthy or abnormal development found in the developmental stages literature, a risk and resilience perspective presents a dynamic, bio-ecological, and transactional conceptualization of child development (Luthar et al., 2000).

Risk, protection, and resilience are the central concepts in a risk and resilience model. Risk factors are "influences that increase the chances for harm, or more specifically, influences that increase the probability of onset, digression to a more serious state, or maintenance of a problem condition" (Fraser, Kirby, & Smokowski, 2004, p. 14). Protective factors act to modify risk, either by directly reducing a disorder or dysfunction or by moderating the relationship among risk factors and problems or disorders, often called "buffering" effects (Fraser, Richman, & Galinsky, 1999). Promotive factors, on the other hand, exert positive effects regardless of risk exposure (Jenson & Fraser, 2006). Finally, resilience can be understood as the successful impact of protective factors on ameliorating or reducing risk factor outcomes and is usually defined as "the ability to function competently despite living or having lived in adversity" (Schofield & Beek, 2005, p. 1283) or the "successful adaptational response to high risk" (Fraser et al., 1999). The notion of risk and resilience throughout the following stages of development is used to organize the findings:

1. Infancy (approximately 0-3): Developmental changes occur the most rapidly in this stage, such as language development, solidification of an attachment relationship, growth, and ambulation. Developmental delays, motor deficits, and poor neuro-development are some of the potential impairments that characterize this stage as a period of extreme vulnerability.
2. Early Childhood (approximately 4-5): This stage is characterized by significant progress in language, cognitive, social, and emotional development. "Early childhood can be conceptualized as a time of increased competence, but continued vulnerability. Preschool children in the child welfare system can use language and play to reveal their maltreatment experience, but are sufficiently young that their ability to self-protect is limited" (Wulczyn et al., 2005, p. 34).
3. Middle Childhood (approximately 6-12): This stage is characterized by increased competence to take on additional roles and responsibilities and the development of broader social networks. This stage is also marked by increased behavioral self-regulation and identity development. Although increased competence might reduce vulnerability to maltreatment, this stage has been identified as a period when mental health issues emerge.
4. Adolescence (approximately 13-18): This stage is often characterized by complex changes across multiple developmental domains, including identity creation, primacy of peer group relations, and movement towards independence. Academic, mental health, and social functioning are often the indicators of wellness for this age group.

While well-being is not limited to concepts of risk and resilience, the definition of well-being used in this literature review relies heavily on the presence of, or potential for the development of, strengths and resilience. These include internal aspects (e.g., subjective life satisfaction and positive self-concept), external aspects (e.g., social connections), and biomedical and developmental aspects (e.g., physical health and intellectual ability). "Indicators" of health, stages of development, and the multidimensionality of well-being inform this ecological and holistic approach. Consequently, findings are presented by developmental stage; within each stage, findings are discussed within the domains of well-being that are most pertinent to that developmental stage. This approach is particularly suited to child welfare practice because it provides a theoretical foundation for intervention and service planning, including the processes of "increasing felt security, building self-esteem, promoting competence, and working towards a range of often modest developmental goals that nevertheless reduce risk and increase resilience" (Schofield & Beek, 2005, p. 1284). Furthermore, the equal importance assigned to strengths and risks restores balance to the past deficit-based models used to assess children and youth.

LITERATURE REVIEW SEARCH CRITERIA AND STRATEGY

This review used pre-determined search terms and search sources to identify research literature within a given topic and to minimize the potential for selection bias. Using specified search terms delineated by search category (e.g., domain of interest, characteristics of interest, etc.) in multiple combinations, we searched numerous social science and academic databases through the University of California library. In addition, we conducted overall internet searches and also searched the websites of research institutes and organizations specializing in systematic reviews, conference proceedings databases, dissertation databases, and internet databases (see Appendix A for description of search strategy). The references in literature reviews and research studies were searched to identify additional sources. Only English language citations were pursued.

To illustrate the magnitude of the child assessment literature, an initial search with the key words "child or youth" and "assessment" in one database yielded 2,109 results. While it is beyond the scope of this review to provide a comprehensive evaluation of all child assessment tools, this review provides an in-depth examination of those instruments that are most pertinent to child welfare and most consistent with the federal mandates. The criteria for inclusion and the recommendation of promising instruments include: (1) instruments that provide comprehensive assessments of child and youth well-being; (2) instruments that assess for child and youth strengths and competence; (3) instruments that have been normed with a child welfare population or appear to be appropriate for child welfare use; and (4) instruments that have demonstrated sound psychometric properties. Thus, the criteria for exclusion of instruments include: (1) instruments that assess psychiatric dysfunction and assign DSM diagnoses; and (2) instruments that focus on risk or deviance such as instruments that predict juvenile criminality. Two-hundred sixty-nine instruments were reviewed; given that most of these instruments are specialized for administration in professional settings other than child welfare, those presented below were determined to be of most use to a child welfare worker. Some of the instruments that have been excluded from this review but are used in related fields and may be encountered by child welfare workers are summarized in Appendix B.

MAJOR FINDINGS

Infancy and Early Childhood (Ages 0-5)

For infants and young children, the assessment of well-being reflects the normal developmental process in the four general domains summarized in Figure 1: (1) language development and communication; (2) intellectual ability and cognitive functioning; (3) physical development and motor skills; and (4) socio-emotional functioning (Capute & Accardo, 1996). Global measures of well-being focus on the continuum of functioning in each of these areas. Until children are old enough to verbally communicate, assessment occurs in the form of behavioral observation and reports from parents, care providers, or teachers. In general, child welfare workers are interested in identifying potential problems in order to refer the child to early intervention services.

The measurement of infant well-being is often the collaborative work of an interdisciplinary team of professionals and the family, particularly for infants born with a disability or at-risk. In infants and young children, the focus is on nutrition, immunization, and physical care along with signs of potential physical or sexual abuse and neglect. Normal developmental milestones are the markers by which delayed or insufficient development are judged and may lead to additional assessments or referrals as the need arises.

While specialized tests can be helpful in assessing infant functioning in different domains of living, a comprehensive evaluation of an infant's well-being should include broader measures of attachment and the infant's social ability (Davies, 2004). Further, assessment should be ongoing and include information about a child's environment. As one component of assessment, instruments can be used to measure both strengths and limitations in the development of an infant in order to identify potential areas for intervention.

FIGURE 1. Domains of Infancy and Early Childhood Assessment

Domain	Sample Components	Measurement Types
Language	Language precursors; vocabulary; concepts; syntax; integrative language skills; phonological awareness; receptive; expressive; speech	-Intelligence tests -Standardized tests of early language -Developmental assessment
Cognition	Fluid reasoning; knowledge; quantitative reasoning; visual-spatial processing; working memory; non-verbal problem solving	-Intelligence tests -General measures of cognition -Developmental assessment
Physical	Normative standards for growth and development; gross motor; fine motor	-Developmental screening & assessment -Specialized instruments -Physical examination
Socio-Emotional	Internalizing and externalizing problem behaviors; regulatory problems; self-help; social competencies	-Behavior screening -Developmental assessment

Instruments that are commonly used to assess infant/ young child functioning and well-being may be specific to infants or toddlers or cross the lifespan into middle childhood or adolescence as summarized in Appendix C. In addition, some instruments focus on one domain of well-being while others cross multiple domains. For example, the Griffiths Scales (Griffiths, 1984) are standardized scales of motor development whereas the Bayley Scales of Infant Development (Bayley, 1993) cross several domains by measuring cognitive, motor, and behavioral development.

The focus of this review is on comprehensive assessment of well-being, therefore the instruments described in detail below are those that best assess multidimensional functioning and developmental competence rather than a single dimension. Of the 87 infant/young child instruments reviewed, the following four met the inclusion criteria: Child Observation Record (High/Scope, 1992), Battelle Developmental Inventory (Newborg et al., 1988), Ages and Stages Questionnaire (Bricker, Squires, & Mounts, 1995), and the Child Development Inventory (Ireton & Glascoe, 1995). These instruments appear in bold type in Appendix C and two are described below.

Child Observation Record (COR). The Child Observation Record (COR) was designed as a developmentally appropriate and culturally sensitive assessment tool of early childhood competencies. Focusing on strengths with the goal of obtaining an accurate picture of the infant or child's developing abilities, the COR assesses the whole child. The COR for Infants and Toddlers is designed for children ages 6 weeks to 3 years and the Preschool Child COR, Second Edition is for children ages 2 1/2 to 6 years and was developed for use in early childhood programs such as Head Start.

The Infant-Toddler COR assesses development in six domains: sense of self, social relations, creative representation, movement, communication and language, and exploration and early logic. Specific items are assessed within each domain. For example, the sense of self category consists of the following items: *expressing initative, distinguishing self from others, solving problems,* and *developing self-help skills.* The preschool version also measures developmental progress in six domains: initiative, social relations, creative representation, music and movement, language and literacy, and mathematics and science. A teacher or care provider who knows the child well can complete the 30-item COR with its 5-point developmental competence scale from lowest (1) to highest (5) level of competency. In studies with urban Head Start children, the COR produced reliable and valid results (Fantuzzo, Hightower, Grim, & Montes, 2002; High/ Scope, 2002; Sekino & Fantuzzo, 2005). Advantages of the COR include: (1) completion of the observations by the teacher or parent/care provider for at least one month rather than a point-in-time assessment, (2) observation in the natural context of a classroom or home environment rather than a doctor's office, and (3) ease of administration.

Ages and Stages Questionnaires (ASQ). The Ages and Stages Questionnaires (ASQ) are completed by a parent or primary caregiver and assess the developmental progress of infants and young children from 4 to 48 months. The ASQ takes approximately 10-15 minutes to complete and parents select the appropriate questionnaire by the age of the child. Each questionnaire consists of 30 items that address five domains: personal-social, gross motor, fine motor, problem solving, and communication. The parent responds to a series of questions in each domain about the child's behavior by responding "yes" (10 points), "sometimes" (5 points) and "not yet" (0 points), with a maximum possible score of 60 points in each domain. Sample questions include "Do you think your child hears well?" and "Does your baby use both hands equally well?" Cut-off scores (two standard deviations below the mean domain score) have been established for referral purposes. The ASQ has been tested with a normative sample as well as samples of children with medical risks and children with environmental risks (e.g., extreme poverty, low maternal education, and parental involvement with Child Protective Services) (Squires, Bricker, & Potter, 1997).

The ASQ has been revised and the psychometric properties have been studied extensively with evidence supporting the general reliability and validity of the instrument (Bricker & Squires, 1989a, 1989b; Squires et al., 1997). Additional information regarding the construct and predictive validity would provide further support of the ASQ (Naar-King, Ellis, & Frey, 2004). An advantage of the ASQ includes the dynamic nature of the questionnaires, allowing an infant and child's developmental status to be tracked over time. The ASQ is also cost-effective, easy to administer, and makes use of reports by individuals who spend most time with the child. Because the ASQ does not require highly trained specialists to administer, the likelihood of repeated measures to monitor a child's progress increases. In addition to the ASQ, the Ages and Stages Questionnaire: Social-Emotional (ASQ: SE; Squires et al., 2001) was developed to assess the social and emotional development needs of infants and young children.

Middle Childhood (Ages 6-12)

As children grow and develop, the assessment of well-being takes on a different meaning from that of infants and young children. As children become more verbal and autonomous, the focus of assessment shifts from heavy reliance on the observations and assessments of parents and care providers to a combination of child and adult data collection. Observation remains an important component however, as children's verbal and communication abilities vary. Less emphasis is placed on basic developmental and cognitive abilities and more emphasis is placed on the child's interaction with the social world. Consequently, the conceptualization of well-being in middle childhood involves the assessment of socio-emotional functioning and general social competence, academic achievement, peer relationships and social skills, a developing sense of identity, and the nature of social support.

Figure 2 summarizes the focus of assessment in middle childhood. The instruments that assess language ability in middle childhood continue to measure developmental progress from early childhood. By middle childhood, the comprehension of basic syntax and grammar structures is developed and children are learning to make connections between cognitive processes and communication (Davies, 2004). Language ability is directly related to a child's ability to navigate the social world, a significant developmental task in middle childhood. Similar to language ability, intellectual functioning and cognition is measured as a continuation of the progress made in early childhood. Many of the traditional tests of cognitive ability, such as the Stanford-Binet (Roid, 2003), are used in middle childhood. Unique to middle and later childhood, however, are measures of academic functioning and aptitudes that assess academic progress. The Children's Skills Test (SmarterKids,

FIGURE 2. Domains of Middle Childhood Assessment

Domain	Sample Components	Measurement Types
Language & Communication	Basic syntax; grammatical structures; receptive; expressive; speech	-Intelligence tests -Standardized tests of early language -Assessment of delays
Cognitive Ability & Academics	Fluid reasoning; knowledge; quantitative reasoning; visual-spatial processing; working memory; academic achievement and skills	-Intelligence tests -General measures of cognition -Standardized academic tests
Physical Health & Development	Normative standards for growth and development; risk-taking behaviors related to health	-Physical examination -Self-report surveys of behaviors
Socio-Emotional	Social competence; internalizing and externalizing problem behaviors; self-concept; identity development; self-regulation; coping; peer relationships; social skills; self-esteem	-Behavior checklists/ screening tools -Self-report surveys

1998), for example, measures achievement in math, language arts, science, and social studies. Such instruments are useful in obtaining information about whether a child has achieved the basic academic skills for a particular grade level.

Physical development remains an important factor in middle childhood, as young people develop and grow in relationship to progress based on normative health care standards. As young children near puberty and adolescence, assessment of physical well-being begins to include risk-taking behaviors that contribute to poor health, such as cigarette smoking and unsafe sexual activity.

The majority of instruments in middle childhood feature aspects of socio-emotional competence. In general, basic social and emotional competence is considered crucial for a child's ability to relate to others and develop a strong and healthy sense of identity. Therefore, psychological constructs such as self-esteem and self-concept are presumed to be indicators of child well-being. Certain constructs, such as self-regulation, are associated with behavior patterns that can become problematic. For example, poor impulse control and sensation-seeking are risk factors for adolescent substance abuse (Jenson, Anthony, & Howard, 2006).

Assessments of socio-emotional competence have traditionally been used for psychological research rather than for assessment or treatment. However, multidimensional assessments of socio-emotional competence are used in clinical, school, and community-based settings. For example, the Social Adjustment Inventory for Children and Adolescents (SAICA; John, Gammon, Prusoff, & Warner, 1987) assesses adaptive functioning in the outcome areas of activities, peer relations, family relations, and academic performance. Also, the Elementary

School Success Profile (ESSP; Bowen, 2006) is a notable example of a multidimensional instrument that uses an ecological perspective of neighborhood, school, friends, and family to assess factors related to health and well-being.

Given the large number of single domain and risk-focused behavioral instruments in middle childhood, no instrument fully met the inclusion criteria of comprehensive *and* strengths based assessment of well-being. Of the 99 middle childhood instruments reviewed, three met most of the criteria and are described below. These instruments appear in bold type in Appendix D.

Behavioral and Emotional Rating Scale–Second Edition (BERS-2). The Behavior and Emotional Rating Scale (BERS; Epstein & Sharma, 1998) and the Behavioral and Emotional Rating Scale–Second Edition (BERS–2; Epstein, 2004) were developed in response to the need for standardized measures for assessing emotional and behavioral strengths in children and youth. Behavioral and emotional rating scales tend to rely on a deficit model of assessment and the BERS is one of the few instruments to incorporate a strengths-based orientation to assessment. The BERS offers parents, care providers, and teachers a more comprehensive picture of the child by describing positive functioning skills. The BERS was designed for use in child welfare agencies, school settings, mental health clinics, and juvenile justice programs and has been tested with school-aged children ranging from 5 to 18 years of age. The BERS consists of 52 items that address the following five domains: interpersonal strength (e.g., reacts to disappointment in a calm manner), family involvement (e.g., participates in family activities), intrapersonal strength (e.g., demonstrates a sense of humor), school functioning (e.g., pays attention in class), and affective strength (e.g., acknowledges painful feelings) (Epstein, Hertzog, & Reid, 2001). The BERS-2 allows for three perspectives to be evaluated via parental observation (Parent Rating Scale), child self-report (Youth Rating Scale), and teacher or other professional observation (Teacher Rating Scale). Responses to statements about how much a characteristic is representative of the child are on a 4-point Likert scale and include 0 = not at all like the child, 1 = not much like the child, 2 = like the child, and 3 = very much like the child. The BERS also includes open-ended questions designed to elicit information about the unique strengths of the child.

The BERS has strong psychometric properties that have been confirmed in multiple studies (Epstein, Harniss, Pearson, & Ryser, 1999; Epstein et al., 2001; Epstein, Ryser, & Pearson, 2002). Given the wide age range for the BERS, establishing separate age-based norms is warranted (Dumont & Rauch, 1998). With its focus on strengths related to assessment and intervention, the BERS can be useful in child welfare settings for pre-referral assessment as well as evaluation of the effectiveness of an intervention over time. The BERS takes only 10 minutes to administer and is scored manually.

Clinical Assessment Package for Assessing Clients' Risks and Strengths (CASPARS). The Clinical Assessment Package for Assessing Clients' Risks and Strengths (CASPARS; Gilgun, 1999) is a set of five instruments designed to assess assets and risks in children and families experiencing a range of adjustment issues and problematic behaviors. The CASPARS instruments assess strengths and risks in the following five areas: (1) emotional expressiveness (14 items); (2) family relationships (20 items); (3) family's embeddedness in the community (13 items); (4) peer relationships (16 items); and (5) sexuality (13 items). The instruments are completed by practitioners in a two-step evaluative process: practitioners first decide whether an individual demonstrates an asset or risk on a particular item and then rate the asset and risk as high, medium, or low. Sample items include the following: (1) "Child has a person in the family and/or community who facilitates appropriate expression of feelings" and (2) "Neighborhood has resources for children: playgrounds, recreation programs, libraries."

Psychometric properties of these instruments were evaluated with a sample of 146 children and their families; ninety-two of the children were in foster care or residential treatment or had experienced at least one out-of-home-placement in the past. Internal consistency and inter-rater reliability were found to be strong and content and construct validity were found to be good to adequate. The advantages of these instruments include: consistency with the goal of assessing well-being, brevity, ease of use and scoring, ability to demonstrate progress over time, and useful assessments for treatment planning and evaluation. The CASPARS instruments have only recently been developed, however, and have not been rigorously evaluated. The initial study of the CASPARS' psychometric properties and applicability to child welfare populations is promising but additional studies are needed to confirm these findings (Gilgun, 1999).

Social Skills Rating System. The Social Skills Rating System (SSRS; Gresham & Elliott, 1990) is a self-report, multi-rater instrument that provides a comprehensive picture of the social behaviors of children and youth in grades 3-12. The SSRS has three subscales related to (1) social skills (cooperation, empathy, assertion, self-control, responsibility), (2) problem behaviors (externalizing problems, internalizing problems, hyperactivity), and (3) academic competence (reading and mathematics performance, general cognitive functioning, motivation, and parental support). The SSRS is completed by a teacher, parent, and student for use in assessing problematic social behaviors and is suitable for service planning and intervention.

The SSRS was standardized on a national sample of over 4,000 children and provides separate norms for boys and girls as well as for students with disabilities. The advantages of the SSRS include the use of multiple raters who know the child, ease of administration and scoring, and strong psychometric properties. In a study of urban Head Start children, the preschool version of the SSRS demonstrated reliability and construct validity (Fantuzzo, Manz, & McDermott, 1998).

Adolescence (Ages 13-18)

As individuals progress from middle childhood to adolescence, the assessment of their well-being becomes increasingly complex. The appraisals of adolescent developmental competencies and the global health indicators rely less on observable and objective characteristics and more on subjective appraisals of internal life (i.e., thoughts, emotions, and perceptions), social adaptation, and role acquisition. While identity formation and awareness of the social world typically emerge during the period of middle childhood, these developments gain primacy as adolescents become more sophisticated in their psychological, emotional, and social development. Additionally, academic achievement and preparation for adult roles and responsibilities represent major markers of adolescent well-being. Consequently, the majority of adolescent assessment instruments address one or more domains related to personal, social, and general achievement competencies.

Given the nature of instruments available, as well as the developmental considerations for adolescent populations, the domains summarized in Figure 3 represent the four general areas of adolescent well-being assessment: (1) personal competence/emotional well-being; (2) social well-being; (3) environmental context and participation; and (4) cognitive/intellectual well-being (Zill & Coiro, 1992). Examining well-being in these domains represents one part of comprehensive adolescent assessment and other types of information (school and medical records) are needed to form a complete profile of adolescent well-being. Appendix E summarizes the instruments that are frequently used to assess adolescent well-being.

FIGURE 3. Domains of Adolescent Assessment

Domain	Sample Components	Measurement Types
Personal Competence/Emotional	Identity; sense of self; self-esteem; self-concept; self-image; self-efficacy; positive outlook	-Self-report surveys -Standardized tests
Social	Social networks; social interaction; peer relationships; social competence; social support; coping; social skills	-Self-report surveys -Standardized tests
Environmental Context	Prevalence of violence; community disorganization; opportunities for self-fulfillment and participatory activities	-Self-report surveys -Neighborhood or community level data
Cognitive/Intellectual	Academic achievement; reasoning and problem solving skills; decision-making	-Academic reports -Standardized tests -Self-report surveys

Although numerous instruments have been developed for the purpose of assessing a single domain of adolescent well-being, very few instruments include multiple domains with demonstrated reliability and validity. Of the 83 adolescent instruments reviewed, fourteen met the criteria however, their appropriateness depends on the purpose of assessment. For example, only three instruments (bold type in Appendix E) identified in this structured review process can be categorized as comprehensive assessment measures for clinical/treatment planning purposes: *Child and Adolescent Social and Adaptive Functioning Scale* (Price, Spence, Sheffield, & Donovan, 2002), *4-D Strengths-Based Assessment Tools for Youth in Care* (Gilgun, 2004), and *Family, Friends, and Self Form* (Simpson & McBride, 1992). The instrument that appears to be most relevant to child welfare practice is described below.

Individual Assessment

Family, Friends, and Self (FFS) Form. The Family, Friends, and Self (FFS) Form is a 60-item self-report questionnaire designed to measure the social relationships and psychological adjustment of youth. Although this measure was originally developed to monitor drug and alcohol use, school problems, and legal involvement of adolescents, the scales appear to be useful for assessment of youth at risk (Corcoran & Fischer, 2000). The FFS provides a comprehensive assessment of youth involving three domains with ten underlying dimensions: (1) Family settings and relationships (warmth, control, and conflict); (2) Peer activities and involvement (trouble, peer activity, familiarity with parents, and conventional involvement); and (3) Self-esteem and environment (environmental satisfaction, school satisfaction and self-esteem). For example, the youth responds to questions such as "Is there a feeling of togetherness in your family?" and "Do you spend a lot of your free time with friends?" on a 5-point Likert scale ranging from Never (0) to Almost Always (4).

The FFS was normed with 154 clients (mean age = 15.4 years) in a statewide substance abuse program; the FFS scales have further been tested with over 1500 youth from diverse ethnic/racial backgrounds. Overall, the FFS has stable psychometric properties; factor analysis has demonstrated a sound factor structure, the subscales have excellent internal consistency, and the FFS appears to have good predictive validity in terms of demonstrating significant correlations between subscales and counselor diagnosis of drug problems. Although the FFS appears to be a brief, easy to score, multidimensional, and psychometrically sound instrument that may be appropriate for use in settings other than drug programs, its reliability with youth in the child welfare system and its ability to predict outcomes other than drug use have yet to be determined.

RESILIENCE AND COPING ASSESSMENT

Three instruments–*Adolescent Coping Orientation for Problem Experiences* (Patterson & McCubbin, 1987); *Resiliency Scale* (Jew, Green, & Kroger, 1999); and *Resilience Scale* (Wagnild & Young, 1987)–two of which are described below, assess general resilience and coping skills that are related to adolescent well-being.

Adolescent Coping Orientation for Problem Experiences (A-COPE). The Adolescent Coping Orientation for Problem Experiences (A-COPE) is designed to assess the behaviors that adolescents display when managing problems or difficult situations related to themselves or family members. The A-COPE instruments can be used for educating adolescents about their coping style, pre-post assessment of stress management programs, and treatment planning for adolescents struggling to manage the demands of life transitions (Patterson & McCubbin, 1987). The 54-item self-report questionnaire assesses twelve different coping behaviors and patterns: (1) ventilating feelings; (2) seeking diversions; (3) developing self-reliance; (4) developing optimism; (5) developing social support; (6) solving family problems; (7) seeking spiritual support; (8) investing in close friends; (9) seeking professional support; (10) engaging in demanding activity; (11) being humorous; and (12) relaxing. Sample items include "Try to help other people solve their problems" and "Talk to a friend about how you feel."

The A-COPE has been used with numerous adolescent populations; subscales of the A-COPE have fair to good internal consistency and reliability data from the Young Adult-COPE (a slightly modified version of the A-COPE) show excellent internal consistency and good stability. Validity of the measure appears to be acceptable and predictive validity for illicit substance use is fair but other outcomes have not been assessed. The applicability of this measure for adolescents in the child welfare system needs to be determined. Nevertheless, the A-COPE appears promising as a multidimensional, relevant, and psychometrically sound instrument for assessing the coping and well-being of adolescents.

Resiliency Scale. The 35-item Resiliency Scale is a self-report questionnaire developed from the cognitive appraisal theory of resiliency conceptualized by Mrazek and Mrazek (Jew et al., 1999). It includes twelve skills and abilities that resilient people use to cope with stress, including information seeking and decisive risk-taking. The Resiliency Scale consists of three subscales: (1) future orientation (19 items), (2) active skill acquisition (10 items), and (3) independence/risk-taking (6 items). Items such as "Look forward to the future" and "Like helping others" are rated by respondents on a 5-point Likert scale ranging from "strongly disagree" to "strong agree." The scale was developed using three adolescent populations including 9th grade students from lower to middle socioeconomic statuses, 7th to 12th grade students in a rural area, and residents in an adolescent psychiatric treatment facility. High internal consistencies were found for each of the subscales and correlations with other similar measures (such as the A-COPE) demonstrated moderate convergent validity. The measure was also able to effectively discriminate between institutionalized and non-institutionalized adolescents as well as between at-risk and not-at-risk students based on self-reports. This instrument shows promise for identifying adolescents who may be at risk but further research is needed before the Resiliency Scale can be endorsed for screening purposes.

INDEPENDENT LIVING SKILLS ASSESSMENT

Several tools have been developed to assess independent living skills (ILS) in youth in out-of-home placement or receiving child welfare services; these include the Daniel Memorial Independent Living Skills System (DMILA; Daniel Memorial, 2006) the Ansell-Casey Life Skills Assessment (ACLSA; Casey Family Programs, 2005), The Life Skills

Inventory: Summary Report Form (Ansell & The Independent Living Skills Center South Bronx Human Development Organization, Inc., 1987), and the Independent Living Skills Assessment Tool (Blostein & Eldridge, 1988). The majority of these tools have either not established and/or reported their psychometric properties or have demonstrated poor overall reliability and validity (Nollan et al., 2000). For example, although the DMILA is one of the most widely used instruments in the national foster care system (Hahn, 1994), a recent evaluation of its psychometric properties demonstrates weak reliability and validity (Georgiades, 2005). The results from this initial psychometric evaluation suggest that further evaluation and revision of the factor structure and item content of the DMILA are needed before it can be endorsed as a valid and reliable measure of a youth's preparedness for transition to adulthood. The ACLSA, however, focuses on independent living skills, demonstrates strong psychometric properties, and is relevant to child welfare services.

Ansell-Casey Life Skills Assessment (ACLSA). The ACLSA is a strengths-based measure of life skills and behaviors generally viewed as necessary for living successfully in the community upon emancipation from out-of-home care (Nollan et al., 2000). Applications of the ACLSA in the child welfare setting include identifying acquired life skills, setting goals for skills not yet learned, and evaluating program effectiveness. Although the ACLSA was designed for youth in out-of-home care, the ACLSA is appropriate for life skills assessment regardless of the youth's living circumstances.

Four versions of the ACLSA are available: ACLSA-I for ages 8-9 (37 items); ACLSA-II for ages 10-12 (56 items): ACLSA-III for ages 13-15 (81 items), and ACSLA-IV for ages 16 and above (118 items). Additionally, a short form can be administered for youth ages 11-18 (18 items). All versions of the ACLSA assess life skills in the following domains: social development, educational/vocational development, physical development, moral development, and money/housing/transportation. Specific items in the moral development domain, for example, include "Refuses illegal, dangerous, or hurtful activities" and "Respects others' views, lifestyles, and attitudes." The ACLSA is administered both to youth and caregivers; youth respond to items on a 3-point Likert scale, with response options ranging from "not like me" to "very much like me," while caregivers respond to items with response options ranging from "not like the youth" to "very much like the youth."

Advantages of the ACLSA include initial psychometric evidence, ease of access (free for public use) and administration (pencil and paper and a Web-based version). As a strengths-based and multidimensional measure of life skills with multiple developmentally appropriate versions, the ACLSA appears to be an especially useful tool for child welfare workers. However, evaluation of the reliability and validity of the most recent versions of the ACLSA should be conducted to ensure that revisions have not affected their psychometric characteristics. Furthermore, additional types of reliability and validity data should be collected; for example, predictive validity would be especially important to assess for this kind of measure.

POPULATION SURVEY/PROGRAM EVALUATION

As illustrated by the major findings, global measures of child and adolescent well-being that are appropriate for use by child welfare practitioners are limited. Most of the comprehensive instruments that address multiple well-being domains, especially those that are specific to middle childhood and adolescence, have not been tested on child welfare populations and/or evaluations of their psychometric properties are in preliminary stages. The majority of well-validated and widely-used assessments of child and youth well-being have been developed for the purposes of program planning and evaluation where data are aggregated to assess and guide program implementation. The seven instruments summarized in Figure 4 are comprehensive assessments of child and adolescent well-being and examples of population surveys and program evaluation measures that are not intended for case or clinical decision-making.

The analysis of service outcomes for a child population related to the overall well-being of children and youth is essential for the informed development of agency-level program planning (Altshuler & Poertner, 2002). While the instruments in Figure 4 have been developed for the purposes of evaluating client populations, they can also offer individual level indications of a child's well-being as part of a more extensive and thorough assessment (Lyons, Doueck, Koster, Witzky, & Kelly, 1999).

IMPLICATIONS FOR PRACTICE

The ability to assess child and youth well-being is hindered by a number of factors. A lack of consensus about how well-being should be defined and subsequently measured can lead to inconsistent use of the term across disciplines and studies. In addition, the historical emphasis

FIGURE 4. Population Survey and Program Evaluation Instruments

Instrument[1]	Description	Domains/ Subscales
Child Health and Illness Profile (CHIP)	Standardized measure documenting health in groups of children or adolescents; tested in child welfare population as a measure of well-being.	Satisfaction; discomfort; resilience; risks; achievement; and disorders
Communities That Care Youth Survey	Designed to collect data on the epidemiology of risk and protection among community youth populations for prevention purposes.	Broad risk and protective factors in community, school, family, peer, and individual domains; health and behavior outcomes
Healthy Kids Resilience Assessment (HKRA)	Optional module of the California Healthy Kids Survey intended to serve as a tool for local and state education agencies and researchers; assesses a variety of external and internal factors associated with positive youth development.	Caring relationships; high expectations; meaningful participation; social competence; autonomy and sense of self; and sense of meaning and purpose
Individual Protective Factors Index (IPFI)	Developed to measure adolescent resiliency; tool for evaluating prevention programs for youth.	Social bonding; personal competence; and social competence
Quality of Life Profile- Adolescent Version (QOLPAV)	Generic quality of life instrument to assess psychosocial aspects of well-being and comprehensive health.	Being (physical, psychological, spiritual); belonging (physical, social, community); and becoming (practical, leisure, growth)
Search Institute Profiles of Student Life: Attitudes and Behaviors	Designed to assess developmental assets in groups of youth for the purposes of informing intervention strategies.	External assets (i.e., health-promoting features of the environment); internal assets (i.e., personal commitments, values, and competencies)
Youth Asset Survey (YAS)	Developed to assess and compare prevalence of youth assets across populations.	Family communication; peer role models; future aspirations; responsible choices; community involvement; cultural respect; good health practices; use of time; nonparental adult role models

[1] *Child Health and Illness Profile* (Starfield et al., 1995); *Communities That Care Survey* (Arthur, Hawkins, Pollard, Catalano, & Baglioni, 2002); *Healthy Kids Resilience Assessment* (Constantine, Benard, & Diaz, 1999); *Individual Protective Factors Index* (Springer & Phillips, 1997); *Quality of Life Profile- Adolescent Version* (Raphael, Rukholm, Brown, HillBailey, & Donato, 1996); *Search Institute Profiles of Student Life: Attitudes and Behaviors* (Leffert et al., 1998); *Youth Asset Survey* (Oman et al., 2002).

on the assessment of individual characteristics in isolation of a child's environment, as well as the focus on risk, has overshadowed efforts to examine the strengths and competencies of children and youth. Lastly, as the results of this structured literature review indicate, the majority of measures assessing global well-being in children and youth have not yet attained the level of reliability and validity that are associated with instruments that assess maltreatment risk and family systems. The field of well-being assessment is largely at a formative stage.

The instruments presented in this structured review are representations of the status of the field and thus embody an improvement on previous deficit-focused measures. The instruments also reflect the measurement challenges related to studying well-being. From a risk and resilience perspective, measures of well-being show promise when conceptualizing child development as dynamic, bio-ecological, and transactional and balancing the assessment of risk and protective factors. A number of lessons can be identified for child welfare practice.

First, consideration of the *developmental process of a child* is essential in the assessment of well-being. What constitutes well-being in infancy versus middle childhood varies considerably; a one-size-fits-all approach to assessment fails to consider this complexity. Effective service planning can occur when developmentally appropriate instruments are employed. Furthermore, while global assessments of well-being in infancy and early childhood are relatively well-established, the complexity of the socio-emotional aspects of well-being in older children makes it difficult to develop similarly well-grounded instruments. Efforts to develop well-being instruments for middle childhood and adolescence should consider the need for multiple informants, assessment of subjective factors related to self-perception, and the impact of social networks on children and youth.

Second, assessment of child and youth well-being may have several purposes at the client as well as the service level. In the processing of a case, for example, child well-being assessment can be particularly useful during *critical decision-making points* such as: (1) temporary removal and disposition, (2) out-of-home placement considering reunification, (3) permanent placement hearing, and (4) transition and emancipation. Child well-being assessment may also be influential in the *prevention* of abuse or neglect for the referred child (i.e., reoccurrence) as well as for other children in the family (i.e., occurrence). On a broader scale, individual level well-being assessments can be aggregated to *inform policy and program development*, as well as to identify needs in specific communities.

Third, the demands of child welfare practice require that global well-being instruments be *inexpensive and available, relatively brief, and easy to administer and score*. Further, instruments must yield practical results that can be translated into effective practice or policy strategies. The broad nature of well-being can be seen from the range of instruments resulting from this structured review. Further psychometric testing and evaluation for use in child welfare practice will strengthen the promising global instruments.

Finally, assessment of child and youth well-being is multidimensional and therefore single domain instruments cannot capture this complexity. Even comprehensive well-being assessments need to be interpreted along with other indicators of well-being. *When used in conjunction with medical and school records as well as existing risk and safety measures, a strengths-based assessment of child well-being can offer something sorely missing in the assessment of children.* Such measures have the potential to "complete the evaluation triangle" between safety, permanency, and well-being in child welfare practice and policy (Altshuler & Gleeson, 1999, p. 143) by restoring balance in a heavily risk-focused process.

When considering the lessons discussed above, the assessment of well-being in child welfare practice can have a number of advantages for the child and family, worker, and the broader service system. Figure 5 provides a framework for discussing these advantages by capturing the convergence of individual child and youth well-being assessment in the different stages of a child welfare case. A promising instrument from each developmental stage was selected as an example. First, the assessment can *serve as a baseline indicator* by providing a measure of the child's status at initial stages of case-processing. A baseline measure allows the worker to compare the child's well-being at intake to later points of intervention and follow-up. Such information is useful in *tracking progress* for the child and the family. Second, assessment of child well-being can *steer intervention and service planning*. As one component of a broader family assessment, an emphasis on the well-being of the child can inform needed services and interventions for a child at different points in the process. Third, individual child assessments *contribute to a larger database of information assessing outcomes*. As depicted in Figure 5, the outcomes may be related to specific needs of the child and relevant interventions or broad service outcomes such as safety, permanency, and well-being. Outcomes are specific to the individual child or youth and therefore intentionally left blank in Figure 5.

Assessments of child well-being also have advantages for the family and the child welfare worker. For example, when joining with the parent(s) to reach the common goal of child well-being, the worker can conduct assessment processes *with* the family rather than *to* the family. This legitimation of the *partnership with the family* can help combat obstacles a worker might encounter. Furthermore, the assessment of child well-being can *enhance worker satisfaction*. In the midst of necessary risk and safety assessments, well-being assessment offers a unique perspective on the strengths and assets of the child and family. The ability

FIGURE 5. Child and Youth Well-Being Assessment in Child Welfare Practice

	Disposition	Reunification	Permanent Placement	Emancipation	CHILD WELFARE OUTCOMES: Safety, Permanency, Well-Being
Infancy/ Early Childhood	Ages and Stages Questionnaire	Ages and Stages Questionnaire	Ages and Stages Questionnaire		
Middle Childhood	Behavior and Emotional Rating Scale-2nd Ed.	Behavior and Emotional Rating Scale-2nd Ed.	Behavior and Emotional Rating Scale-2nd Ed.		
Adolescence	Behavior and Emotional Rating Scale-2nd Ed.	Behavior and Emotional Rating Scale-2nd Ed.	Behavior and Emotional Rating Scale-2nd Ed.	Ansell-Casey Life Skills Assessment	
CHILD NEEDS					

to see a child's development unfold can offer glimpses of progress and change. Both the worker and the parent may learn new things about the child in the shared assessment process.

Lastly, child well-being assessment has some practical advantages for the worker in court presentations. A well-being assessment can help a worker *organize observed behavior* by synthesizing necessary pieces of information. An objective assessment of well-being can further substantiate narrative reports of well-being, thereby increasing credibility in court. Finally, child well-being assessments contribute to the overall comprehensiveness of a worker's report. By anticipating questions, a comprehensive assessment of well-being may reduce the need for outside psychological tests.

REFERENCES

Achenbach, T. M. (1991). *Manual for the Youth Self-Report and 1991 Profile.* Burlington, VT: Department of Psychiatry, University of Vermont.

Adelman, H. S., Taylor, L., & Nelson, P. (1989). Minors' dissatisfaction with their life circumstances. *Child Psychiatry and Human Development, 20,* 135-147.

Altshuler, S. J., & Gleeson, J. P. (1999). Completing the evaluation triangle for the next century: Measuring child "well-being" in family foster care. *Child Welfare, 78*(1), 125-147.

Altshuler, S. J., & Poertner, J. (2002). The Child Health and Illness Profile-Adolescent Edition: Assessing well-being in group homes or institutions. *Child Welfare, 81*(3), 495-513.

Angold, A., & Costello, E. J. (2000). The Child and Adolescent Psychiatric Assessment (CAPA). *Journal of the American Academy of Child & Adolescent Psychiatry, 39,* 39-48.

Angold, A., Costello, E. J., Loeber, R., Messer, S. C., Pickles, A., Winder, F. et al. (1995). Development of a short questionnaire for use in epidemiological studies of depression in children and adolescents: Factor composition and structure across development. *International Journal of Methods in Psychiatric Research, 5*(4), 251-262.

Ansell, D. & The Independent Living Skills Center South Bronx Human Development Organization, Inc. (1987). *Life Skills Inventory: Summary Report Form.* New York: South Bronx Human Development Organization.

Arthur, M., Hawkins, J., Pollard, E., Catalano, R. F., & Baglioni, A. J. (2002). Measuring risk and protective factors for substance use, delinquency, and other adolescent problem behaviors: The Communities That Care Survey. *Evaluation Review, 26*(6), 575-601.

Asher, S. R., Hymel, S., & Renshaw, P. D. (1984). Loneliness in children. *Child Development, 55,* 1456-1464.

Bayley, N. (1993). *Bayley scales of infant development, 2nd edition manual.* San Antonio, TX: The Psychological Corporation.

Behar, L. B. (1977). The Preschool Behavior Questionnaire. *Journal of Abnormal Child Psychology, 5*(3), 265-275.

Beidel, D. C., Turner, S. M., & Fink, C. M. (1996). Assessment of childhood social phobia: Construct, convergent, and discriminative validity of the social phobia and anxiety inventory for children (SPAI-C). *Psychological Assessment, 8*(3), 235-240.

Bird, H. R., Canino, G. J., Davies, M., Ramirez, R., Chavez, L., Duarte, C. et al. (2005). The Brief Impairment Scale (BIS): A multidimensional scale of functional impairment for children and adolescents. *Journal of the American Academy of Child & Adolescent Psychiatry, 44*(7), 699-707.

Bird, H. R., Shaffer, D., Fisher, P., Gould, M. S., Staghezza, B., & Chen, J. V. (1993). The Columbia Impairment Scale (CIS): Pilot findings on a measure of global impairment for children and adolescents. *International Journal of Methods in Psychiatric Research, 3,* 167-176.

Bledsoe, J. C. (1967). Self-concept of children and their intelligence, achievement, interest, and anxiety. *Child Education, 43,* 436-438.

Block, J., & Block, J. H. (1969). *The California Child Q-Sort.* Berkeley, CA: Department of Psychology, University of California at Berkeley.

Blostein, S., & Eldridge, W. D. (1988). *The Independent Living Skills Assessment Tool (ILSAT).* Final Report. Ohio Department of Human Services (ODHS).

Bolea, A. S., Felker, D. W., & Barnes, M. D. (1971). A pictorial self-concept scale for children in K-4. *Journal of Educational Measurement 8*(3), 223-224.

Bowen, N. K. (2006). Psychometric properties of the elementary school success profile for children. *Social Work Research, 30*(1), 51-63.

Bracken, B. A. (1992). *Multidimensional Self-Concept Scale (MSCS).* Lutz, FL: Psychological Assessment Resources Inc.

Bricker, D., & Squires, J. (1989a). The effectiveness of parental screening of at-risk infants: The Infant Monitoring Questionnaires. *Topics in Early Childhood Special Education, 9*(3), 67-85.

Bricker, D., & Squires, J. (1989b). Low cost system of using parents to monitor the development of at-risk infants. *Journal of Early Intervention, 13,* 50-60.

Bricker, D., Squires, J., & Mounts, L. (1995). *Ages and Stages Questionnaire: A parent-completed, child monitoring system.* Baltimore, MD: Paul H. Brookes.

Briere, J. (1996). *Trauma Symptom Checklist for Children*. Odessa, FL: Psychological Assessment Resources.

Brigance, A. H. (1991). *BRIGANCE Diagnostic Inventory of Early Development, Revised Edition (BDIED-R)*. North Billerica, MA: Curriculum Associates.

Briggs-Gowan, M. J., Carter, A. S., Irwin, J. R., Wachtel, K., & Cicchetti, D. V. (2004). The Brief Infant-Toddler Social and Emotional Assessment: Screening for Social-Emotional Problems and Delays in Competence. *Journal of Pediatric Psychology, 29*(2), 143-155.

Brodzinsky, D. M., Elias, M. J., Steiger, C., Simon, J., Gill, M., & Hitt, J. C. (1992). Coping Scale for children and youth: Scale development and validation. *Journal of Applied Developmental Psychology, 13*, 195-214.

Brown, L., & Alexander, J. (1991). *Self-esteem Index (SEI)*. Lutz, FL: Psychological Assessment Resources, Inc.

Butcher, J. N., Williams, C. L., Graham, J. R., Kaemmer, B., Archer, R. P., Tellegen, A. et al. (1992). *Minnesota Multiphasic Personality Inventory-Adolescent*. Minneapolis: University of Minnesota Press.

Capute, A. J., & Accardo, P. J. (1996). A neurodevelopmental perspective on the continuum of developmental disabilities. In A.J. Capute, P.J. Accardo, & J. Pasquale (Eds.), *Developmental disabilities in infancy and childhood* (pp. 7-41). Baltimore, MD: Brooks Publishing Co.

Carter, A. S., & Briggs-Gowan, M. J. (2000). *Manual of the Infant-Toddler Social-Emotional Assessment*. New Haven, CT: Yale University.

Casey Family Programs (2005). Ansell-Casey Life Skills Assessments (ACLSA). Retrieved August 9, 2006 from http://www.caseylifeskills.org/pages/assess/assess_index.htm

Constantine, N. A., Bernard, B., & Diaz, M. D. (1999). *A new survey instrument for measuring protective factors and resilience traits in youth: The Healthy Kids Resilience Assessment*. Oakland, CA: WestEd.

Coopersmith, S. (2002). Revised Coopersmith Self-Esteem Inventory manual. Redwood, CA: Mindgarden, Inc.

Corcoran, K., & Fischer, J. (2000). *Measures for clinical practice: A sourcebook, 3rd edition*. New York: The Free Press.

Damon, W. (2004). What is positive youth development? *The Annals of the American Academy of Political and Social Science, 591*, 13-24. Research National Conference.

Daniel Memorial (2006). *Independent Living Skills (ILS) System*. Retrieved July 27, 2006 from http://www.danielkids.org/sites/web/store/order.cfm?productID=59

Davies, D. (2004). *Child development: A practitioner's guide, 2nd ed.* New York: The Guilford Press.

Derogatis, L. R., & Melisaratos, N. (1983). The Brief Symptom Inventory: An introductory report. *Psychological Medicine, 13*(3), 595-605.

DuBois, D. L., Felner, R. D., Brand, S., Phillips, R. S.., & Lease, A. M. (1996). Early adolescent self-esteem: A developmental-ecological framework and assessment strategy. *Journal of Research on Adolescence, 6*, 543-579.

Dumont, R., & Rauch, M. (1998). Behavioral and Emotional Rating Scale [Test review]. NASP Communiqué, 28(7).

Dunn, L. M., & Dunn, L. M. (1981). *Peabody Picture Vocabulary Test- Revised Manual*. Circle Pines, MN: American Guidance Service.

Educational and Industrial Testing Service (EdITS). (2004). *Tests of Achievement in Basic Skills*. San Diego, CA: Author.

Elliott, C. D. (1990). *DAS: Administration and Scoring Manual*. San Antonio, TX: The Psychological Corporation.

Ellis, R. H., Wilson, N. Z., & Foster, F. M. (1984). Statewide treatment outcome assessment in Colorado: the Colorado Client Assessment Record (CCAR). *Community Mental Health Journal, 20*(1), 72-89.

Epstein, M. H. (2004). Assessing the Emotional and Behavioral Strengths of Children. *Reclaiming Children and Youth: Journal of Emotional and Behavioral Problems, 6*(4), 250-252.

Epstein, M. H., Cullinan, D., Ryser, G., & Pearson, N. (2002). Development of a scale to assess emotional disturbance. *Behavioral Disorders, 28*(1), 5-22.

Epstein, M. H., Harniss, M. K., Pearson, N., & Ryser, G. (1999). The Behavioral and Emotional Rating Scale: Test-retest and inter-rater reliability. *Journal of Child and Family Studies, 8*(3), 319-327.

Epstein, M. H., Hertzog, M. A., & Reid, R. (2001). The behavioral and emotional rating scale: Long term test-retest reliability. *Behavioral Disorders, 26*(4), 314-320.

Epstein, M. H., Ryser, G., & Pearson, N. (2002). Standardization of the behavioral and emotional rating scale: Factor structure, reliability, and criterion validity. *Journal of Behavioral Health Services & Research, 29*(2), 208-216.

Epstein, M. H., & Sharma, J. (1998). *Behavioral and emotional rating scale: A strength-based approach to assessment*. Austin, TX: PRO-ED.

Fantuzzo, J. W., Hightower, D., Grim, S., & Montes, G. (2002). Generalization of the Child Observation Record: A validity study for diverse samples of urban, low-income preschool children. *Early Childhood Research Quarterly, 17*, 106-125.

Fantuzzo, J. W., Manz, P. H., & McDermott, P. (1998). Preschool version of the Social Skills Rating System: An empirical analysis of its use with low-income children. *Journal of School Psychology, 36*, 199-214.

Fantuzzo, J., Suttonsmith, B., Coolahan, K. C., Manz, P. H., Canning, S., & Debnam, D. (1995). Assessment of Preschool Play Interaction Behaviors in Young Low-Income Children–Penn Interactive Peer Play Scale. *Early Childhood Research Quarterly, 10*(1), 105-120.

Fenson, L., Dale, P. S., Reznick, J. S., Thal, D., Bates, E., Harters, J. P. et al. (1993). *The MacArthur Communication Development Inventories: User's Guide and Technical Manual*. San Diego: Singular Publishing Group.

Finney, S. J., Pieper, S. L., & Barron, K. E. (2004). Examining the psychometric properties of the Achievement Goal Questionnaire in a general academic context. *Educational and Psychological Measurement, 64*(2), 365-382.

Fitts, W. H. (1965). *Manual: Tennessee Self-Concept Scale*. Los Angeles, CA: Western Psychological Services.

Folio, M. R., & Fewell, R. R. (2000). *Peabody Developmental Motor Scales, 2nd Edition*. Austin, TX: ProEd.

Fraser, M. W., Kirby, L. D., & Smokowski, P. R. (2004). Risk and resilience in childhood. In M. W. Fraser (Ed.), *Risk and resilience in childhood: An ecological perspective* (2nd ed., pp. 13-66). Washington, DC: NASW Press.

Fraser, M. W., Richman, J. M., & Galinsky, M. J. (1999). Risk, protection, and resilience: Towards a conceptual framework for social work practice. *Social Work Research, 23*(3), 131-143.

French, D., Christie, M. J., Goddhew, A., & Sowden, A. (1993). The reliability and validity of the Childhood Asthma Questionnaires as measures of quality-of-life for 4-7 year and 8-11-year-olds. *American Review of Respiratory Disorders, 147*, A463.

Gardner, M. (1989). *Tests of Academic Achievement Skills- Reading, Arithmetic, Spelling.* San Francisco, CA: Health Publishing Company.

Georgiades, S. (2005). Initial internal consistency evidence on the Daniel Memorial Independent Living Assessment: A research note. *Children and Youth Services Review, 27*(8), 921- 930.

Gilgun, J. F. (1999). CASPARS: New tools for assessing client risks and strengths. *Families in Society–the Journal of Contemporary Human Services, 80*(5), 450-459.

Gilgun, J. F. (2004). The 4-D Strengths-Based Assessment Instruments for Youth, Their Families, and Communities. *Journal of Human Behavior in the Social Environment, 10*(4), 51-73.

Gilgun, J. F., Klein, C., & Pranis, K. (2000). The significance of resources in models of risk. *Journal of Interpersonal Violence, 15*(6), 631-650.

Goodman, R. (2001). Psychometric properties of the Strengths and Difficulties Questionnaire. *Journal of the American Academy of Child & Adolescent Psychiatry, 40*(11), 1337-1345.

Gresham, F. M., & Elliott, S. N. (1990). *Social Skills Rating System.* Circle Pines, MN: American Guidance Service, Inc.

Griffiths, R. (1984). *The abilities of young children. A comprehensive system of mental measurement for the first eight years of life.* London, UK: The test agency LTD.

Hahn, A. (1994). The use of assessment procedures in foster-care to evaluate readiness for independent living. *Children and Youth Services Review, 16*(3-4), 171-179.

Haley, S. M., Coster, W., Ludlow, L. H., Haltiwanger, J. T., & Andrellos, P. J. (1992). *Pediatric Evaluation of Disability Inventory (PEDI): Development, standardization and administration manual.* Boston, MA: Trustees of Boston University.

Harrison, P. L. (1990). *AGS Early Screening Profiles.* Circle Pines, MN: American Guidance Service.

Harter, S. (1985). *Manual for the Self-Perception Profile for Children.* Denver, CO: University of Denver.

Harter, S. (1988). *Manual for the Self-Perception Profile for Adolescents.* Denver, CO: University of Denver.

Hedrick, D., Prather, E., & Tobin, A. (1984). *Sequenced Inventory of Communication Development.* Los Angeles: Western Psychological Services.

Heppner, P. P., & Petersen, C. H. (1982). The development and implications of a personal problem-solving inventory. *Journal of Counseling Psychology, 29*, 66-75.

High/Scope Educational Research Foundation. (1992). *High/Scope Child Observation Record (COR) for Ages 2 1/2-6 [Assessment instrument].* Ypsilanti, MI: High/Scope Press.

High/Scope Educational Research Foundation. (2002). Appendix A: Statistical findings for the Preschool Child Observation Record (COR). Retrieved July 27, 2006 from http://www.highscope.org/Book-Pages/PCOR_evidence.pdf

Hodges, K. (1990). *Child and Adolescent Functional Assessment Scale.* Ypsilanti, MI: Eastern Michigan University, Department of Psychology.

Huebner, E.S. (1991). Initial development of the Student's Life Satisfaction Scale. *School Psychology International, 12*, 231-240.

Huebner, E. S. (1994). Preliminary Development and Validation of a Multidimensional Life Satisfaction Scale for Children. *Psychological assessment, 6*(2), 149-158.

Inderbitzen, H. M., & Foster, S. L. (1992). The Teenage Inventory of Social Skills: Development, reliability, and validity. *Psychological Assessment, 4*(4), 451-459.

Ireton, H., & Glascoe, F. P. (1995). Assessing children's development using parents reports–the Child Development Inventory. *Clinical Pediatrics, 34*(5), 248-255.

Jenson, J. M., Anthony, E. K., & Howard, M. O. (2006). Policies and programs for adolescent substance abuse. In J. M. Jenson and M. W. Fraser (Eds.), *Social policy for children and families: A risk and resilience perspective* (pp. 195-229). Thousand Oaks: Sage Publications.

Jenson, J. M., & Fraser, M. W. (2006). A risk and resilience framework for child, youth, and family policy. In J. M. Jenson & M. W. Fraser (Eds.), *Social policy for children & families: A risk and resilience perspective* (pp. 1-18). Thousand Oaks: Sage Publications.

Jew, C. L., Green, K. E., & Kroger, J. (1999). Development and validation of a measure of resiliency. *Measurement and Evaluation in Counseling and Development, 32*(2), 75-89.

John, K., Gammon, G. D., Prusoff, B. A., & Warner, V. (1987). The Social Adjustment Inventory for Children and Adolescents (SAICA): Testing of a new semi structured interview. *Journal of the American Academy of Child and Adolescent Psychiatry, 26*(6), 898-911.

Kaufman, J., Birmaher, B., Brent, D., Rao, U., Flynn, C., Moreci, P., et al. (1997). Schedule for Affective Disorders and Schizophrenia for School-Age Children-Present and Lifetime Version (K-SADS-PL): Initial reliability and validity data. *Journal of the American Academy of Child & Adolescent Psychiatry, 36*(7), 980-988.

Kaufman, A. S., & Kaufman, N. L. (2004). *Kaufman Assessment Battery for Children, 2nd Edition Manual.* Circle Pines, MN: AGS.

Kohn, M., & Rosman, B. L. (1972). Social Competence Scale and Symptom Checklist for Preschool Child-Factor Dimensions, Their Cross-Instrument Generality, and Longitudinal Persistence. *Developmental Psychology, 6*(3), 430-444.

Kovacs, M. (1992). *The Children's Depression Inventory (CDI). Manual.* Toronto, Ontario, Canada: Multi-Health Systems, Inc.

Lachar, D., & Gruber, C. P. (1993). Development of the Personality Inventory for Youth: A self-report companion to the Personality Inventory for Children. *Journal of Personality Assessment, 61*(1), 81-98.

LaGreca, A. M., Dandes, S. K., Wick, P., Shaw, K., & Stone, W. L. (1988). Development of the Social Anxiety Scale for Children: Reliability and concurrent validity. *Journal of Clinical Child Psychology, 17*, 84-91.

Landgraf, J. M., Abetz, L., & Ware, J. E. (1996). *The CHQ User's Manual.* Boston, MA: The Health Institute, New England Medical Center.

Lang, M., & Tisher, M. (1978). *Childrens Depression Scale: Research Edition.* Melbourne: The Australian Council for Educational Research Limited.

Lee, D. Y., Hallbert, E. T., Slemon, A. G., & Haase, R. F. (1985). An assertiveness scale for adolescents. *Journal of Clinical Psychology, 41*, 51-57.

Leffert, N., Benson, P. L., Scales, P. C., Sharma, A. R., Drake, D. R., & Blyth, D. A. (1998). Developmental assets: Measurement and prediction of risk behaviors among adolescents. *Applied Developmental Science, 2*(4), 209-230.

Leslie, L. K., Gordon, J. N., Ganger, W., & Gist, K. (2002). Developmental delay in young children in child welfare by initial placement type. *Infant Mental Health Journal, 23*(5), 496-516.

Leslie, L. K., Hurlburt, M. S., Landsverk, J., Rolls, J. A., Wood, P. A., & Kelleher, K. J. (2003). Comprehensive assessments for children entering foster care: A national perspective. *Pediatrics, 112*(1), 134-142.

Luthar, S. S., Cicchetti, D., Becker, B., Von Eye, A., Schuster, C., Roosa, M. W., et al. (2000). The construct of resilience: A critical evaluation and guidelines for future work. *Child Development, 71*(3), 543-575.

Lyons, P., Doueck, H. J., Koster, A. J., Witzky, M. K., & Kelly, P. L. (1999). The Child Well-Being Scales as a clinical tool and a management information system. *Child Welfare, 78*(2), 241-258.

Malecki, C. K., & Elliot, D. S. (1999). Adolescents' ratings of perceived social support and its importance: Validation of the Student Social Support Scale. *Psychology in the Schools, 36*(6), 473-483.

Marsh, H. W. (1990). *Self-Description Questionnaire-II Manual.* Cambelltown, NSW, Australia: University of Western Sydney.

Marsh, H. W. (1992). *Manual for the Self-Description Questionnaire-III.* Cambelltown, NSW, Australia: University of Western Sydney.

Matson, J. L., Rotatori, A. F., & Helsel, W. J. (1983). Development of a rating scale to measure social skills in children: The Matson Evaluation of Social Scales with Youngsters (MESSY). *Behavior Research and Therapy, 21*(4), 335-340.

McInerney, D. M., & Sinclair, K. E. (1991). Cross cultural model testing: Inventory of school motivation. *Educational and Psychological Measurement, 51*, 123-133.

Merrell, K. W. (1993). Using behavior rating-scales to assess social skills and antisocial-behavior in school settings: Development of the School Social-Behavior Scales. *School Psychology Review, 22*(1), 115-133.

Miller, L. J. (1993). *FirstSTEP: Screening Test for Evaluating Preschoolers.* San Antonio, TX: Developmental Technologies.

Miller, L. J., & Roid, G. H. (1994). *Toddler and Infant Motor Evaluation.* San Antonio, TX: Harcourt Assessment, Inc.

Muris, P. (2001). A brief questionnaire for measuring self-efficacy in youths. *Journal of Psychopathology and Behavioral Assessment, 23*(3), 145-149.

Murphy, J. M., Pagano, M. E., Ramirez, A., Anaya, Y., Nowlin, C., & Jellinek, M. S. (1999). Validation of the Preschool and Early Childhood Functional Assessment Scale (PECFAS). *Journal of Child and Family Studies, 8*(3), 343-356.

Naar-King, S., Ellis, D. A., & Frey, M. A. (Eds.). (2004). *Assessing children's well-being: A handbook of measures.* Mahwah, NJ: Lawrence Erlbaum Associates, Inc.

Naglieri, J., LeBuffe, P., & Pfeiffer, S. (1994). *Devereux Scales of Mental Disorders (DSMD).* San Antonio, TX: The Psychological Corporation.

Naglieri, J., McNeish, T. J., & Bardos, A. N. (1991). *Draw A Person: Screening Procedure for Emotional Disturbance.* Austin, TX: PRO-ED.

Newborg, J., Stock, J. R., Wnek, L., Guidubaldi, J., Svincki, J., Dickson, J., et al. (1988). *Battelle Development Inventory and recalibrated technical data and norms: Screening test examiner's manual* (2nd ed.). Allem, TX: DLM, Inc.

Nollan, K. A., Wolf, M., Ansell, D., Burns, J., Barr, L., Copeland, W. et al. (2000). Ready or not: Assessing youths' preparedness for independent living. *Child Welfare, 79*(2), 159-176.

Oman, R. F., Vesely, S. K., Mcleroy, K. R., Harris-Wyatt, V., Aspy, C. B., Rodine, S. & Marshall, L. (2002). Reliability and validity of the youth asset survey (YAS). *Journal of Adolescent Health, 31*(3), 247-256.

Park, N. (2004). Character strengths and positive youth development. *Annals of the American Academy of Political and Social Science, 591*, 40-54.

Patterson, J. M., & McCubbin, H. I. (1987). Adolescent coping style and behaviors: Conceptualization and measurement. *Journal of Adolescence, 10*(2), 163-186.

Piers, E. V., Harris, D. B., & Herzberg, D. (1999). *Piers-Harris Children's Self-Concept Scale* (2nd ed.). Los Angeles, CA: Western Psychological Services.

Price, C. S., Spence, S. H., Sheffield, J., & Donovan, C. (2002). The development and psychometric properties of a measure of social and adaptive functioning for children and adolescents. *Journal of Clinical Child and Adolescent Psychology, 31*(1), 111-122.

Procidano, M. E., Heller, K. (1983). Measures of perceived social support from friends and from family: Three validation studies. *American Journal of Community Psychology, 11*, 1-24.

Raphael, D., Rukholm, E., Brown, I., HillBailey, P., & Donato, E. (1996). The quality of life profile–Adolescent version: Background, description, and initial validation. *Journal of Adolescent Health, 19*(5), 366-375.

Reynell, J., & Huntley, M. (1985). *Reynell Developmental Language Scales (Second revision).* Windsor, England: NFER-Nelson.

Reynolds, C. R., & Kamphaus, R. W. (1992). *Behavior Assessment System for Children manual.* Circle Pines, MN: American Guidance Service.

Rohrbeck, C. A., Azar, S. T., & Wagner, P. E. (1991). Child Self-Control Rating Scale: Validation of a child self-report measure. *Journal of Clinical Child Psychology, 20*(2),179-183.

Roid, G. H. (2003). *Stanford-Binet Intelligence Scales, 5th edition.* Itasca, IL: Riverside.

Rosenberg, M. (1989). *Society and the adolescent self-image (Revised Ed.).* Middletown, CT: Wesleyan University Press.

Russell, D. J., Rosenbaum, P. L., Avery, L. M., & Lane, M. (2002). *Gross Motor Function Measure (GMFM-66 and GMFM-88) User's Manual.* London: Mac Keith Press.

Saleebey, D. (2006). *The strengths perspective in social work practice* (4th ed.). Boston, MA: Allyn and Bacon.

Schofield, G., & Beek, M. (2005). Risk and resilience in long-term foster-care. *The British Journal of Social Work, 35*(8), 1283-1301.

Sekino, Y., & Fantuzzo, J. (2005). Validity of the child observation record: An investigation of the relationship between COR dimensions and social-emotional and cognitive outcomes for head start children. *Journal of Psychoeducational Assessment, 23*(3), 242-261.

Shaffer, D., & Fisher, P. (1997). *NIMH- Diagnostic Interview Schedule for Children. Child Informant.* New York: New York State Psychiatric Institute.

Shaffer, D., Gould, M. S., Brasic, J., Ambrosini, P., Fisher, P., & Bird, H. R. (1983). Children's Global Assessment Scale (CGAS). *Archives of General Psychiatry, 40*(1), 1228-1231.

Silverman, W. K., Fleisig, W., Rabian, B., & Peterson, R. A. (1991). Childhood Anxiety Sensitivity Index. *Journal of Clinical Child Psychology, 20*(2), 162-168.

Simpson, D. D., & McBride, A. A. (1992). Family, Friends, and Self (FFS) Assessment Scales for Mexican-American Youth. *Hispanic Journal of Behavioral Sciences, 14*(3), 327-340.

SmarterKids. (1998). *The Children's Skills Test.* Needham, MA: Author.

Sparrow, S. S., & Balla, D. A. (1998). *Vineland Social-Emotional Early Childhood Scales/Vineland SEEC.* Circle Pines, MN: American Guidance Service, Inc.

Sparrow, S. S., Balla, D. A., & Cicchetti, D. V. (1984). *Vineland Adaptive Behavior Scales: Interview edition, survey form manual.* Circle Pines, MN: American Guidance Service.

Spirito, A., Stark, L. J., & Williams, C. (1988). Development of a brief coping checklist for use with pediatric populations. *Journal of Pediatric Psychology, 13*, 555-574.

Springer, F., & Phillips, J. L. (1997). *Individual Protective Factors Index (IPFI): A measure of adolescent resiliency.* Folsom, CA: EMT Associates.

Squires, J., Bricker, D., Heo, K., & Twombly, E. (2001). Identification of social-emotional problems in young children using a parent-completed screening measure. *Early Childhood Research Quarterly, 16*(4), 405-419.

Squires, J., Bricker, D., & Potter, L. (1997). Revision of a parent-completed developmental screening tool: Ages and Stages Questionnaires. *Journal of Pediatric Psychology, 22*(3), 313-328.

Starfield, B., Riley, A. W., Green, B. F., Ensminger, M. E., Ryan, S. A., Kelleher, K. et al. (1995). The Adolescent Child Health and Illness Profile - a population-b measure of health. *Medical Care, 33*(5), 553-566.

Taylor, K. M., & Betz, N. E., (1983). Applications of self-efficacy theory to the understanding and treatment of career indecision. *Journal of Vocational Behavior, 22*, 63-81.

The Psychological Corporation. (2002). *WPPSI-III Technical and Interpretive Manual.* San Antonio, TX: Author.

Ungar, M. (2004). The importance of parents and other caregivers to the resilience of high-risk adolescents. *Family process, 43*(1), 23-41.

U. S. Department of Health and Human Services, Administration for Children, Youth, and Families. (1997-2007). *National Survey of Child and Adolescent Well-Being.* Washington, D.C.

U. S. Department of Health and Human Services, Administration for Children, Youth, and Families. (1998). PI-98-02 Adoption and Safe Families Act of 1997. Retrieved May 25, 2006 from http://www.acf.hhs.gov/programs/cb/laws_policies/policy/pi/pi9802.htm

U. S. Department of Health and Human Services. (2006). *Comprehensive Family Assessment Guidelines for Child Welfare.* Washington, DC: Administration for Children and Families Children's Bureau.

Valla, J., Bergeron, L., & Smolla, N. (2000). The Dominic-R: A pictorial interview for 6-to 11-year-old children. *Journal of the American Academy of Child and Adolescent Psychiatry,39*(1), 85-93.

Varni, J. W., Seid, M., & Kurtin, P. S. (2001). PedsQL (TM) 4.0: Reliability and validity of the Pediatric Quality of Life Inventory (TM) Version 4.0 generic core scales in healthy and patient populations. *Medical Care, 39*(8), 800-812.

Wagnild, G., & Young, H. (1993). Development and psychometric evaluation of the Resilience Scale. *Journal of Nursing Measurement, 1*, 165-178.

Williamson, D. E., Birmaher, B., Ryan, N. D., Shiffrin, T. P., Lusky, J. A., Protopapa, J. et al. (2003). The Stressful Life Events Schedule for Children and Adolescents: Development and validation. *Psychiatry Research, 119*(3), 225-241.

Wirt, R. D., Lachar, D., Klinedinst, J. E., Seat, P. D., & Broen, W. E. (1977). *Multidimensional evaluation of child personality: A manual for the Personality Inventory for Children.* Los Angeles: Western Psychological Services.

Wulczyn, F., Barth, R. P., Yuan, Y. T., Harden, B. J., & Landsberk, J. (2005). *Beyond common sense: Child welfare, child well-being, and the evidence for policy reform.* New Brunswick, NJ: Aldine Transaction.

Zill, N., & Coiro, M. J. (1992). Assessing the condition of children. *Children and Youth Services Review, 14*(1-2), 119-136.

Zimet, G. D., Zimet, S. G., Dahlem, N. W., & Farley, G. K. (1988). The Multidimensional Scale of Perceived Social Support. *Journal of Personality Assessment, 52*(Spring), 30-41.

Zimmer, M. H., & Panko, L. M. (2006). Developmental status and service use among children in the child welfare system–A national survey. *Archives of Pediatrics & Adolescent Medicine, 160*(2), 183-188.

Zimmerman, I. L., Steiner, V. G., & Pond, R. E. (2002). *Preschool Language Scale, 4th Edition.* San Antonio, TX: The Psychological Corporation.

APPENDIX A
BASSC Search Protocol

Search Terms

VAR1
Protective Factor*
Resilien*
Coping skill*
Well-being
Strength-based
Efficac*
Competenc*
Asset*

VAR2
Infant*
Child*
Youth
Adolescen*

VAR3
Foster*
Child welfare

VAR4
Assessment*
Instrument*
Scale*
Inventor*
Measure*
Psychometric*

VAR5
Peer*
Famil* (only for four VAR)
School*
Relationship*
Develop*
Social support*

Databases

Academic databases for books and articles

Pathfinder or Melvyl
ArticleFirst
ERIC
Expanded Academic ASAP
Family and Society Studies Worldwide
PAIS International
PsychInfo
Social Science Citation Index
Social Services Abstracts
Social Work Abstracts
Sociological Abstracts

APPENDIX A (continued)

Systematic Reviews

Campbell Collaboration–C2-Spectre & C2-Ripe
Children and Family Research Center
Cochrane Library
ESRC Evidence Network
NHS Centre for Reviews & Dissemination
Social Care Institute for Excellence

Research Institutes

Brookings Institute
Manpower Demonstration Research Corporation
Mathematica Policy Research, Inc.
Urban Institute
RAND
GAO
National Academy of Sciences
Chapin Hall
CASRC (San Diego)

Conference Proceedings

PapersFirst (UCB Database)
Proceedings (UCB Database)

Internet

Google Scholar

Administration for Children and Families, DHHS, Resources for Measuring Services & Outcome in Head Start Programs Serving Infants & Toddlers:
http://www.acf.hhs.gov/programs/opre/ehs/perf_measures/reports/resources_measuring/res_meas_toc.html

Violence Institute of New Jersey at UMDNJ:
http://www.umdnj.edu/vinjweb/research_projects/instrument_inventory/instrument_inventory.html

http://www.lib.berkeley.edu/SOCW/socw_instruments.html

APPENDIX B
Excluded Instruments

1. Brief Symptom Inventory (BSI; Derogatis & Melisaratos, 1983)
2. California Child Q-Sort (CCQ) (Block & Block, 1969)
3. Child and Adolescent Functional Assessment Scale (CAFAS; Hodges, 1990)
4. Child and Adolescent Psychiatric Assessment (CAPA; Angold & Costello, 2000)
5. Child Behavior Checklist (CBCL; Achenbach, 1991)
6. Childhood Anxiety Sensitivity Index (CASI; Silverman, Fleisig, Rabian, Peterson, 1991)
7. Children's Depression Inventory (CDI; Kovacs, 1992)
8. Children's Depression Scale (CDS; Lang & Tisher, 1978)
9. Children's Global Assessment Scale (CGAS; Shaffer et al., 1983)
10. Brief Impairment Scale (Bird et al., 2005)
11. Colorado Client Assessment System Record (CCAR; Ellis, Wilson, & Foster, 1984)
12. Columbia Impairment Scale (Bird et al., 1993)
13. Devereux Scales of Mental Disorder (Naglieri, LeBuffe, & Pfeiffer, 1994)
14. Diagnostic Interview Schedule for Children (DISC; Shaffer & Fisher, 1997)
15. Draw-A-Person: Screening Procedure for Emotional Disturbance (DAP: SPED; Naglieri, McNeish, & Bardos, 1991)
16. Dominic-R (Valla, Bergeron, & Smolla, 2000)
17. Minnesota Multiphasic Personality Inventory-Adolescent (MMPI-A; Butcher et al., 1992)
18. Moods and Feelings Questionnaire (MFQ; Angold et al., 1995)
19. Personality Inventory for Children (PIC; Wirt, Lachar, Klinedinst, Seat, & Broen, 1977)
20. Personality Inventory for Youth (PIY; Lachar & Gruber, 1993)
21. Preschool Behavior Questionnaire (PBQ; Behar, 1977)
22. Scale for Assessing Emotional Disturbance (SAED; Epstein, Cullinan, Ryser, & Pearson, 2002)
23. Schedule for Affective Disorders and Schizophrenia for School-Age Children (K-SADS; Kaufman et al., 1997)
24. Social Anxiety Scale for Children (SASC; La Greca, Dandes, Wick, Shaw, & Stone, 1988)
25. Social Phobia and Anxiety Inventory for Children (SPAI-C; Beidel, Turner, & Fink, 1996)
26. Stressful Life Events Schedule (SLES; Williamson et al., 2003)
27. Teacher Report Form (TRF; Achenbach, 1991)
28. Trauma Symptom Checklist for Children (TSCC; Briere, 1996)
29. Youth Self Report (YSR; Achenbach, 1991)

APPENDIX C
Infant and Young Child Instruments

	Age Group I/P= Infant/Preschool C= Child A= Adolescent	Language Development & Communication	Intellectual Ability & Cognitive Functioning	Physical Development & Motor Skills	Socio-Emotional Competence
1. Preschool Language Scale-4 (PLS-4; Zimmerman et al., 2002)	I/P	X			
2. Reynell Developmental Language Scales (RDLS; Reynell & Huntley, 1985)	I/P	X			
3. Sequenced Inventory of Communication Development (Hedrick et al., 1984)	I/P	X			
4. MacArthur Communicative Development Inventory (MDCI; Fenson et al., 1993)	I/P	X			
5. Peabody Picture Vocabulary Test -Revised (Dunn & Dunn, 1981)	I/P	X			
6. Wechsler Preschool and Primary Scale of Intelligence, 3rd Edition (WPPSI-III; The Psychological Corporation, 2002)	I/P, C	X	X		
7. Stanford-Binet Intelligence Scale, 5th Edition (SB5; Roid, 2003)	I/P,C,A		X		
8. Kaufman Assessment Battery for Children, 2nd Edition (KABC-II; Kaufman & Kaufman, 2004)	I/P, C, A		X		
9. Differential Abilities Scale (DAS; Elliott, 1990)	I/P,C		X		
10. Griffiths Scales of Motor Development (Griffiths, 1984)	I/P			X	
11. Peabody Developmental Motor Scales, 2nd Edition (Folio & Fewell, 2000)	I/P			X	
12. Gross Motor Function Measure (Russell et al., 2002)	I/P			X	
13. Toddler and Infant Motor Evaluation (T.I.M.E.; Miller & Roid, 1994)	I/P			X	
14. Pediatric Evaluation of Disability Inventory (PEDI; Haley et al., 1992)	I/P			X	

	Age Group I/P= Infant/Preschool C= Child A= Adolescent	Language Development & Communication	Intellectual Ability & Cognitive Functioning	Physical Development & Motor Skills	Socio-Emotional Competence
15. Brief Infant-Toddler Social and Emotional Assessment (BITSEA; Briggs-Gowan et al., 2004)	I/P,C				X
16. Infant-Toddler Social and Emotional Assessment (ITSEA; Carter & Briggs-Gowan, 2000)	I/P,C				X
17. Preschool and Early Childhood Functional Assessment Scale (PECFAS; Murphy et al., 1999)	I/P,C				X
18. Social Skills Rating System- PreSchool Version (SSRS; Gresham & Elliott, 1900)	I/P				X
19. Vineland Social-Emotional Early Childhood Scale (SEEC; Sparrow & Balla, 1998)	C				X
20. Bayley Scales of Infant Development (Baley, 1993)	I/P,C		X	X	
21. Vineland Adaptive Behavior Scales (Sparrow et al., 1984)	I/P,C,A	X		X	X
22. Battelle Developmental Inventory (BDI; Newborg et al., 1988)	**I/P,C**	**X**	**X**	**X**	**X**
23. Brigance Diagnostic Inventory of Early Development, Revised Edition (BDIED-R; Brigance, 1991)	I/P,C	X	X	X	
24. Child Development Inventory (CDI; Ireton & Glascoe, 1995)	**I/P,C**	**X**	**X**	**X**	**X**
25. Child Observation Record (COR; High/Scope, 1992)	**I/P,C**	**X**	**X**	**X**	**X**
26. Early Screening Profiles (ESP; Harrison, 1990)	I/P,C	X	X	X	X
27. FirstSTEP Screening Test for Evaluating Prechoolers (FirstSTEP; Miller, 1993)	I/P,C	X	X	X	X
28. Ages and Stages Questionnaire (ASQ; Bricker et al., 1995)	**I/P,C**	**X**	**X**	**X**	**X**

APPENDIX D
Middle Childhood Instruments

	Age Group I/P= Infant/Preschool C= Child A= Adolescent	Language & Communication	Cognitive Ability & Academic Achievement	Physical Health & Development	Socio-Emotional Competence
1. Children's Skills Test (SmarterKids, 1998)	C		X		
2. Tests of Achievement in Basic Skills (TABS; EdITS, 2004)	C		X		
3. Tests of Academic Achievement Skills (Gardner, 1989)	C		X		
4. Childhood Asthma Questionnaire (French et al., 1993)	C			X	
5. Multidimensional Self-Concept Scale (MSCS; Bracken, 1992)	C				X
6. Pictorial Self-Concept Scale (PSCS; Bolea at al., 1971)	C				X
7. Piers-Harris Self-Concept Scale, 2nd Edition (Piers et al., 1999)	C				X
8. Self-Perception Profile for Children (SPPC; Harter, 1985)	C				X
9. Child Self-Control Rating Scale (CSCRS; Rohrbeck et al., 1991)	C				X
10. Coping Scale for Children and Youth (CSCY; Brodzinsky et al., 1992)	C,A				X
11. Kidcope (Spirito et al., 1988)	C,A				X
12. Kohn Social Competence Scale (Kohn & Rosman, 1972)	C				X
13. Loneliness and Social Dissatisfaction Questionnaire (LSDS; Asher et al., 1984)	C				X
14. Penn Interactive Peer Play Scale (PIPPS; Fantuzzo et al., 1995)	C				X

	Age Group I/P= Infant/Preschool C= Child A= Adolescent	Language & Communication	Cognitive Ability & Academic Achievement	Physical Health & Development	Socio-Emotional Competence
15. Self-Esteem Inventory-Revised (SEI; Coopersmith, 2002)	A	X			
16. Self-Esteem Index (SEI; Brown & Alexander, 1991)	C,A				X
17. Social Skills Rating System (SSRS; Gresham & Elliott, 1990)	**C,A**		X		X
18. Clinical Assessment Package for Assessing Client Risks and Strengths (CASPARS; Gilgun, 1999)	**C,A**		X		X
19. Matson Evaluation of Social Skills for Youngsters (MESSY; Matson et al., 1983)	C				X
20. Social Adjustment Inventory for Children & Adolescents (SAICA; John et al., 1987)	C,A				X
21. Elementary School Success Profile (ESSP; Bowen, 2006)	C				X
22. Behavioral and Emotional Rating Scale (BERS; Epstein & Sharma, 1998)	**C,A**				X
23. Multidimensional Student's Life Satisfaction Scale (MSLSS; Huebner, 1994)	C,A				X
24. Strengths & Difficulties Questionnaire (SDQ; Goodman, 2001)	C,A				X
25. School Social Behavior Scales, 2nd Edition (SSBS-2; Merrell, 1993)	C				X
26. Behavior Assessment System for Children (BASC; Reynolds & Kamphaus, 1992)	I/P,C,A				X
27. Child Health & Illness Profile (CHIP; Starfield et al., 1995)	C		X	X	X
28. Child Health Questionnaire (CHQ; Landgraf et al. 1996)	C,A		X	X	X
29. Pediatric Quality of Life (PedsQL™; Varni et al., 2001)	I/P, C, A		X	X	X

APPENDIX E
Adolescent Instruments

	Age Group I/P= Infant/Preschool C= Child A= Adolescent	Self-Esteem/Self-Concept	Self-Efficacy	Life Satisfaction	Social Competence/ Communication Skills	Perceived Social Support	Perceived Academic/ General Achievement	Problem-Solving/Decision-Making
1. Rosenberg Self-Esteem Scale (RSE; Rosenberg, 1989)	A	X						
2. Self-Esteem Questionnaire (SEQ; DuBois et al., 1996)	C,A	X						
3. Bledsoe Self-Concept Scale (BSCS; Bledsoe, 1967)	A	X						
4. Multidimensional Self-Concept Scale (MSCS; Bracken, 1992)	A	X			X			
5. Self-Perception Profile for Adolescents (SPPA; Harter, 1988)	A	X			X		X	
6. Self-Description Questionnaire (SDQII; SDQIII; Marsh 1990, 1992)	A	X			X		X	
7. Tennessee Self-Concept Scale (TSCS; Fitts, 1965)	A	X		X	X			
8. Career Decision-Making Self-Efficacy Scale (CDMSES; Taylor & Betz, 1983)	A		X					X
9. Self-Efficacy Questionnaire for Children (SEQ-C; Muris, 2001)	A		X					
10. Student's Life Satisfaction Scale (SLSS; Huebner, 1991)	C,A			X				
11. Perceived Life Satisfaction Scale (PLSS; Adelman et al., 1989)	A			X				
12. Assertiveness Scale for Adolescents (ASA; Lee, 1985)	A				X			
13. Teenage Inventory of Social Skills (TISS; Inderbitzen & Foster, 1992)	A				X			
14. Child and Adolescent Social Support Scale (CASSS; Malecki et al., 1999)	C					X		

	Age Group I/P= Infant/Preschool C= Child A= Adolescent	Self-Esteem/Self-Concept	Self-Efficacy	Life Satisfaction	Social Competence/ Communication Skills	Perceived Social Support	Perceived Academic/ General Achievement	Problem-Solving/Decision-Making
15. Social Support Scale for Children (SSSC; Harter, 1985)	C,A					X		
16. Multidimensional Scale of Perceived Social Support (MSPSS; Zimet et al., 1988)	A					X		
17. Perceived Social Support from Family and Friends (PSS-FA & PSS-FR; Procidano & Heller, 1983)	A					X		
18. Achievement Goal Questionnaire (AGQ; Finney et al., 2004)	A						X	
19. Inventory of School Motivation (ISM; McInerney & Sinclair, 1991)	A						X	
20. Problem-Solving Inventory (PSI; Heppner & Peterson, 1992)	A							X
21. 4-D: Strengths-Based Assessment Tools for Youth in Care (4 -D; Gilgun, 2004)	A		X		X	X	X	X
22. Family, Friend, and Self Form (FFS; Simpson & McBride, 1992)	A	X		X	X	X	X	
23. Child and Adolescent Social and Adaptive Functioning Scale (CASAFS; Price et al., 2002)	A		X		X	X	X	
24. Adolescent-Coping Orientation for Problem Experiences (A-COPE; Patterson & McCubbin, 1987)	A		X	X	X	X	X	X
25. Resiliency Scale (Jew et al., 1999)	A		X	X	X	X		X
26. Resilience Scale (Wagnild & Young, 1993)	A		X	X				X
27. Ansell-Casey Life Skills Assessment (ACLSA; Casey Family Programs, 2005)	C,A		X		X	X	X	X

Understanding and Measuring Child Welfare Outcomes

Amy D'Andrade, PhD
Kathy Lemon Osterling, PhD
Michael J. Austin, PhD

SUMMARY. The new "Children's and Family Services Reviews" (CFSR) process focuses on the effectiveness of services to children and families by measuring client outcomes. This article reviews the research literature related to child welfare outcomes in order to provide a context for federal accountability efforts. It also summarizes the 2001 federal mandate to hold states accountable for child welfare outcomes and describes California's response to this mandate. Implications of the outcomes literature review and measurement problems in the CFSR process suggest CSFR measures do not always capture meaningful outcomes. Recommendations for change are made.

Amy D'Andrade is Research Director and Michael J. Austin is Professor; both are affiliated with Bay Area Social Services Consortium, School of Social Welfare, University of California, Berkeley. Kathy Lemon Osterling is affiliated with School of Social Work, San Jose State Univesity, San Jose, CA.

KEYWORDS. Child welfare, federal outcomes, safety, permanence, well-being

INTRODUCTION

Efforts to use data to monitor and improve social services are not new. As far back as 1930s, there were calls for accountability for social services (Courtney, Needell & Wulczyn, 2004). More recently, the Government Performance and Reporting Act of 1993 required federal agencies to establish performance goals and monitor performance results for all federal programs (Kautz, Netting, Huber, Borders & Davis, 1997). In addition, the Social Security Amendments of 1994 required the Department to "promulgate regulations for reviews of states' child and family services" (Administration for Children and Families, n.d.[b]). Finally, the Adoption and Safe Families Act of 1997 required the federal government to develop a set of outcome measures for public child welfare programs (USGAO, 2004).

This article reviews the research literature related to child welfare outcomes in order to provide a context for federal accountability efforts. It also summarizes the 2001 federal mandate to hold states accountable for child welfare outcomes and describes California's response to this mandate. The federal outcomes and this structured review of the literature focus on client outcomes: namely, outcomes for children as they move in and out of state child welfare systems. The data on the efficiency and effectiveness of specific child welfare programs (e.g., independent living, therapeutic foster care, kinship care, domestic violence or substance abuse treatment) are not included in this review.

The most frequently cited child welfare outcomes in the research literature and in federal and state accountability efforts fall into three broad domains: (1) safety, (2) permanency, and (3) well-being. The outcomes for safety include protecting children from abuse and neglect and maintaining them safely in their own homes. In the permanency domain, outcomes assess whether children in out-of-home care have permanency and stability in their living situations. The outcomes related to well-being include education, physical health, and mental health of children while they are in care and upon emancipation from the system.

OUTCOMES AS REFLECTED IN RESEARCH LITERATURE

The search of the literature for findings related to child welfare safety, permanency and well-being outcomes involve the use of specific search terms for accessing social science and academic databases available through the University of California library. In addition, the search included websites specializing in systematic reviews, publications of research institutes, databases for conference proceedings, dissertation databases, and general internet searches. When child, family or case characteristics have been found to be associated with the outcomes, these are described as well.

Safety Indicators

Child safety is a priority for the child welfare system. The measures of child safety that are assessed in the research literature include: (1) *maltreatment recurrence*, or the rate at which children experience maltreatment subsequent to an initial investigated event of maltreatment; (2) *maltreatment in out-of-home care*, or the rate at which children experience maltreatment while placed in foster care; and (3) *re-entry to foster care*, the rate at which children experience placement into foster care subsequent to reunification with their parents. The research findings related to these indicators are described below.

Maltreatment Recurrence: The findings related to maltreatment recurrence vary depending on the definition of "recurrence" and the time span of the observation period following the initial referral. When "recurrence" is defined as a subsequent referral or report to the child welfare system, studies have found that about one quarter of children experience maltreatment recurrence within 18 months of the initial referral (English, Marshall, Brummel & Orme, 1999; Fuller & Wells, 2003). When "recurrence" is defined as a subsequent *substantiated* referral or report to the child welfare system, a smaller proportion of referred children experience recurrence (Depanfilis & Zuravin, 2002; Depanfilis & Zuravin, 1999; English, Marshall, Brummell & Orme, 1999; Lipien & Forthofer, 2004; Terling, 1999) and that proportion grows as more time elapses from the initial referral (Depanfilis & Zuravin, 2002; Depanfilis & Zuravin, 1999; Terling, 1999).

The child factors found to be associated with an increased likelihood of child maltreatment recurrence include younger age (Drake, Johnson-Reid, Way & Chung, 2003; Fuller, Wells, & Cotton, 2001; Lipien & Forthofer, 2004; Marshall & English, 1999), health, mental health, and/or developmental problems (Depanfilis & Zuravin, 2002; Marshall & English, 1999. Additionally, Asian/Pacific Islander children appear to have lower recurrence rates than children of other racial/ethnic backgrounds (Fluke, Yuan & Edwards, 1999). The risk factors related to parents include substance abuse (Fuller & Wells, 2003), criminal history (Fuller & Wells, 2003), domestic violence (Depanfilis & Zuravin, 2002), childhood abuse (Marshall & English, 1999), lack of social support (Depanfilis & Zuravin, 2002), and poverty (Jones, 1998). Families with multiple children (Depanfilis & Zuravin, 2002; Marshall & English, 1999) and single parent-families (Fuller, Wells, & Cotton, 2001) have been found to be more likely than other types of families to have a subsequent substantiated report of child maltreatment. Finally, the risk of maltreatment recurrence increases if the initial report is substantiated (Lipien & Forthofer, 2004) and increases with each subsequent maltreatment incident (Fluke et al., 1999; Fuller et al., 2001; Terling, 1999).

Maltreatment in Out-of-Home Care: The federal statistics do not describe what proportion of children in foster or group care nationwide have been maltreated. However, a federal report indicates that less than 1% of perpetrators of maltreatment in 2003 were foster parents or residential staff, with neglect being the most common form of maltreatment reported (U.S. Department of Health and Human Services, 2005). When former foster youth are queried, over 30% report that they experienced some form of child maltreatment while in care; neglect again is the most commonly reported type of maltreatment (Annie E. Casey Foundation, 2005). The studies examining incidence of maltreatment in care have found that between 8 and 120 children per 1000 in care are victims of substantiated maltreatment and the rate varies by placement type (Spencer & Knudsen, 1992).

Re-Entry to Foster Care: A substantial portion of children who are reunified with their parents subsequently re-enter care within one to two years. About 13-14% of them re-enter care within one year (Jones, 1998; Needell, Webster, Cuccarro-Alamin, Armijo, Lee, Levy, Shaw, Dawson, Piccus, Magruder, Kim, Conley, Henry, Korinek, Paredes & Smith, 2005), about 20% of them re-enter care within two to three years (Courtney, 1995; Courtney et al., 1997; Festinger, 1996), and the proportion increases as more time elapses since reunification (Frame et al., 2000; Wulczyn, 1991).

A number of child, parent, and case characteristics have been found to be associated with re-entry into care. Infants (Courtney, 1995; Courtney, Piliavin & Wright, 1997; Frame, Berrick, & Brodowski, 2000; Wells & Guo, 1999), African American children (Courtney,

1995; Courtney et al., 1997; Jones, 1998; Wells & Guo, 1999), and children with health problems (Courtney, 1995; Jones, 1998) have been found to have a greater likelihood of re-entry. Parents who are poor (Courtney, 1995), who have a history of criminal activity (Frame et al., 2000), substance abuse problems (Frame et al., 2000), or limited social supports (Festinger, 1996) are more likely to have their children re-enter care. Lastly, children placed with kin prior to reunification (Courtney, 1995; Courtney et al., 1997; Frame et al., 2000; Wells & Guo, 1999) and who experience more placement moves while in care (Courtney, 1995; Courtney et al., 1997; Wells & Guo, 1999) are more likely to re-enter care.

PERMANENCY INDICATORS

The second primary goal of the child welfare system is permanency; namely, reunifying children with their parents or finding them adoptive homes as quickly as possible. While children remain in care, an important aspect of permanency is the degree of stability they experience in the form of fewer placement changes. The research findings related to permanency indicators are described below.

Reunification: Although national data suggest that over half of children exiting care in 2001 were reunified (U.S. Department of Health and Human Services, 2003), rates of reunification in longitudinal studies generally reflect lower rates of reunification that vary between 23-48% of children entering care after 1-2 years (Berrick, Needell, Barth & Jonson-Reid, 1998; Courtney, McMurty & Zinn, 2004; Needell et al., 2005; Wells & Guo, 2003; Wells & Guo, 2004). The rate of reunification varies based on the time period under investigation, with a higher proportion of cases reunifying as more time elapses from entry into care (Barth, 1997; Courtney, 1994; Harris & Courtney, 2003; McMurty & Lie, 1992; Wells & Guo, 1999).

The research on factors affecting reunification have identified a variety of child, family and case characteristics that appear to affect the likelihood of reunification. In general, the research suggests that younger children (Courtney & Wong, 1996; Smith, 2003a), children of color (Courtney & Wong, 1996; Wells & Guo, 1999), and children with health and emotional/behavioral problems (Courtney, 1994; Landsverk, Davis, Ganger, Newton, & Johnson, 1996) are less likely to reunify than children without those characteristics. While poor families are less likely to reunify than those who are not poor (Courtney & Wong, 1996; Smith, 2003a), moving from welfare to employment also appears to decrease the likelihood of reunification (Wells & Guo, 2003). The children from two-parent homes appear more likely to be reunified than children from one-parent homes (Harris & Courtney, 2003; Wells & Guo, 1999). In terms of parental characteristics, the presence of maternal mental health problems (Wells & Gou, 2004) and homelessness (Courtney, McMurty & Zinn, 2004) decrease the likelihood of reunification. Children initially placed as a result of neglect have been found to be less likely to reunify than children placed for other reasons (Courtney & Wong, 1996; Harris & Courtney, 2003; Wells & Guo, 1999; Wells & Guo, 2003), and children placed with kin reunify more slowly than children placed with non-kin (Courtney & Wong, 1996; Harris & Courtney, 2003). Some studies have found families receiving services are more likely to reunify than those not receiving these services (Courtney & Wong, 1996; Smith, 2003a).

Adoption: The national data indicate that among children exiting care in 2001, 18% were adopted (U.S. Department of Health and Human Services, 2003). The national data also suggest that a sizable portion of children wait long periods in out-of-home care before adoption. The research using longitudinal data has generally found lower adoption rates than those reported in federal exit cohort data, with rates varying from about 2% after 2-31/2 years (Courtney, 1994 Needell et al., 2005; Berrick et al., 1998), to 9-20% after 6 years (Barth, 1997; Berrick et al., 1998; McMurty & Lie, 1992). The child characteristics associated with a decreased likelihood of adoption include male gender (Kemp & Bodonyi, 2002; Kemp & Bodonyi, 2000), younger age (Barth, 1997; Courtney & Wong, 1996; Kemp & Bodonyi, 2002; Smith, 2003b), non-white ethnicity (Barth, 1997; Courtney & Wong, 1996; Kemp & Bodonyi, 2002; Smith, 2003b), health problems or disabilities (Courtney & Wong, 1996; Smith, 2003b), and placement with kin (Courtney & Wong, 1996; Smith, 2003b). Some research suggests demographics such as urban residence (Courtney & Wong, 1996) and state of residence (Smith, 2003b) may affect the likelihood of adoption as well.

Placement Stability: The studies of placement stability often use different definitions of stability and different time periods for observation. In general, research suggests that the more time children spend in out-of-home care, the more placements they experience. After 1-2 1/2 years, about 20-40% of children still in care experience three or more placements (Berrick et al., 1998; Palmer, 1996; Pardeck, 1984; Needell et al., 2005) and after 3-4 years, about 40-50% of children still in care have had three or more placements (Berrick et al., 1998; Fernandez, 1999; Usher, Randolph, & Gogan, 1999). There are a number of factors associated with placement disruptions, including such child factors as male gender and African American ethnicity (Webster, Barth & Needell, 2000), older age (James, Landsverk & Slyman, 2004; Smith, Stormshak, Chamberlain & Whaley, 2001; Webster et al., 2000; Wulczyn, Kogan & Harden, 2003), and child behavior problems (Barber, Delfabbro & Cooper, 2001; Newton, Litrownik, & Landsverk, 2000; Palmer, 1996). Children placed as a result of neglect (Barber et al., 2001; Webster et al., 2000) and children placed with kin (Webster et al., 2000; Wulczyn et al., 2003) tend to have more placement stability than children without those characteristics.

Well-Being Indicators

Enhancing child and family well-being is a third goal of the child welfare system. Physical health, mental health and educational problems among children in the child welfare system have been fairly well documented in the research literature, although differing research methodologies present some challenges in interpreting findings. Many studies use data collected at one point in time, which may over-sample children who have been in the child welfare system for long periods, possibly inflating rates of mental, physical and educational problems. Some studies suggest that children come into the child welfare system with numerous problems and it is often difficult to determine if problems are improved or exacerbated by experiences in out-of-home care.

Physical and Mental Health Issues: Children entering the child welfare system appear to have a number of physical health problems (Chernoff, Combs-Orme, Risley-Curtis & Heisler, 1994; Hochstadt, Jaudes, Zimo, & Schachter, 1987), in addition to relatively high rates of developmental delays (Chernoff et al., 1994; Leslie, Gordon, Ganger & Gist, 2002) and emotional and behavioral problems (Clausen, Landsverk, Ganger, Chadwick & Litrownik, 1998; Halfon, Berowitz & Klee, 1992; Harman, Childs, & Kelleher, 2000; Landsverk, Davis, Ganger, Newton, & Johnson, 1996; McIntyre & Kessler, 1986).

Educational Issues: The research consistently notes the educational deficits among children in foster care. A substantial portion of these children have repeated a grade, and/or receive SED services (Chernoff et al., 1994; Flynn & Biro, 1998). Children in the child welfare system have been found to be more likely than other children to have low levels of engagement in school, to be suspended or expelled, to change schools, and to receive lower grades (Eckenrode, Laird & Doris, 1993;

Flynn & Biro, 1998; Kortenkamp & Ehrle, 2002; Wodarski, Kurtz, Gaudin & Howing, 1990).

Preparation for Independent Living. Annually, approximately 20,000 youth are discharged from the foster care system to "independent living" (U. S. General Accounting Office, 1999). Available research suggests that foster youth who "age out" of the system face serious challenges, such as difficulty accessing health insurance and mental health services (Courtney, Piliavin, Grogan-Kaylor, & Nesmith, 2001; Merdinger, Hines, Lemon, & Wyatt, in press; Reilly, 2003), incarceration (Courtney et al., 2001; Reilly, 2003), housing instability and homelessness (Cook, 1994; Courtney et al., 2001), and low high school completion/GED rates (Barth, 1990; Blome, 1997; Cook, 1994; Courtney et al., 2001; Festinger, 1983; Mech, 1994; Reilly, 2003; Zimmerman, 1982).

THE FEDERAL REVIEW PROCESS

While previous federal review and accountability processes focused almost entirely on the accuracy and completeness of case files and other records, the new federal "Children's and Family Services Reviews" (CFSR) process focuses on the effectiveness of services to children and families by measuring client outcomes. The CFSR process was launched in 2001; all 50 states, plus the District of Columbia and Puerto Rico, have now completed their CSFR reviews.

The review process has three phases. First, administrative data are summarized to assess certain quantitative indicators for each state. Second, an on-site review is conducted of a sample of 50 cases (half are foster care cases, and half in-home services cases) from three sites (Administration for Children and Families, May, 2002). Reviewers spend one week reviewing cases and interviewing agency stakeholders (such as judges or advocates) and case-specific stakeholders (such as parents, workers, and children) (U.S. General Accounting Office, April 2004) in order to determine whether each case is in "substantial conformity" with seven overall outcomes (U.S. Department of Health and Human Services, 2003). If the state is found to be out of compliance on any of the outcomes based on both the administrative data and the on-site review process, the third phase involves the development of a program improvement plan. After a two-year implementation period, changes in the outcomes are assessed. If agreed upon targets have not been met by that time, financial penalties are assessed (Administration for Children and Families, August 2001).

A total of 26 different indicators are used to assess the seven outcomes. Of these indicators, 3 rely on the administrative data only, 20 rely on the on-site data only, and 3 rely on both the on-site review and administrative data sources. Figure 1 provides a summary of the federal CSFR outcomes, the indicators used to measure each outcome, and the sources of information for evaluating the indicator.

The federal government has established the minimum performance level that a state must attain in order to be in "substantial conformity" with the outcomes. For outcomes based solely upon administrative data, a state must meet or exceed the standard established by the federal government. The standards are set at the point at which approximately 25% of states had performed better and 75% had performed worse in AFCARS and NCANDS submissions (Administration for Children and Families (a); Courtney, Needell & Wulczyn, 2004). Figure 2 displays the measures for the six administrative data indicators as well as the national standards. For outcomes based solely upon on-site case review data, 90% of cases reviewed in the state must be found to be in "substantial conformity." For those outcomes based on both on-site reviews and administrative data, both requirements must be met.

No state has achieved substantial conformity on all the outcomes. Figure 3 shows the number and proportion of jurisdictions achieving substantial conformity on the seven outcomes. California did not meet any of the national standards for the administrative data indicators, and was not in substantial conformity with any of the seven outcomes. As of January 2004 no penalties had been applied, but potential penalties range from $91,492 for North Dakota to $18,244,430 for California (U.S. General Accounting Office, April 2004).

Measurement Issues

The federal government and many state officials report that the CSFR process is valuable. In the 2004 GAO survey, 26 of 36 responding states either generally or completely agreed with results of their final CSFR report, even though none of the states achieved substantial conformity with all the outcomes. As a result of the process, some states reported improved relationships with community stakeholders, as well as increased public and legislative attention being given to important child welfare issues (USGAO, 2004).

However, a number of measurement issues regarding the federal outcomes have been raised. State officials in all five states visited by the GAO office in 2004 expressed concerns that AFCARS and NCANDS

FIGURE 1. Federal Outcomes, Indicators, and Data Source

Domain	Outcome	Indicator	Case Reviews	Admin Data
SAFETY	Children are protected from abuse and neglect	1. Timeliness of investigations of reports	x	
		2. Recurrence of maltreatment	x	x
		3. Incidence of abuse or neglect in foster care		x
	Children are safely maintained in their homes	4. Services to family to protect children/prevent removal	x	
		5. Current risk of harm to child	x	
PERMANENCY	Children have permanency and stability in their living arrangements	6. Foster care re-entries	x	x
		7. Stability of foster care placement	x	x
		8. Permanency goal for child	x	
		9. ILS (2001); reunification, guardianship or permanent placement with relative (2002-2004)	x	
		10. Achievement of adoption	x	
		11. Permanency goal of "other planned living arrangement"	x	
		12. Time to reunification		x
		13. Time to adoption		x
	Continuity of family relationship is preserved	14. Proximity of current placement	x	
		15. Placement with siblings	x	
		16. Visiting with parents and siblings	x	
		17. Relative placement	x	
		18. Current relation of child in care with parents	x	
		19. Preserving connections	x	
WELL-BEING	Families have enhanced capacity to provide for children's needs	20. Needs and services of child, parents, foster parents	x	
		21. Child and family involvement in case planning	x	
		22. Worker visits with child	x	
		23. Worker visits with parents	x	
	Children receive appropriate services to meet educational needs	24. Educational needs of child	x	
	Children receive adequate services to meet their physical and mental health needs	25. Physical health of child	x	
		26. Mental health of child	x	

data, upon which administrative data indicators are based, were not reliable. In addition, researchers have argued that administrative and case review data indicators may not be good measures of the phenomena of interest.

Administrative Data Indicators: The administrative data indicators have a number of measurement problems. First, these indicators do not capture important aspects of child welfare processes, such as the rate of

FIGURE 2. Administrative Data Indicator Measures and National Standards

Indicator	Measurement	National Standard
Recurrence of maltreatment	Of all victims of substantiated child abuse or neglect during the first six months of the period under review, what % had another substantiated or indicated report within 6 months.	6.1%
Incidence of abuse or neglect in foster care	For all children in foster care during the period under review, what % were the subject of substantiated or indicated maltreatment by a foster parent or facility staff	0.57%
Foster care re-entries	For all children who entered foster care during the year under review, what % of them re-entered care within 12 months of a prior episode.	8.6%
Stability of foster care placement	Of all children who have been in foster care less than 12 months from the time of the latest removal, what % had no more than 2 placement settings.	86.7%
Time to reunification	Of all children reunified with their parents at time of discharge from foster care, what % were reunified in less than 12 months from the time of the latest removal from home.	76.2%
Time to adoption	Of all children who exited foster care during the year under review to a finalized adoption, what % did so in less than 24 months from the time of the latest removal from home.	32.0%

reunification and adoption. None of the six indicators relate to family and child well-being or to emancipated youth. Similarly, some do not capture the experience of important subsets of children. For example, placement stability is a far greater problem for youth who have been in care for longer periods, yet the related indicator captures the phenomenon only for children in care for 12 months or less.

Second, the indicators do not take into account the dynamic nature of the child welfare system. Changes in one outcome can affect other outcomes (Courtney, Needell & Wulczyn, 2004; Goerge, Wulczyn & Harden, 1996; Tilbury, 2004; Usher, Wildfire & Gibbs, 1999; Wells & Johnson, 2001). For example, decreasing the time to reunification is problematic if the re-entry rate increases as a result. Outcomes need to be considered in the context of other outcomes.

Third, the indicators do not take into account differences between states. According to Goerge et al., "...states exhibit a rather stunning degree of diversity..." (Goerge, Wulczyn & Harden, 1996, p. 25). These differences can include caseload dynamics (caseload population counts), use of kin placements, rate of entry, racial/ethnic populations, poverty, ethnicity, age and other variables that are likely to influence the outcomes. However, all states are required to meet the national standards, regardless of these differences.

Fourth, the indicators are limited by the format of the datasets from which they are drawn, and do not capture longitudinal caseload dynamics. As a result, indicators that require a longitudinal view, such as re-entry, cannot be adequately captured. Currently, the re-entry indicator represents *the portion of current entries to care that are re-entries*, a statistic that does not convey information about the rate at which cases re-enter care.

Fifth, several indicators rely upon exit cohorts to describe case phenomena. Exit cohorts are likely to be biased in important ways, since they exclude all youth who do not leave care. As a result, indicators derived from exit cohorts will tend to misrepresent the proportion of cases achieving permanency outcomes within the time frames (Courtney, Needell & Wulczyn, 2004). Exit cohorts are also heavily influenced by population dynamics, such as the number of children entering or exiting care per year. When these dynamics shift, length of stay estimates based on exit cohorts will change as well, even if nothing in the system has occurred that would affect them (Wulcyzn, Kogan & Dilts, 2001). These problems are intensified when indicators based upon exit cohorts are used to measure change over time. Research studies have demonstrated that performance trends differ markedly according to whether an entry or an exit cohort is used to assess change, even occasionally heading in opposite directions (Courtney, Needell & Wulczyn, 2004).

Lastly, there are concerns regarding the amount of improvement the federal government will be requiring states to make on the administrative indicators in order to avoid financial penalties. To determine how much states should be required to improve on each administrative indicator, the federal government treated the data submissions of the 52 jurisdictions as a sample, then derived the "sampling error." This sampling error is the amount by which states must improve. However, the variability within the 52 jurisdiction sample is likely to be substantially greater than the variability of an individual state's performance over time, particularly if the state is large. Applying the sampling error derived from the 52 sample to every individual state is inappropriate and places a much greater burden upon larger states.

On-Site Review Indicators: A primary concern regarding the on-site reviews is the small sample size of 50 cases, half of which are in-home services cases and half foster care cases. While small samples can sometimes adequately reflect patterns that exist in a population, this is likely only when the sample is randomly selected. Moreover, because not every one of the cases in the sample has relevance for each indicator assessed in the on-site review, sometimes as few as one or two cases are used to evaluate a state's performance (USGAO, 2004). For example, in Wyoming only 2 cases were relevant to assess the on-site indicator of time-to-adoption. In one of these cases, reviewers determined that appropriate efforts had not been made to achieve the outcome. As a result, the state was assessed as "needing improvement" in this area (USGAO,

2004). In California, 49 cases from three sites–Los Angeles, San Mateo, and Stanislaus–(Administration of Children and Families (c), n.d.) represented over 100,000 children receiving services in California.

A second concern is that in spite of the small sample, data from the on-site record reviews and interviews are heavily weighted in the CSFR process: 23 of the 26 indicators are based upon data from on-site reviews. Additionally, impressions arising from interviews and focus groups may be distorted when some participants are more vocal, even if the experiences they describe are not common. According to a state official in Arizona, one vocal participant in a focus group or interview can have an unreasonably large effect. "Those single comments too often become part of the case (review) report" (Stack, 2005, p.18).

California's Accountability Efforts

California passed legislation AB 636 in 2001 in response to both the federal outcomes reporting requirements and the limitations of the indicators as performance measures. The "Child Welfare System Improvement and Accountability Act" of 2001 introduces an accountability system designed to facilitate continuous improvements in each county. Beginning in January 2004, "California Child and Family Service Reviews" were initiated in each of California's 58 counties. These include a set of administrative performance indicators (see Figure 4). While a subset of these parallel the federal CFSR administrative data indicators, another subset goes beyond the federal effort by using California's own database, the Child Welfare Services Case Management System (CWS/CMS). CWS/CMS data are shared with the Center for Social Services Research at the University of California at Berkeley where it can be reconfigured and analyzed longitudinally. This longitudinal database can be used to generate outcomes that reflect the performance of the system and changes in that performance over time (CDSS, n.d.).

The California and federal accountability efforts differ in several important respects. First, the California approach is more comprehensive, utilizing more administrative data indicators including measures related to well-being and emancipating youth. Secondly, these measures are more carefully constructed. For example, the federal indicator assessing maltreatment recurrence includes all children who experienced an initial referral. However, children who were removed at the time of the initial referral are much less likely to experience a subsequent referral, as they are now in state custody; therefore, one California indicator related to this area excludes these children from consideration. Third, California's data are con-

FIGURE 3. Number and Proportion of States Achieving Substantial Conformity on Outcomes

Domain	Outcome	# of states	%
Safety	Children are protected from abuse and neglect	6	12%
	Children are safely maintained in their homes	6	12%
Permanency	Children have permanency and stability in their living arrangements	0	0%
	Continuity of family relationship is preserved	7	14%
Well-Being	Families have enhanced capacity to provide for children's needs	0	0%
	Children receive appropriate services to meet educational needs	16	31%
	Children receive adequate services to meet their physical and mental health needs	1	2%

figured longitudinally, allowing accurate estimates of outcomes like re-entry to foster care. And fourth, indicators assessing the proportion of cases attaining permanency outcomes within certain time frames are based upon *entry* cohorts. Entry cohorts provide better estimates of change over time than do exit cohorts.

Lastly, the state did not establish any particular standards and counties are not expected to meet a particular performance goal (with the single exception of the measure monthly worker visits with children that requires a level of 90% compliance). Instead, counties identify areas for improvement based on their performance on the measures. To enhance their understanding of problem areas, counties conduct "peer quality reviews." Relevant cases are randomly selected and interviews are conducted with the social workers involved with the case, clients, and other personnel. This process generates qualitative information that "provides an in-depth analysis of case results and promotes information sharing that helps build the capacity of social workers and other staff" (CDSS, n.d.). This strategy eliminates direct comparisons of outcomes between counties that may have very different economic and demographic characteristics.

IMPLICATIONS AND RECOMMENDATIONS

This review of the child welfare research literature provides a context for assessing federal and state measurement and accountability efforts. However, researchers and federal administrators have framed outcomes differently. While federal reports and outcomes use exit cohorts to de-

FIGURE 4. California 636 Administrative Indicators

Area	
Safety	Of all children with substantiated allegation within first 6 months of study period, what % had another substantiated allegation within 6 months? (Federal indicator #2)
	Of all children with a substantiated allegation during the 12 month study period, what % had a subsequent substantiated allegation within 12 months?
	Of all children with a first substantiated allegation during the 12 month study period, what % had a subsequent substantiated allegation within 12 months?
	Of all children with an inconclusive or substantiated allegation during the 12 month period who were not removed, what % had a subsequent substantiated allegation within 12 months?
	Of all children in foster care, what % had substantiated allegation by a foster parent? (Federal indicator #3)
	What % of child abuse and neglect referrals in the study quarter have resulted in an in-person investigation [stratified by immediate and 10 day]?
	Of all children who required a monthly social worker visit, how many received them?
Permanency	For all children who entered foster care during the year under review, what % of them re-entered care within 12 months of a prior episode? (Federal indicator #6)
	For all children entering foster care for the first time and staying in care for 5 or more days during the 12 month period, and reunified within 12 months of entry, what % re-entered care within 12 months?
	Of all children who have been in foster care less than 12 months from the time of the latest removal, what % had no more than 2 placement settings? (Federal indicator #7)
	For all children entering foster care for the first time and staying in care for 5 or more days during the 12 month period, and were in care for 12 months, what % had no more than 2 placements?
	Of all children reunified with their parents at time of discharge from foster care, what % were reunified in less than 12 months from the time of the latest removal from home? (Federal indicator #12)
	Of all children entering foster care for the first time and staying in care for 5 or more days during the 12 month study period, what % were reunified within 12 months?
	Of all children who exited foster care during the year under review to a finalized adoption, what % did so in less than 24 months from the time of the latest removal from home? (Federal indicator #13)
	Of all children entering foster care for the first time and staying in care for 5 or more days, what % were adopted within 24 months?
Well-being	For all children in care at the point-in-time of interest, of those with siblings in care, what % were places with some or all siblings [stratified by all/some]?
	For all children entering foster care for the first time (5 days+) during the 12 month study period, what % were in each placement type? [stratified by first placement, predominant placement, point-in-time]?
	Of those children identified as American Indian, what % were placed with relatives, non-relative Indian, and non-relative Indian families?

termine the proportion and timelines of cases that reunify or are adopted, researchers have not used this sampling strategy due to the biases involved. This makes it difficult to assess whether the national standards are reasonable in the context of the historical achievements of the system. However, a number of conclusions can be drawn from the research literature on child welfare outcomes.

First, there is clearly plenty of room for improvement in child welfare outcomes, and the federal government's effort to assess outcomes is an important step in the right direction. Second, some of the important outcomes that researchers have been studying over the last few decades are not captured by the current federal administrative data outcome indicators (e.g., the proportion of cases overall that reunify or are adopted, or placement stability for children in long-term care). Third, a myriad of factors appear to influence each outcome, suggesting that comparisons between states could be misleading if these factors are not taken into account. And fourth, while the outcomes of youth in care and emancipating from the system related to well-being are generally poor, this area is not emphasized in the federal review process.

Additionally, the measurement problems in the federal review process have several implications. First, the distortion from using estimates based upon exit cohorts (combined with the questionable reliability of the data from the on-site reviews due to the small sample size) suggest that conclusions about state performance drawn from these data sources *could very well be erroneous.* As a result, heavy fines could be levied inappropriately. The potential consequences for California are substantial; the state stands to lose more than 18 million dollars, more than any other state (USGAO, 2004).

Secondly, because the understanding gained from these data could be inaccurate, "corrective action" taken by a state to improve outcomes could negatively affect the true outcomes being sought (Courtney, Needell & Wulczyn, 2004). Since financial penalties will be imposed if targets are not met, states have a strong incentive to achieve the targets even if these efforts do not necessarily serve the best interests of children and families (Courtney, Needell & Wulczyn, 2004). For example, in order to reach the re-entry target, an agency might reunify fewer families, since fewer reunified families results in fewer re-entries. Similarly, current practices that benefit children might negatively affect the outcomes (USGAO, 2004). For example, successful efforts to move children currently in long-term foster care into adoptive homes would negatively affect a state's performance on the adoptions indicator as currently defined; any child adopted after having been in care *over* 24 months will reduce the proportion of those adoptions that are completed *within* 24 months.

With the CSFR review process, the federal government has chosen to hold states accountable for what can be counted, even though these measures do not always capture meaningful outcomes. To correct the situation, three changes related to administrative indicators are recommended: First, administrative indicators should be redefined based upon entry cohorts and longitudinal data, rather than exit cohorts and point-in-time samples, so that a more accurate depiction of case processes can be obtained. Second, additional administrative data indicators (based upon longitudinal entry cohorts) should be incorporated into the review process in order to capture important aspects of child welfare case, such as the proportion of cases reunified, adopted, and still in care at certain points in time). Third, national standards for administrative indicators should be eliminated. Given the diversity in states' characteristics, they should only be compared against themselves. If this is not possible, estimates could be risk-adjusted. For example, while incorporating all relevant risk factors would be impossible, it would not be difficult to use some basic demographics like age and race to adjust performance estimates (Courtney, Needell & Wulczyn, 2004).

Additionally, states should ensure their data systems allow for a longitudinal view of child welfare cases. While the changes to SACWIS systems that would be necessary to facilitate this change may involve some costs to states, they would not be difficult to undertake (Courtney, Needell & Wulczyn, 2004). States would also be well-advised to develop their own accountability systems based upon longitudinal data in order to better understand their own performance and make corresponding program and policy adjustments as well as be prepared to defend their performance should findings from the federal CSFR process differ from their own assessments.

The measurement concerns regarding the administrative indicators arise from the limitations of AFCARS and NCANDS data. These databases do not link files for children from year to year, a structure that does not allow a longitudinal consideration of children's experiences (Courtney, Needell & Wulczyn, 2004). Ultimately, AFCARS and NCANDS datasets need to be overhauled so that the federal government can gain more accurate understanding of state processes and achievements (Courtney, Needell & Wulczyn, 2004). Until AFCARS and NCANDS are reconstituted, states should be allowed to utilize other data sources in their CFSR assessments and these should be considered before final CFSR determinations are made (USGAO, 2004).

On-site case review and interview data should not be used to assess state performance, unless a true random sample of a reasonable size can be drawn. If this is not possible, a small, non-random sample might be useful as a way to explore possible explanations for outcomes seen in administrative data.

Lastly, federal and state legislatures need to devote resources to helping public child welfare agencies carry out their responsibilities for accountability (Courtney, Needell & Wulczyn, 2004). States need the ability to configure data so that it conveys meaningful information for management and accountability efforts. This requires the resources to hire personnel with the capacity to conceptualize and calculate appropriate measures of systems improvements. These resources are needed so that states can evaluate and improve the outcomes of services to children and families.

REFERENCES

Administration for Children and Families (a). *Background Paper: Child and Family Services Reviews National Standards.* Available at: http://www.acf.hhs.gov/programs/cb/hotissues/background.htm

Administration for Children and Families (b). *Child Welfare Final Rule: Executive summary.* Available at: http://www.acf.hhs.gov/programs/cb/laws/execsumm.htm

Administration of Children and Families (c). *Executive Summary - Final Report: California Children and Families Services Review.* Available at: http://www.acf.hhs.gov/programs/cb/cwrp/executive/caes.pdf

Administration for Children and Families. *Information Memorandum,* August, 2001.

Administration for Children and Families. *Information Memorandum,* May, 2002.

Annie E. Casey Foundation (2005). *Improving family foster care: Findings from the Northwest foster care alumni study.* Available at: http://www.aecf.org/

Barber, J. G., Delfabbro, P. H., & Cooper, L. L. (2001). The predictors of unsuccessful transition to foster care. *Journal of Child Psychology and Psychiatry, 42*(6), 785-790.

Barth, R. (1990). On their own: The experiences of youth after foster care. *Child and Adolescent Social Work Journal, 7*(5), 419-440.

Barth, R. P. (1997). Effects of age and race on the odds of adoption versus remaining in long-term foster care. *Child Welfare, 76*(2), 285-308.

Berrick, J.D., Beedell, B., Barth, R.P., & Jonson-Reid, M. (1998). *The tender years: toward developmentally sensitive child welfare services for very young children.* New York, NY: Oxford University Press.

Blome, W. (1997). What happens to foster kids: Educational experiences of a random sample of foster care youth and a matched group of non-foster care youth. *Child and Adolescent Social Work Journal, 14*(1), 41-53.

California Department of Social Services. State of California Program Improvement Plan. Available at: http://www.dss.cahwnet.gov/cfsr/res/pdf/PIP/PIPoverview.pdf #xml

Chernoff, R., Combs-Orme, T., Risley-Curtiss, C., & Heisler, A. (1994). Assessing the health status of children entering foster care. *Pediatrics, 93*(4), 594-601.

Clausen, J. M., Landsverk, J., Ganger, W., Chadwick, D., & Litrownik, A. (1998). Mental health problems of children in foster care. *Journal of Child and Family Studies, 7*(3), 283-296.

Cook, R. J. (1994). Are we helping foster care youth prepare for their future? *Children and Youth Services Review, 16*(3), 213-229.

Courtney, M. E. (1994). Factors associated with the reunification of foster children with their families. *Social Service Review, 68,* 81-109

Courtney, M. E. (1995). Reentry to foster care of children returned to their families. *Social Service Review, 69,* 226-241.

Courtney, M. E., McMurty, S. L., & Zinn, A. (2004). Housing problems experienced by recipients of child welfare services. *Child Welfare, 83*(5), 393-422.

Courtney, M.E., Needell, B., Wulczyn, F. (2004). Unintended consequences of the push for accountability: The case of national child welfare performance standards. *Child and Youth Services Review, 26,* 1141-1154.

Courtney, M. E., Piliavin, I., Grogan-Kaylor, A., & Nesmith, A. (2001). Foster youth transitions to adulthood: A longitudinal view of youth leaving care. *Child Welfare, 80*(6), 685-717.

Courtney, M. E., Piliavin, I., & Wright, B. R., (1997). Transitions from and returns to out-of-home care. *Social Service Review, 71*(4), 652-668.

Courtney, M. E. & Wong, Y. I. (1996). Comparing the timing of exits from substitute care. *Children and Youth Services Review, 18*(4/5), 307-334.

Depanfilis, D., & Zuravin, S. J. (1999). Epidemiology of child maltreatment recurrences. *Social Service Review, 73,* 218-240.

Depanfilis, D., & Zuravin, S. J. (2002). The effect of services on the recurrence of child maltreatment. *Child Abuse and Neglect, 26,* 187-205.

Drake, B., Johnson-Reid, M., Way, I., Chung, S. (2003). Substantiation and recidivism. *Child Maltreatment, 8*(4), 248-260.

Eckenrode, J., Laird, M. & Doris, J. (1993). School performance and disciplinary problems among abused and neglected children. *Developmental Psychology, 29*(1), 53-62.

English, D. J., Marshall, D. B., Brummel, S., & Orme, M. (1999). Characteristics of repeated referrals to child protective services in Washington State. *Child Maltreatment, 4*(4), 297-397.

Fernandez, E. (1999). Pathways in substitute care: Representation of placement careers of children using event history analysis. *Children and Youth Services Review, 21*(3), 177-216.

Festinger, T. (1983). *No one ever asked us: A postscript to foster care.* New York: Columbia University Press.

Festinger, T. (1996). Going home and returning to foster care. *Children and Youth Services Review, 18*(4/5). 383-402.

Fluke, J. D. Yuan, Y. Y., & Edwards, M. (1999). Recurrence of maltreatment: An application of the National Child Abuse and Neglect Data System (NCANDS). *Child Abuse and Neglect, 23*(7), 633-650.

Flynn, R. J., & Biro, C. (1998). Comparing developmental outcomes for children in care with those of other children in Canada. *Children and Society, 12,* 228-233.

Frame, L., Berrick, J. D., Brodowski, M. L. (2000). Understanding reentry to out-of-home care for reunified infants. *Child Welfare, 79*(4), 339-369.

Fuller, T. L., & Wells, S. J. (2003). Predicting maltreatment recurrence among CPS cases with alcohol and other drug involvement. *Children and Youth Services Review, 25*(7), 553-569.

Fuller, T. L., Wells, S. J., & Cotton, E. E. (2001). Predictors of maltreatment recurrence at two milestones in the life of a case. *Children and Youth Services Review, 23*(1), 49-78.

George, R., Wulczyn, F. & Harden, A. (1996). New comparative insights into states and their foster children. *Public Welfare, 54*(3), 12-25.

Halfon, N., Berowitz, G. & Klee, L. (1992). Mental health services utilization by children in foster care. *Pediatrics, 89,* 951-960.

Harman, J. S., Childs, G. E., & Kelleher, K. J. (2000). Mental health care utilization and expenditures by children in foster care. *Archives of Pediatrics and Adolescent Medicine, 154,* 1114-1117.

Harris, M. S., & Courtney, M. E. (2003). The interaction of race, ethnicity, and family structure with respect to the timing of family reunification. *Children and Youth Services Review, 25*(5/6), 409-429.

Hochstadt, N. J., Jaudes, P. K., Zimo, D. A., & Schachter, J. (1987). The medical and psychosocial needs of children entering foster care. *Child Abuse and Neglect, 11,* 53-62.

James, S., Landsverk, J., & Slyman, D. J. (2004). Placement movement in out-of-home care: Patterns and predictors. *Children and Youth Services Review, 26,* 185-206.

Jones, L. (1998). The social and family correlates of successful reunification of children in foster care. *Children and Youth Services Review, 20*(4), 305-323.

Kautz, J.R., Netting, F.E., Huber, R., Borders, K., & Davis, T.S. (1997). The Government Performance and Results Act of 1993: Implications for Social Work Practice. *Social Work, 42*(4), 364-373.

Kemp, S. P., & Bodonyi, J. M. (2002). Beyond termination: Length of stay and predictors of permanency for legally free children. *Child Welfare, 81*(1), 59-85.

Kemp, S. P., & Bodonyi, J. M. (2000). Infants who stay in foster care: Child characteristics and permanency outcomes of legally free children first placed as infants. *Child and Family Social Work, 5,* 95-106.

Kortenkamp, K., & Ehrle, J. (2002). *The well-being of children involved with the child welfare system: A national overview.* Washington DC: The Urban Institute.

Landsverk, J., Davis, I., Ganger, W., Newton, R. & Johnson, I. (1996). Impact of child psychosocial functioning on reunification from out-of-home placement. *Children and Youth Services Review, 18*(4/5), 447-462.

Leslie, L. K., Gordon, J. N., Ganger, E., & Gist, K. (2002). Developmental delay in young children in child welfare by initial placement type. *Infant mental health, 23*(5), 496-516.

Lipien, L., & Forthofer, M. S. (2004). An event history analysis of recurrent child maltreatment reports in Florida. *Child Abuse and Neglect, 28,* 947-966.

Marshall, D. B., & English, D. J. (1999). Survival analysis of risk factors for recidivism in child abuse and neglect. *Child Maltreatment, 4*(4), 287-296.

McIntyre, A., & Kessler, T. Y. (1986). Psychological disorders among foster children. *Journal of Clinical Child Psychology, 15*(4), 297-303.

McMurty, S. L. & Lie, G. Y. (1992). Differential exit rates of minority children in foster care. *Social Work Research and Abstracts, 28*(1), 42-48.

Mech, E. (1994). Foster youth in transition: Research perspectives on preparation for independent living. *Child Welfare, 73,* 603-623.

Merdinger, J. L., Hines, A. M., Lemon, K. M., & Wyatt, P. (2005). Pathways to college for former foster youth: Understanding factors that contribute to educational success. *Child Welfare 84* (6), 867-896.

Needell, B., Webster, D., Cuccaro-Alamin, S., Armijo, M., Lee, S., Lery, B., Shaw, T., Dawson, W., Piccus, W., Magruder, J., Kim, H., Conley, A., Henry, C., Korinek, P., Paredes, C., & Smith, J. (2005). *Child Welfare Services Reports for California.* Available at <http://cssr.berkeley.edu/CWSCMSreports/>

Newton, R. R., Litrownik, A. J., & Landsverk, J. A. (2000). Children and youth in foster care: Disentangling the relationship between problem behaviors and number of placements. *Child Abuse and Neglect, 24*(10), 1363-1374.

Palmer, S. E. (1996). Placement stability and inclusive practice in foster care: An empirical study. *Children and Youth Services Review, 18*(7), 589-601.

Pardeck, J. T. (1984). Multiple placements of children in foster family care: An empirical analysis. *Social Work, 29,* 506-509.

Reilly, T. (2003). Transition from care: Status and outcomes of youth who age out of foster care. *Child Welfare, 82*(6), 727-745.

Smith, B. D. (2003a). How parental drug use and drug treatment compliance relate to family reunification. *Child Welfare, 82*(3), 335-365.

Smith, B. D. (2003b). After parental rights are terminated: Factors associated with exiting foster care. *Children and Youth Services Review, 25*(12), 965-985.

Smith, D. K., Stormshak, E., Chamberlain, P., Whaley, R. B. (2001). Placement disruptions in treatment foster care. *Journal of Emotional and Behavioral Disorders, 9*(13), 200-210.

Spencer, J. W., & Knudsen, D. D. (1992). Out-of-home maltreatment: An analysis of risk in various settings for children. *Children and Youth Services Review, 14,* 485-492.

Stack, B.W. (2005). Child welfare's harsh test. *Youth Today, 14*(5), p. 18.

Terling, T. (1999). The efficacy of family reunification practices: Reentry rates and correlates of reentry for abused and neglected children reunited with their families. *Child Abuse and Neglect, 23*(12), 1359-1379.

Tilbury, C. (2004). The influence of performance measurement on child welfare policy and practice. *British Journal of Social Work,34*, 225-241.

U.S. Department of Health and Human Services (2003). *The AFCARS Report.* Available at: http://www.acf.hhs.gov/programs/cb.

U.S. Department of Health and Human Services (2005). *Maltreatment 2003.* Washington DC: Author.

U.S. General Accounting Office (1999). *Foster Care: Effect of Independent Living Program services unknown.* Report No. GAO/HEHS-00-13. Washington DC: Author.

U.S. General Accounting Office (2004). *Child and family service reviews: better use of data and improved guidance could enhance HHS's oversight of state performance.* GAO-04-333.

Usher, C. L., Randolph, K. A., & Gogan, H. C. (1999). Placement patterns in foster care. *Social Service Review, 73,* 22-37.

Usher, C.L., Wildfire, J.B., & Gibbs, D.A. (1999). Measuring performance in child welfare: secondary effects of success. *Child Welfare, 78*(1), 31-51.

Webster, D., Barth, R. P., & Needell, B. (2000). Placement stability for children in out-of-home care: A longitudinal analysis. *Child Welfare, 79*(5), 614-631.

Wells, K., & Guo, S. (1999). Reunification and reenty of foster children. *Children and Youth Services Review, 21*(4), 273-294.

Wells, K. & Guo, S. (2003). Mothers' welfare and work income and reunification with children in foster care. *Children and Youth Services Review, 25*(3), 203-224.

Wells, K. & Guo, S. (2004). Reunification of foster children before and after welfare reform. *Social Service Review, 78,* 74-96.

Wells, S. J. & Johnson, M.A.(2001). Selecting outcomes measures for child welfare settings: lessons for use in performance measurement. *Children and Youth Services Review, 23*(2), 169-199.

Wodarski, J. S., Kurtz, P. D., Gaudin, J. M., & Howing, P. T. (1990). Maltreatment and the school-age child: Major academic, socioemotional, and adaptive outcomes. *Social Work, 35*(6), 506-513.

Wulczyn, F. (1991). Caseload dynamics and foster care reentry. *Social Service Review, 65,* 133-156.

Wulcyzn, F., Kogan, J., Dilts, J. (2001). The effect of population dynamics on performance measurement. *Social Service Review, 75* (2), 292-317.

Wulczyn, F., Kogan, J., & Harden, B. J. (2003). Placement stability and movement trajectories. *Social Service Review, 77,* 212-237.

Zimmerman, R. (1982). *Foster care in retrospect.* New Orleans, LA: Tulane University Press.

Substance Abuse Interventions for Parents Involved in the Child Welfare System: Evidence and Implications

Kathy Lemon Osterling, PhD
Michael J. Austin, PhD

SUMMARY. As child welfare systems across the country face the problem of parental substance abuse, there is an increasing need to understand the types of treatment approaches that are most effective for substance-abusing parents in the child welfare system–the majority of whom are mothers. This structured review of the literature focuses on evidence related to two areas: (1) individual-level interventions designed to assist mothers and women in addressing their substance abuse problems, and (2) system-level interventions designed to improve collaboration and coordination between the child welfare system and the alcohol and other drug system. Overall, research suggests the following program components may be effective with substance-abusing women with children: (1) Women-centered treatment that involves children, (2) Specialized health and mental health services, (3) Home visitation services, (4) Concrete assistance, (5) Short-term targeted interventions, and (6) Comprehensive programs that integrate many of these components.

Kathy Lemon Osterling is affiliated with School of Social Work, San Jose State University, San Jose, CA. Michael J. Austin is Mack Professor of Nonprofit Management, Staff Director, Bay Area Social Services Consortium, School of Social Welfare, University of California, Berkeley, Berkeley, CA 94720.

Research also suggests that promising collaborative models between the child welfare system (CWS) and the alcohol and other drug (AOD) system typically include the following core elements: (1) Out-stationing AOD workers in child welfare offices, (2) Joint case planning, (3) Using official committees to guide collaborative efforts, (4) Training and cross-training, (5) Using protocols for sharing confidential information, and (6) Using dependency drug courts. Although more rigorous research is needed on both individual-level and system-level substance abuse interventions for parents involved in the child welfare system, the integration of individual-level interventions and system-level approaches is a potentially useful practice approach with this vulnerable population.

KEYWORDS. Parental substance abuse, intervention, child welfare, alcohol and other drug

INTRODUCTION

Parental substance abuse is a serious problem for the child welfare system. Estimates suggest that between 50 percent to 80 percent of child welfare cases involve a parent with a substance abuse problem (Bellis, Broussard, Herring, Wexler, Moritz, & Benitez, 2001; Famularo, Kinscherff, & Fenton, 1992; Murphy, Jellinek, Quinn, Smith, Poitrast, & Goshko, 1991, U.S. General Accounting Office [USGAO], 1998). Nationally, it is estimated that 8.3 million children live with at least one parent who has a substance abuse problem (Substance Abuse and Mental Health Services Administration, ([SAMHSA] 1996). Estimates also indicate that 4.3 percent of pregnant women use illegal drugs during pregnancy and 9.8 percent of pregnant women use alcohol during pregnancy, with 4.1 percent being binge drinkers (SAMHSA, 2003). Research suggests that children in the child welfare system who have parents with substance abuse problems are at risk for a variety of poor outcomes; they are more likely to experience an out-of-home placement, they have lengthier stays in out-of-home placement, and they are more likely to have adoption as a case plan (U.S. Department of Health and Human Services [USDHHS], 1997).

As child welfare systems across the country face the problem of parental substance abuse, there is an increasing need to understand the types of treatment approaches that have been found to be effective for parents with substance abuse problems. Research suggests that compliance with substance abuse treatment is related to faster reunification (Smith, 2003), however less is known about the actual effectiveness of substance abuse interventions for parents in the child welfare system, and the types of outcomes associated with differing treatment approaches. In addition, strong collaboration between the child welfare system (CWS) and the alcohol and other drug (AOD) system can play an important role in ensuring access to substance abuse treatment for parents involved in the child welfare system, as well as treatment coordination between systems. As such, this review of the literature focuses on evidence related to both individual level substance abuse interventions, as well as system-level collaborative approaches that may be effective with this population.

Impact of Parental Substance Abuse on Child and Family Functioning

Research suggests that parental substance abuse is associated with a variety of problems related to child and family functioning. Studies indicate that parental substance abuse increases the risk of poor child developmental outcomes in several domains, including complications at birth, lower cognitive functioning, physical and mental health problems, and problems with social adaptation (Bauman & Levine, 1986; Conners, Bradley, Whiteside Mansell, Liu, Roberts, Burgdorf et al., 2004; McMahon & Luthar, 1998; McNichol & Tash, 2001; Werner, 1986). There is also evidence that children with a family history of substance abuse have an increased risk for substance abuse themselves (Merikangas, Stolar, Stevens, Goulet, Preisig, Fenton et al., 1998).

Problems in family functioning are also associated with parental substance abuse. Maternal substance abuse has been linked with increased punitiveness toward children (Hien & Honeyman, 2000; Miller, Smyth, & Mudar, 1997), increased rigidity and overcontrol in parenting (Burns, Chethik, Burns, & Clark, 1991), authoritarian parenting attitudes (Bauman & Levine, 1986), and parenting stress (Kelley, 1998). Some research indicates that parents with substance abuse problems have a greater likelihood of neglectful or abusive behaviors toward their children (Chaffin, Kelleher, & Hollenberg, 1996; Kelleher, Chaffin, Hollenberg, & Fisher, 1994; Wasserman & Leventhal, 1993; Williams-Petersen, Myers, McFarland Degen, Knisely, Elswick, Schnoll, 1994). However, although there is evidence suggesting that parental substance abuse is associated with problems in parenting and family functioning, other research indicates that mothers who use drugs may also be strongly attached and committed to their children (Baker & Carson, 1999; Kearney, Murphy, & Rosenbaum, 1994).

INDIVIDUAL-LEVEL FACTORS AFFECTING TREATMENT

Unique Needs of Women in Substance Abuse Treatment

Although both mothers and fathers are equally likely to abuse drugs or alcohol, mothers make up the majority of substance-abusing parents in the child welfare system (U.S. Department of Health and Human Services [USDHHS], 1999). Research suggests that women who abuse alcohol or other drugs typically experience different circumstances than men and have unique needs that should be considered in the design of substance abuse interventions (Abbott, 1994, Reed, 1987). Overall, studies indicate that women with substance abuse problems experience a high incidence of socioeconomic problems, criminal justice system involvement, histories of victimization, and mental and physical health problems (Conners, Bradley, Whiteside Mansell, Liu, Roberts, Burgdorf, et al., 2004).

Socioeconomic Problems

Studies have found unemployment rates among women entering substance abuse treatment to range from 89 percent to 92 percent (Clark 2001; Conners, et al., 2004). Other studies have found homelessness rates to range from 25 percent to 58 percent (Chavkin, Paone, Friedman, & Wilets, 1993; Clark, 2001; El-Bassel, Gilbert, Schilling, & Wada, 2000; Grella, 1999; Saunders, 1993). Public assistance use ranges from 48 percent to 96 percent (Clark, 2001; Dore & Doris, 1998; Knight, Hood, Logan, & Chatham, 1999). And one study found that among woman in residential substance abuse treatment, 88 percent had incomes below the poverty line (Knight et al., 1999).

Criminal Justice System Involvement

Women in substance abuse treatment also tend to have a history of arrest, incarceration, or other involvement in the criminal justice system. Studies suggest that the majority of women in substance abuse treatment have been arrested at least once; arrest rates range from 66 percent to 90 percent (Clark, 2001; Conners et al., 2004; Knight et al., 1999; Whitesdale-Mansell, Crone & Conners, 1998). Incarceration rates range from 22 percent to 46 percent (Chavkin et al., 1993; El-Bassel et al., 2000). Moreover, current or past criminal justice system involvement (e.g. convictions, parole, probation, incarceration) ranges from 52 percent to 80 percent (Clark, 2001; Conners et al., 2004; Porowski, Burgdorf, & Herrell, 2004; Stevens & Arbiter, 1995).

Current and Past Histories of Abuse and Victimization

One of the most consistent findings from studies on women in substance abuse treatment is the high prevalence of abuse and victimization. Studies have found high rates of childhood abuse among women in substance abuse treatment. Overall childhood abuse rates range from 30 percent to 57 percent (Conners et al., 2004; Dore & Doris, 1998; El-Bassel et al., 2000; Saunder, 1993; Whitesdale-Mansell et al., 1998). Rates of ever-having-been sexually abused (e.g., rape, incest) range from 20 percent to 95 percent (Chavkin, et al., 1993; Dore & Doris, 1998; Ladwig & Andersen, 1989; Knight et al., 1999; Stevens & Arbiter, 1995). Rates of ever-having-been physically abused (including spousal abuse) range from 40 percent to 90 percent (Clark, 2001; Dore & Doris, 1998; Knight et al., 1999; Saunders, 1993; Stevens & Arbiter, 1995; Whitesdale-Mansell et al., 1998). Rates of emotional abuse range from 73 percent to 93 percent (Knight et al., 1999; Whitesdale-Mansell et al., 1998).

Physical and Mental Health Problems

Rates of physical health problems among women in substance abuse treatment range from 60 percent to 67 percent (Connners et al., 2004; Porowski et al., 2004). Rates of mental health problems range from 49 percent to 58 percent (Chavkin et al., 1993; Porowski et al., 2004). Additionally, one study found that nearly 30 percent of the mothers in a substance abuse program had attempted suicide (Conners et al., 2004). Other research has found that substance-abusing women are more likely than their male counterparts to have a psychiatric diagnosis (Grella, 1997; SAMHSA, 1997).

Special Vulnerability of Substance-Abusing Mothers in the Child Welfare System

Research suggests that substance-abusing mothers involved in the child welfare system may be especially vulnerable. Compared to substance-abusing mothers not involved in the child welfare system, child welfare system-involved mothers tend to be younger, unemployed, have less education, are less likely to be married, are more likely to have a chronic mental illness, are more likely to have more children, are more likely to use methamphetamines, and are more likely to have unsatisfactory exits from treatment (Shillington, Hohman, & Jones, 2001). Other research also suggests that substance-abusing mothers in the child welfare system are more likely than their non-child welfare system involved counterparts to have unsatisfactory exits from treatment (Hohman, Shillington, & Grigg Baxter, 2003).

SYSTEM-LEVEL FACTORS AFFECTING TREATMENT

Collaboration Between the Child Welfare and Alcohol and Other Drug Systems

In addition to individual-level interventions, researchers, practitioners and policy makers have begun to identify the issue of collaboration between alcohol and other drug (AOD) systems and the child welfare system (CWS) as a key factor in substance abuse treatment for parents in the CWS. Poor collaboration between systems can lead to fragmented service delivery. Several scholars have described numerous barriers to collaboration between AOD systems and the CWS (Hunter, 2003; McAlpine, Marshall, Harper Doran, 2001; USDHHS, 1999, Young, Garnder, & Dennis, 1998). These barriers include: (1) differences in how the two systems define the client, (2) differing time line constraints, (3) different training and education of practitioners, (4) funding barriers and shortages of available treatment, (5) problems related to confidentiality mandates, and (6) differences in defining successful outcomes.

Differences in Defining the Client

AOD systems and the CWS have historically defined the client in different ways. Child welfare systems typically consider the client to be first and foremost the child and then secondarily the family; whereas AOD systems typically define the client as the individual who is abusing drugs or alcohol (Hunter, 2003). As a result, the child welfare system is primarily concerned with the safety and well-being of the child within the family. In contrast, AOD systems typically do not consider children or the adults' status as a parent as necessarily relevant to addressing their problems with drugs or alcohol (Young et al., 1998). Instead, the individual's use of drugs or alcohol is the primary focus of intervention. These differing definitions of the client can act as a barrier to collaboration; both systems may see themselves as the primary service provider and the two systems may struggle with different treatment goals depending on who is viewed as the client (USDHSS, 1999).

Differences in Case Goals

The potentially conflicting value and treatment orientations of the AOD system and the CWS may also be reflected in different case goals for parents and children. In general, substance abuse treatment programs are concerned with assuring that clients decrease or eliminate their drug use and the negative consequences of drug use related to criminal behavior or health problems (Feig, 1998; USDHHS, 1999). The well-being of the family or child of the client is generally not a primary goal of treatment. However, the CWS is primarily concerned with the safety and well-being of the child and ensuring a timely permanent placement, with birth parents or in an alternate setting (USDHHS, 1999). While the goals of each system may compliment one another, they may also conflict. For instance, Feig (1998) notes that removing a child from the home may help ensure the child's safety and well-being and help create a permanent living situation, but may also cause a parent to drop out of substance abuse treatment.

Time Line Constraints

Young et al. (1998) note that substance-abusing parents involved with the child welfare system typically face "four clocks" that can act as a barrier to collaboration between the AOD system and the CWS. These four clocks include: (1) *Child welfare time limits* mandated by the Adoption and Safe Families Act (ASFA) which stipulate that a permanency hearing must be held after 12 months of out-of-home care, (2) *Treatment time lines* also affect substance-abusing parents in the child welfare system. The long-term nature of substance abuse treatment and the occurrence of relapses may conflict with child welfare time limits requiring substance-abusing parents to be drug-free for a certain amount of time prior to reunification (USDHHS, 1999), (3) *Welfare time limits* mandated by the Temporary Assistance to Needy Families (TANF) polices mandate a 24 month TANF time limit requiring parents to be engaged in work activities. For parents involved in TANF and the CWS, this may interfere with their treatment needs, as well as their ability to provide for their children if their welfare benefits are cut, and 4) The *developmental time trajectory* of children can also serve as a time constraint. It may be detrimental to children's development to be separated from their parents for long periods of time, yet, the AOD system typically views substance abuse treatment as a long-term process.

These four time-line constraints can cause conflicts between the AOD system and the CWS. While the AOD system may view long-term treatment as typical, the relatively short time lines imposed by ASFA and TANF policies, as well as the developmental needs of children, may create a number of challenges to effective collaboration.

Differences in Training and Education

The differences in training and education between the AOD system and the CWS may also act as a barrier to collaboration. Young et al. (1998) note that education on substance abuse interventions is generally lacking in CWS training, and that those working in the AOD system may not be aware of CWS practices. In addition, training within the two systems does not generally include information on cross-system collaboration.

Funding Barriers and Shortages of Available Treatment

Funding barriers between the two systems can also create problems with collaboration; Young et al. (1998) suggest that both systems may seek to safeguard their own funding sources by seeking reimbursements from the other. Moreover, court mandates and the restrictions set forth by the managed care system may cause both systems to be faced with difficulties in controlling their own resources. These external restrictions may make collaboration more difficult because ensuring treatment for some clients may not be in the control of either system. In addition, there is also an overall shortage of resources in both fields. SAMHSA (1997, as cited in USDHHS, 1999) reports that only 37 percent of substance-abusing mothers with children received some form of substance abuse treatment in 1994-1995, compared with 48 percent of substance-abusing fathers.

Problems Surrounding Confidentiality Mandates

Both AOD systems and the CWS are bound by federal and state regulations governing the types of client information that can be shared or released. Although these regulations are intended to protect the privacy and rights of clients and children, they can also create a barrier to collaboration between the two systems. Typically, substance abuse treatment programs are not allowed to discuss information about a client with other service systems, and child welfare agencies are generally not allowed to release information about children or families (Feig, 1998, USDHHS, 1999). However, collaboration between the two fields could be improved by sharing information on children and families. For instance, the USDHHS (1999) suggests that sharing information between AOD systems and the CWS can help to ensure that: (1) clients are fully assessed and their needs are understood, (2) desired case outcomes are consistent between the two systems so that agencies are not working toward conflicting goals, and (3) resources are used efficiently to prevent duplication of services.

Overall, both individual-level interventions and system-level collaborative approaches are important for successful treatment of parents with substance abuse problems in the CWS. Effective individual-level interventions can assist parents in the child welfare system to address their substance abuse problems, while effective system-level collaborative interventions can help streamline access to services and ensure treatment coordination between service providers. This review of the literature describes evidence related to core program components within both individual-level interventions and system-level collaborative approaches.

METHODS

The methods for this review involved the selection of studies based on an explicit search protocol that included identification of the population, interventions, and outcomes of interest, as well as the use of pre-determined search terms, databases to be searched, and an inclusion and exclusion criteria. This review focused on two overall areas: (1) individual-level substance abuse interventions, and (2) system-level collaborative approaches between the child welfare and alcohol and other drug systems.

Search Protocol for Individual-Level Substance Abuse Interventions

The population of interest for the individual-level substance abuse intervention review included parents with substance abuse problems who are involved in the child welfare system and women with and without children who are experiencing substance abuse problems. Information on outcomes related to the child welfare system were specifically targeted, including outcomes related to family reunification and permanency, however all outcomes included in the research are described. All substance abuse interventions targeted to parents involved in the child welfare system and women with substance abuse problems were eligible for review.

Inclusion criteria for individual-level interventions included studies using experimental or quasi-experimental methods. The experimental studies used a randomized controlled trial research design in which participants were randomly assigned to an intervention condition or a control condition. Randomized controlled trials are typically considered to represent the highest level of evidence because the randomization process generally eliminates possible differences between the two groups. Quasi-experimental studies included in this study either used a pre and post outcome design or a non-equivalent control group design. In the pre and post outcome design, outcome measures taken prior to the intervention are compared to those after the completion of the intervention. This is considered a less rigorous design than a randomized control trial because it is impossible to say definitively whether the intervention caused changes between pre and post or whether changes are due to some other unmeasured factor. A non-equivalent control group design compares an intervention group to some other group who either did not receive the intervention or received less of the intervention. Because the groups are not randomly assigned the possible differences between measures may be related to pre-existing differences between the two groups.

For individual-level interventions, the studies that were excluded from review included those that described interventions or program approaches that included no data on outcomes, studies that provided only descriptive data with no outcome data, studies that did not have an exclusive focus on women, women with children, or parents in the child welfare system, studies that provided no description of the intervention, studies that focused on adolescent mothers, and studies that reported preliminary results for which a subsequent evaluation provided full results.

Search Protocol for System-Level Collaborative Approaches Between the CWS and AOD System

The population of interest for the system-level collaborative review included all workers and clients involved in the child welfare and alcohol and other drug systems. Because empirical information on system-level collaborative practice approaches between the child welfare and alcohol and other drug systems is extremely limited, explicit inclusion and exclusion criteria for literature generated from the collaborative models search was not possible. Similarly, although outcomes of interest related to improved treatment access and effectiveness were included in the search protocol, the lack of any empirical information related to collaborative practice approaches between the CWS and AOD system made it impossible to assess outcomes. As a result, a broad search protocol was used in which all materials relevant to the topic area were reviewed. This broad approach was chosen in an effort to identify potentially effective collaborative practice approaches that could be implemented and further evaluated in local agencies.

SEARCH STRATEGY

Twelve academic databases available from the University of California were searched including those related to psychology, sociology, social work, and social services. Systematic review websites (e.g., Cochrane and Campbell Collaborations) were also searched, as were research institute databases, conference proceedings, dissertation abstracts, professional evaluation listservs and overall internet searches. In addition, a snowball method was also used in which additional materials were identified from primary reference lists of other studies. For instance a systematic review of the effectiveness of substance abuse treatment for women by Ashley, Marsden and Brady (2003) was used to identify several studies focusing on women and women with children.

RESULTS

Individual-Level Substance Abuse Interventions

Forty-seven studies focused on micro-level substance abuse interventions were identified through the structured review process. Table 1 presents an overview of all studies included in this review. A synthesis of this research suggests that outcomes for women with children in substance abuse treatment are enhanced by the inclusion of the following program components: (1) woman-centered treatment that involves children, (2) specialized health and mental health services, (3) home visitation, (4) concrete assistance (e.g., transportation, child care, assistance linking with substance abuse treatment), (5) short-term targeted interventions, and (6) comprehensive programs that integrate many of these components. Figure 1 summarizes these interventions and their outcomes.

Woman-Centered Treatment Involving Children

Fifteen studies were identified that investigated outcomes related to the effectiveness of woman-centered treatment and treatment that involved children. Overall, research suggests that women in woman-only treatment centers tend to have greater treatment retention and completion than those in mixed-gender programs (Egelko, Galanter, Dermatis, & DeMaio, 1998; Grella, 1999; Stevens, Arbiter, & Glider, 1989; Stranz & Welch, 1995). Women-only treatment is also associated with greater sobriety (Dahlgren & Willander, 1989; deZwart, 1991; Egelko et al., 1998; Rosett, Weiner, Zuckerman, McKinlay & Edelin, 1980; Stevens & Arbiter, 1995), greater likelihood of employment (Dahlgren & Willander, 1989; Stevens & Arbiter, 1995), decreased arrest rates, decreased use of government assistance and increased likelihood of having custody of children (Stevens & Arbiter, 1995). Although most identified studies suggest that woman-centered treatment may be more effective than mixed gender or traditional treatment, one quasi-experimental study that compared outcomes for women in a 6-week woman-centered residential program to outcomes for women in one of two traditional mixed gender residential programs (one that lasted 3 weeks and one that lasted 1 week) found no differences in drug use, employment status, social support or mental health status (Copeland, Hall, Didcott, & Biggs, 1993).

Other research suggests that better outcomes result when children are living with their mothers while they are in treatment. Studies suggest that women who are allowed to reside in residential treatment with their children experience greater treatment retention and completion than those not residing with their children (Clark, 2001; Hughes, Coletti, Neri, Urmann, Stahl, Sicilian, & Anthony, 1995; Wobie, Eyler, Conlon, Clarke & Behnke, 1997) and also exhibit greater abstinence (Metsch, Wolfe, Fewell, McCoy, Elwood, Wohler-Torres et al., 2001), fewer problems with depression and higher self-esteem (Wobie et al., 1997). Although most identified studies suggest better outcomes when children live with their mothers in treatment, two studies found no differences between women residing with children compared to those

FIGURE 1. Intervention Components and Outcomes

Component	Description	Outcomes
Woman-centered treatment involving children	Treatment programs that involve only women and are targeted toward the unique needs of women, as well as programs that involve children in treatment.	• Increased treatment retention and completion • Greater abstinence • Decreased likelihood of criminal justice system involvement • Increased likelihood of employment • Decreased likelihood of public assistance use • Increased likelihood of child custody • Decreased depression • Higher self-esteem
Health and Mental Health Care	Health care services, particularly prenatal care for pregnant women and mental health interventions such as individual therapy and specialized group therapy.	• Longer gestational periods • Better birth outcomes • Increased treatment retention • Greater abstinence • Greater likelihood of employment • Reduction in high-risk injecting drug use behavior
Home Visitation	Home visits by a nurse or a paraprofessional that focus on providing maternal support, promoting healthy parent-child interaction ,and providing linkages to concrete resources.	• Greater abstinence • Greater attendance at medical appointments • More emotional responsivity to children • More stimulating home environment • Increased likelihood of using reliable form of birth control • Higher rates of having children live with mother • Decreased subsequent pregnancy or birth • Increase in permanent housing • Decrease in incarceration • Decreased likelihood of involvement in the CWS
Concrete Support and Assistance	Services such as child care, transportation, or the provision of counseling workers to facilitate entry into treatment.	• Increased attendance and completion of treatment • Greater abstinence • Increased likelihood of accessing treatment quickly • Fewer days in out-of-home placement among children with substance-abusing parents in the CWS
Short-term and Targeted Interventions	Psychoeducational groups, support groups, contingency management.	• Higher self-esteem • Greater treatment retention • Greater improvements in knowledge concerning assertiveness, communication skills and sexual health • More positive attitudes toward safe sex and being assertive • Greater attendance at prenatal health visits • Better birth outcomes • Lower health care costs
Comprehensive and Holistic Interventions	Combine several program elements into a comprehensive intervention.	• Decreased criminal activity • Decreased neglect of self or children • Decreased socioeconomic problems • Decreased likelihood of being taken advantage of • Decreased suicidality and psychological distress • Decreased out-of-home placements for children • High compliance rates with prenatal care • Good birth outcomes • High treatment retention rates • Greater abstinence • Greater family cohesion • Improved parenting skills • Increased likelihood of enrollment in vocational/education training • Reductions in physical health problems

without their children (Schinka, Hughes, Coletti, Hamilton, Renard, Urmann et al., 1999; Wexler, Cuadrado, & Stevens, 1998).

Health and Mental Health Care

There is some evidence to suggest that substance abuse treatment services that include health care services, especially prenatal care, as well

TABLE 1. Summary of Studies on Interventions for Parents in the Child Welfare System or Mothers and Women in General

Author	Type of Intervention	Location and Time Period	Type of Study	Sample Characteristics	CWS Involvement	Outcomes
Bander et al. (1983)	Outpatient program focusing on individual and group counseling	Hartford, CT, 1977-1979	Quasi-experimental (N=167)	Average age 40 yrs, 56% African American, 31% white, 7% American Indian, 6% Hispanic, 86% unmarried	Not reported	Increased abstinence & increased employment
Bartholomew et al. (1994)	A 6-week sexuality and assertiveness workshop for women	Corpus Christi, Dallas and Houston Texas 1991-1993	Quasi-experimental (N=81)	Average age 35 yrs, 26% Mexican-American, 50% White, 24% African American, 55% not married	Not reported	Higher self-esteem, greater retention in drug treatment
Berkowitz et al. (1998)	Outpatient treatment included comprehensive and holistic services	California 1993-1995	Quasi-experimental (N=460)	Average age 30.4 yrs, 53% White, 29% African American, 14% Hispanic, 2% Native American, 1% Asian	18% referred by CWS or criminal justice system	Decreases in: drug use, criminal activity, fights, neglect to self or children, homelessness, suicidal ideation, and OHP for children
Black et al. (1994)	An 18 month home visiting program	Not reported	Experimental (N=60)	Average age 26.4 yrs, 100% single, specific race/ethnicity information not provided. Sample described as "primarily African American."	Not reported	Increased abstinence and emotional responsiveness to children, higher compliance with medical appointments, and mothers provided more opportunities for stimulation
Carroll et al. (1995)	Targeted to methadone-maintained pregnant women, focused on health and mental health services	New Haven, CT, 1990-1992	Experimental (N=14)	Average age 27.6 yrs., 79% "non-minority," average number of children 1.4	Not reported	Greater number of prenatal visits, longer gestational periods, greater birth weights, no differences in drug use
Chang et al. (1992)	Targeted to methadone-maintained pregnant women, focused on health and mental health services	New Haven, Ct, time period not reported	Quasi-experimental (N=12)	Intervention group: average age 25.8yrs, 16% minority, 83% not married, average number of children 2.2	Not reported	Fewer positive urine toxicology screens, increased prenatal care, longer gestational periods, greater birth weights
Clark (2001)	Residential treatment for women and their children	Multiple sites across the nation, 24 sites participated in evaluation	Quasi-experimental (N=1,847)	Median age 29 years, 49% African American, 32% white, 9% Hispanic, 4% Asian, 4% American Indian/Alaska Native. At admission, 18% did not have custody of child	21% of sample referred by CWS	Better birth outcomes, increased abstinence and employment, women with children living with them had the highest completion rates and the longest stays in treatment
Conners et al. (2001)	Comprehensive and holistic residential treatment	Little Rock, Arkansas, time period not reported	Quasi-experimental (N=62)	Specific demographics not reported	Not reported	Increased abstinence, employment, improvement in parenting skills, poverty status, decreased arrests, improvements in family cohesion

Author	Type of Intervention	Location and Time Period	Type of Study	Sample Characteristics	CWS Involvement	Outcomes
Copeland et al. (1993)	Residential woman-centered treatment	Australia, 1989-1991	Quasi-experimental (N=160)	Intervention group: average age 30.3 yrs, race/ethnicity not reported, 61.3% not married, 53.8% with dependent children	Not reported	No effects found
Dahlgren & Willander (1989)	Woman-only outpatient alcohol treatment	Sweden, 1983-1986	Experimental (N=200)	Not reported	Not reported	Increased abstinence and employment
deZwart (1991)	Alcohol clinic for women only	The Netherlands, 1985	Quasi-experimental (N=44)	Mean age 37.7 yrs., 63% not married, 64% of women had children	Not reported	Increased abstinence
Dore & Doris (1998)	Targeted to CW involved parents, provided concrete support and assistance	Major metropolitan area in the Northeast	Quasi-experimental (N=119)	Average age 31.5 yrs, average of 3 children per home, 100% African American, 98% female, 77% single, never married	100% involved in CWS	Use of child care related to treatment completion. No relationship between treatment completion and child placement
Egelko et al. (1998)	A multisystems gender specific perinatal program	New York City, 1992-1995	Quasi-experimental (N=48)	Intervention group: average age 28.8 yrs, 78% African American, 22% Hispanic, 77% unmarried	Intervention group: 66% had an open CWS case.	Greater abstinence and greater treatment retention
Elk et al. (1998)	Contingency management intervention (CMI) that provided financial incentives for clean drug tests	Location not reported, 1994-1996	Experimental (N=12)	Intervention group: 50% African American, 83% not married	Not reported	Higher compliance with prenatal visits
Elk et al. (1997)	Multidisciplinary, comprehensive and holistic treatment	Houston TX, time period not reported	Quasi-experimental (N=70)	Average age 29 yrs., 54% African American, 37% White, 9% Hispanic, 77% not married	Not reported	High treatment retention rate, compliance with prenatal care and abstinence
Ernst et al. (1999)	Home visitation program	Seattle Washington, 1991-1995	Experimental (N=90)	Intervention group: average age 27.6 yrs, 77% single/separated/ divorced, 45% African American, 30% White, 17% Native American, 8% Other	Not reported	Increased abstinence, use of regular birth control, likelihood of living with child, decreased likelihood of pregnancy
Grant et al. (2003)	Home visitation program	Seattle WA, 1991-1995	Quasi-experimental (N=45)	Not reported	Not reported	Increased abstinence, regular use of family planning, employment, permanent housing, decrease in public assistance, incarceration and subsequent pregnancy
Grella (1999)	Woman-only residential treatment	Los Angeles CA, 1987-1994	Quasi-experimental (N=4,117)	Average age 29.7 yrs., 49.5% African American, 29.3% White, 16.9% Latino, 4.5% Other	Not reported	Greater treatment retention and completion
Author	Type of Intervention	Location and	Type of Study	Sample Characteristics	CWS	Outcomes

171

TABLE 1 (continued)

		Time Period			Involvement	
Hiller et al. (1996)	A 6-week sexuality and assertiveness workshop for women	Houston Texas, 1994	Experimental (N=21)	Intervention group: average age 33 yrs., 73% African American, 18% white, 9% Hispanic	Not reported	Improvements in assertiveness knowledge, communication skills, & sexual health, more positive attitudes toward safer sex
Hughes et al. (1995)	Residential treatment for women	Southeastern U.S., time period not reported	Experimental (N=53)	Intervention group: average age 27.8 yrs, 81% African American, 80% not married, average number of children 3.3	Intervention group 58% referred by CWS	Increased treatment retention
Killeen & Brady (2000)	Residential program for women and their children	Rural South Carolina. Time period not reported	Quasi-experimental (N=63)	Average age 31.5 yrs, 70% African American, 29% white, 1% Hispanic, 75% unmarried	Not reported	Improved parenting skills, child behaviors, & improved scores on an Addiction Severity Index
Knight et al. (1999)	Residential program for women and their children	Fort Worth, TX, 1996-2000	Quasi-experimental (N=41)	54% between 25-34 yrs, 51% African American, 42% white, 7% Hispanic, 71% not married, 88% had at least one child in treatment	20% had an open CWS case	73% of women stayed in treatment 90 days or longer
Laken & Ager (1996)	Concrete support and assistance within an outpatient program	Detroit Michigan, 1990-1992	Quasi-experimental (N=225)	Average age 29.6 yrs, 88.4% African American	Not reported	Retention in the outpatient program was related to receiving transportation to services
Marsh et al. (2000)	Concrete support and assistance for women involved in CWS	Chicago and Rockford, Illinois, 1995-1996	Quasi-experimental (N=148)	Average age 33 yrs, approximately 82% African American, average number of children 3.6	100% involved in CWS	Increased abstinence
McComish et al. (1999)	Weekly grief counseling group included as part of a residential program	Flint Michigan,1994-1996	Quasi-experimental (N=55)	Intervention group: average age 31 yrs, 83% African American, 97% single, average number of children in program with mother 2	Not reported	Increased treatment retention and self-esteem
Metsch et al. (2001)	Residential program for women with children	Key West Florida, 1996-1998	Quasi-experimental (N=36)	Average age 34 yrs, 22.5% were married, 65% Caucasian, 27.5% African American, 7.5% Hispanic	22.5% referred by CWS	Women in program with children had higher abstinence rates than those in program without children
Mullins et al. (2004)	Motivational interviewing	Midwestern city, time period not reported	Experimental (N=71)	Average age 27.1yrs, 73.2% single, never married, 47.9% Caucasian, 32.4% African American, 12.7% Native American, and 7.0% Hispanic	97% had open CWS case	No impact on treatment engagement and retention
O'Neill et al. (1996)	Six-session cognitive behavioral intervention for methadone-maintained pregnant women	Syndey, Australia, 1992-1993	Experimental (N=80)	Average age 26.2 yrs, all currently pregnant, 36% had one other child	Not reported	Reduction in high-risk injecting drug use behavior

Author	Type of Intervention	Location and Time Period	Type of Study	Sample Characteristics	CWS Involvement	Outcomes
Porowski et al. (2004)	Residential program for women and their children	32 sites across the nation. 1996-2001	Quasi-experimental (N=1,181)	Average age 30.3yrs, 40% African American, 32% white, 14% Hispanic. 88% not married/not living with spouse, 54% had three or more children	47% had child in OHP at some time	Increased abstinence, employment, and likelihood of living with children, decreased criminal activity, physical health problems, and likelihood of living with an AOD partner
Potocky & McDonald (1996)	Home visitation program	Midwestern metropolitan area, 1991-1993	Quasi-experimental (N=27)	Average age 26.8 yrs, 75% minority, 70% unmarried, average number of children 3.1	100% referred by CWS	The more services mothers used, the greater the improvement in their child's well-being. 70% of children remained with parents
Roberts & Nishimoto (1996)	An intensive day treatment that was women focused and included concrete support and assistance	Location not reported, 1995	Quasi-experimental (N=369)	33.3% between 31-35 yrs, 94% African American, 3.5% Hispanic, 87% not married	Not reported	Increased treatment retention and completion
Rosett et al. (1980)	Woman-only outpatient treatment program for pregnant women	Boston, MA, 1974-1977	Quasi-experimental (N=138)	Average age 26.2 yrs, 57% African American, 39% White, 4% American Indian, 49.5% living alone	Not reported	Better birth outcomes among women who stopped using alcohol in the third trimester
Saunders (1993)	Residential program for women and their children	Des Moines, Iowa, 1990-1992	Quasi-experimental (N=70)	Average age 28.5 yrs, 73% white, 18% African American, 6.3% Native American, 1% Hispanic. Marital status not reported	32% involved with CWS	Increased abstinence, decreased psychological distress, improved parenting skills
Schinka et al. (1999)	Residential program for women and their children	Florida, 1990-1992	Experimental (N=46)	Average age 27.3 yrs, 81% African American, 69.8% had never been married, average number of children 3.2	57% referred by CWS	Improvements in psychopathology
Schuler et al. (2000)	Home visitation program	Not reported	Experimental (N=171)	Not reported	Not reported	Decreased likelihood of CWS involvement
Smith & Marsh (2002)	Matching substance-abusing women with specific treatment services	Illinois, time period not reported	Quasi-experimental (N=183)	Average age 33 yrs, 83% African American, 11% white, 2% Hispanic	100% had some contact with the CWS	The more services women received, the better the outcomes
Sowers et al. (2002)	A transitional housing program providing comprehensive and holistic interventions	Broward County, Florida, time period not reported.	Quasi-experimental (N=41)	Intervention group: average age 29.5 yrs, 65.4% white, 15.4% African American, 7.7% Hispanic, 3.8% American Indian	Not reported	Decreased likelihood of arrest, increased employment, improvements in overall functioning
Stevens & Arbiter (1995)	Residential treatment for women with children	Tucson, AZ, 1994	Quasi-experimental (N=114)	Average age 28 yrs, 44% white, 25% African American, 22% Hispanic, 9% Native American, 82% not married	33% involved with CWS	At follow-up, the majority of women were employed and had custody of children

TABLE 1 (continued)

Author	Type of Intervention	Location and Time Period	Type of Study	Sample Characteristics	CWS Involvement	Outcomes
Stevens et al. (1989)	Residential treatment for women with children	Tucson AZ, 1981-1985	Quasi-experimental, sample size not reported	Not reported	Not reported	Increased length of stay
Strantz & Welch (1995)	Woman-centered day treatment program	Location not reported, Discharge date 1995	Experimental (N=292)	Average age 30.5 years, specific race/ethnicity not reported, sample described as a "large majority" African American, 69.9% never married, median number of children was 3	82.7% referred by CWS	Increased treatment retention, having custody of child predicted treatment retention
Svikis et al. (1998)	Weekly substance abuse support group	Baltimore, MD, 1989-1990	Quasi-experimental (N=121)	Intervention group: average age 24.9 yrs, 84% African American, 79% not married	Not reported	Increased attendance at prenatal visits, greater birth weights, higher Apgar scores, lower health care costs
Sweeney et al. (2000)	Outpatient program that included maternal and child health care	Providence RI, time period not reported	Quasi-experimental (N=174)	Average age 26.9 yrs., 54% white, 33% African American, 68% had other children. Postpartum group: Mean age 27.6 yrs., 51% white, 39% African American, 87% had other children	Not reported	Women who enrolled during pregnancy had better birth outcomes
Testa et al. (2003)	"Recovery Coaches" to assist CWS-involved parents in participating in substance abuse treatment	Cook County Illinois, 2000-2002	Experimental (N=532)	Intervention group: average age 33 yrs, 73% women, 80% African American, 4% African American, 73% women, 84% African American, 6% Hispanic. Control group: average age 33 yrs,	100% involved in the CWS	Increased likelihood of accessing treatment and obtaining treatment more quickly, children in intervention group experienced less time in placement
Volpicelli et al. (2000)	A psychosocially enhanced treatment program	Not reported	Experimental (N=84)	Intervention group: average age 31.6 yrs, 97.6% African American, 2.4% Hispanic, average number of children 3.83	Not reported	Increased abstinence and treatment retention
Wexler et al. (1998)	Residential program for women and their children	Tucson AZ, 1992-1993	Quasi-experimental (N=83)	Average age 28.3 yrs, 59% white, 22% African American, 13% Hispanic, 6% Native American, 76% not married	Not reported	Increased employment and abstinence, decreased criminality, depression, and psychopathology
Whiteside-Mansell et al. (1998)	Residential program that included comprehensive and holistic interventions	Little Rock, Arkansas, time period not reported	Quasi-experimental (N=95)	Average age 28.8 yrs, 75% African American, 60.9% never married	31.4% involved in CWS	Increased abstinence, decreased likelihood of premature labor and maternal infection
Wobie et al. (1997)	Residential treatment center for women and their children	Orlando, FL, 1993-1996	Quasi-experimental (N=172)	Average age 27.3 yrs., 62% African American, 25% White, 13% Hispanic	Not reported	Women with children residing with them had greater treatment completion, less depression and higher self-esteem

as mental health services may improve outcomes for women and their children. Six studies were identified that examined specific health or mental health substance abuse treatment services. Overall, the research suggests that health interventions, particularly those aimed at prenatal care for pregnant substance-abusing women are associated with longer gestational periods and better birth outcomes (Carroll, Chang, Behr, Clinton & Kosten, 1995; Chang, Carroll, Behr & Kosten, 1992; Sweeney, Schwartz, & Mattis, 2000).

Mental health interventions may also improve outcomes. Research suggests that substance abuse treatment that includes specialized mental health interventions such as individual therapy or specialized group therapy is associated with increased treatment retention (Volpicelli, Markman, Monterosso, Filing, & O'Brien, 2000), greater sobriety (Bander, Stilwell, Fein, & Bishop, 1983; Volpicelli et al., 2000), greater likelihood of employment (Bander et al., 1983), and a reduction in high-risk injecting drug use behavior (O'Neill, Baker, Cooke, Collins, Heather, & Wodak, 1996).

Home Visitation

Other studies suggest that home visitation programs may improve outcomes for substance-abusing mothers. Five studies were identified that evaluated home visitation services for substance-abusing mothers. These interventions typically include home visits by a nurse or a paraprofessional that focus on providing maternal support, promoting healthy parent-child interactions, and providing information and linkages to concrete resources. Overall, research suggests that home visitation programs are associated with greater sobriety (Black, Nair, Kight, Wachtel, Roby, & Schuler, 1994; Ernst, Grant, Streissguth, & Sampson, 1999; Grant, Ernst, Pagalilauan, & Streissguth, 2003), greater attendance at medical appointments, more emotional responsivity to children, a more stimulating home environment (Blair et al., 1994), increased likelihood of using a reliable method of birth control (Ernst et al., 1999), higher rates of having children living with their mother (Ernst et al., 1999; Potocky & McDonald, 1996), decreased subsequent pregnancy or birth, increase in permanent housing, decrease in incarceration (Grant et al., 2003) and a decreased likelihood of involvement in the child welfare system (Schuler, Nair, Black, & Kettinger, 2000).

Concrete Support and Assistance

Some studies have evaluated the effectiveness of interventions that provide concrete support and assistance, such as transportation, child care or the provision of counselors to facilitate entry into treatment. Five studies were identified that evaluated the use of concrete supports and assistance in substance abuse treatment for women. Overall, research suggests that certain supports are associated with improved outcomes, specifically transportation to services is associated with increased treatment attendance (Laken & Ager, 1996) and child care is associated with increased treatment retention and completion (Dore & Doris, 1998; Roberts & Nishimoto, 1996). A combination of supports including transportation, outreach, and child care services has been linked to greater abstinence (Marsh, D'Aunno & Smith, 2000). The use of "Recovery Coaches" to assist parents in the child welfare system in obtaining and participating in substance abuse treatment as well as providing assistance in understanding and negotiating child welfare and court requirements is linked with increased access to treatment, quicker entry into treatment and fewer days in out-of-home placement among children (Testa, Ryan, Louderman, Sullivan, Gillespie, Gianforte et al., 2003).

Short-Term and Targeted Interventions

Some research has focused on the use of short-term and targeted interventions, such as psychoeducational groups, motivational interviewing and contingency management interventions, on outcomes for women in substance abuse treatment. Six studies were identified that investigated short-term and targeted interventions. Research suggests that the use of psychoeducational groups is associated with higher self-esteem (Bartholomew, Rowan-Szal, Chatham, & Simpson, 1994; Hiller, Rowan-Szal, Bartholomew, & Simpson, 1996), greater treatment retention (Bartholomew et al., 1994), greater improvements in knowledge concerning assertiveness, communication skills and sexual health, and more positive attitudes toward safe sex and being assertive (Hiller et al., 1996). Another study on the effects of a grief counseling group found that participation in the group was associated with increased treatment retention and self-esteem (McComish, Greenberg, Kent-Bryant, Chruscial, Ager, Hines et al., 1999). The use of support groups is linked to greater attendance at prenatal visits, better birth outcomes and lower health care costs (Svikis, McCaul, Feng, Stuart, Fox, & Stokes 1998). The use of contingency management interventions (in which incentives are provided for abstinence) is associated with higher compliance with prenatal medical visits. The use of motivational interviewing, a short-term intervention described as client-centered and directed toward decreasing clients' ambivalence about stopping their substance abuse and increasing their motivation for change has been found to be unrelated to treatment retention or completion among substance-abusing women in the child welfare system (Mullins, Suarez, Ondersma, & Page, 2004).

Comprehensive and Holistic Interventions

In addition to the program components noted above, there is also evidence that comprehensive and holistic interventions that combine several of these program elements may be effective with substance-abusing mothers. Ten studies were identified that focus on comprehensive and holistic interventions. Overall, research suggests that the more services substance-abusing women receive, the better the outcomes (Smith & Marsh, 2002). Comprehensive and holistic interventions that combine a variety of services have been linked to decreased criminal activity (Berkowitz, Brindis, & Peterson, 1998; Conners, Bradley, Whiteside-Mansell, & Crone, 2001; Porowski, Burgdorf, & Herrell, 2004; Sowers, Ellis, Washington & Currant, 2002), decreased neglect of self or children, decreased homelessness, decreased likelihood of being taken advantage of, decreased suicidality, decreased out-of-home placement of children (Berkowitz et al., 1998), high compliance rates with prenatal care (Elk, Mangus, LaSoya, Rhoades, Andres, & Grabowski, 1997), good birth outcomes (Elk et al., 1997; Whiteside-Mansell et al., 1998), high treatment retention rates (Elk et al., 1997; Knight et al., 1999), greater abstinence (Conners, Bradley, Saunders, 1993; Whiteside-Mansell, & Crone, 2001; Whiteside et al., 1998), decreased poverty, greater family cohesion (Conners et al., 2001), improved parenting skills (Conners et al., 2001; Killeen & Brady, 2000; Saunders, 1993), increased likelihood of employment (Porowski et al., 2004; Sowers et al., 2002), increased likelihood of enrollment in vocational/educational training, reductions in physical health problems, increased likelihood of living with at least one child (Porowski et al., 2004), and decreases in psychological distress (Saunders, 1993).

Studies Addressing Child Welfare Outcomes

Very few studies identified in this review reported on outcomes related to child welfare system involvement. It is therefore not possible to draw conclusions about which interventions are most effective with substance-abusing parents in the child welfare system. Overall, nine studies were identified that either contained samples exclusively of child welfare parents or included some outcome data related to child welfare outcomes (such as whether children resided with parents after treatment). Figure 2 provides a summary of these program components and the related child welfare outcomes. Three studies assessed home visitation services, three studies assessed concrete support and assistance, two studies assessed comprehensive programs and one study assessed woman-centered treatment. It should be noted that it is possible that other interventions are equally or more effective with substance-abusing parents in the child welfare system, but outcomes related to involvement in the child welfare system have not been assessed.

System-Level Collaborative Approaches Between the CWS and the AOD System

Literature related to system-level collaborative approaches between the child welfare system (CWS) and alcohol and other drug system (AOD) was synthesized to identify core components of promising collaborative models. These core components include: (1) Outstationing AOD workers in child welfare offices, (2) Creating joint case plans between AOD and CWS, (3) Using official committees to guide collaborative efforts, (4) Training and cross-training, (5) Establishing protocols for sharing confidential information, and (6) Using dependency drug courts. Figure 3 provides a summary of the core components of promising collaborative models between the CWS and the AOD system.

Outstationing AOD Workers in Child Welfare Offices

Several collaborative models have placed AOD specialists within child welfare offices to ensure that parents are assessed as quickly as possible, to improve client engagement and retention in treatment, to streamline entry into treatment and to provide consultation to child welfare workers. In general, outstationed AOD workers typically assist child welfare workers in assessing parents, provide treatment referral, engage parents in substance abuse treatment and provide consultation to child welfare workers. The general goal behind outstationing AOD workers in child welfare offices is to provide parents with a smooth entry into the AOD system (McAlpine, Marshall & Doran, 2001; Semidei, Radel, & Nolan, 2001; Young & Gardner, 2002).

FIGURE 2. Summary of Interventions with Child Welfare Outcome Data

Component	Child Welfare Related Outcomes
Home Visitation	• Increased likelihood of maintaining custody of child • Decreased involvement in the child welfare system
Concrete Support and Assistance	• Increased likelihood of accessing treatment • Increased likelihood of timely access to treatment • Children experience fewer days in out-of-home placement
Comprehensive and Holistic Interventions	• Reductions in out-of-home placement
Woman-Centered Treatment	• Increased likelihood of maintaining custody of child

FIGURE 3. Collaborative Model Components

Component	Description and Rationale
Outstationing Alcohol and other Drug Workers in Child Welfare Offices	Placing AOD workers in child welfare offices may help ensure that parents are assessed quickly, improve client engagement and retention in treatment, streamline entry into treatment, and provide CWS workers with consultation on cases involving parental substance abuse.
Joint Case Planning	Joint case plans that are created and monitored by workers in both systems may help reduce conflicting case goals and improve treatment planning.
Official Committees to Guide Collaborative Efforts	Specially appointed committees or task forces that guide collaborative efforts can provide structure and oversight to collaboration and ensure input from both systems.
Training and Cross-Training	Training for CWS workers on substance abuse issues and training AOD workers on child welfare issues can improve understanding of the issues facing both systems.
Protocols for Sharing Confidential Information	Protocols include release of information forms that specify the types of information that can be shared. These protocols can help ensure that clients are fully assessed, that desired outcomes are consistent between the two systems and that resources are used efficiently to prevent duplication of services.
Dependency Drug Courts	Dependency drug courts usually provide judges with the primary role of monitoring the behaviors of parents and implementing rewards and sanctions based on treatment progress. Dependency drug courts may help ensure effective coordination between the CWS, AOD system and the courts so that parents have timely access to treatment, as well as the timely completion of reunification or permanency plans.

Joint Case Planning

The collaboration between the CWS and the AOD system can also be structured through the use of case plans that are jointly created and monitored by both systems (and other systems when appropriate). In general, joint case planning includes the creation of a family-focused case plan that includes input from all involved agencies, including AOD, CWS, the court, and others when appropriate. The case plan is then jointly implemented by the systems involved (Harrell & Goodman, 1999; Young & Gardner, 2002). The process of including input from representatives of the AOD system in case planning is described by Young and Gardner (2002) as a major breakthrough in enhancing effective relations between AOD and CWS services.

Official Committees to Guide Collaborative Efforts

Most collaborative models use specially appointed committees or task forces to guide collaborative efforts. These committees help to establish a closer relationship between AOD and CWS representatives, they ensure input from both systems, and can provide structure and oversight to the collaboration efforts (Young & Gardner, 2002; Semidei et al., 2001).

Training and Cross-Training

Training and cross-training between systems are core elements of most promising collaborative models. Elements involved in training include substance abuse training for all new child welfare workers and in-service training for current workers, as well as the creation of training curriculums developed by both CWS and AOD workers. Trainings often include AOD information for child welfare workers that focuses on basic information related to substance abuse and use, assessment tools, methods to engage clients and how to access treatment, as well as CWS information for AOD workers including an overview of child welfare policies and mandates and the types of services offered to families (McAlpine et al., 2001; Young & Gardner, 2002).

Protocols for Sharing Confidential Information

Most collaborative models identified in this search have established protocols for sharing confidential information between the CWS and

AOD systems. These protocols include release of information forms that specify the types of information that can be shared; clients then must give their written consent on the release of information forms in order for the two systems to share information. Many collaborative models have integrated these protocols into daily practice in order to streamline the sharing of information about client progress (Young & Gardner, 2002).

Dependency Drug Courts

The use of dependency drug courts also represents a collaborative model that is being used in a number of localities. In general, the use of dependency drug courts by the child welfare system is aimed at ensuring effective coordination between the CWS, AOD systems and the courts so that parents have timely access to treatment, as well as the timely completion of reunification or permanency plans (Harrell & Goodman, 1999; Young & Gardner, 2002). Dependency drug courts usually provide judges with the primary role of monitoring the behavior of parents and implementing rewards and sanctions based on treatment progress (Harrell & Goodman, 1999; Young & Gardner, 2002).

CONCLUSION AND IMPLICATIONS

The growing number of substance-abusing parents who come to the attention of the child welfare system has created an urgent need to understand the types of interventions that are most effective with this population. This review of the literature focused on evidence related to individual-level interventions for parents involved in the CWS and mothers and women in general, as well as descriptive information on system-level collaborative approaches between the CWS and the AOD system. At the individual level, experimental and quasi-experimental research suggests the following program components are associated with a variety of positive outcomes: (1) Women-centered treatment that involves children, (2) Specialized health and mental health services, (3) Home visitation services, (4) Concrete assistance (e.g., transportation, child care, assistance linking with substance abuse treatment), (5) Short-term targeted interventions, and (6) Comprehensive programs that integrate many of these components. Although the research on individual-level interventions identified in this review points to the potential effectiveness of these program components, more research using experimental designs is needed to establish effectiveness. In addition, more research is needed to test the effectiveness of individual-level interventions specifically for parents in the child welfare system. Most studies identified in this review did not report on child welfare system involvement, and only nine of the studies in this review reported on outcomes related to the child welfare system.

In addition to individual-level interventions, this review identified key components of promising system-level collaborative approaches between the CWS and the AOD system. Descriptive information suggests that many collaborative models between the CWS and the AOD system contain the following core elements: (1) Outstationing AOD workers in child welfare offices, (2) Joint case planning, (3) Using official committees to guide collaborative efforts, (4) Training and cross-training, (5) Using protocols for sharing confidential information, and (6) Using dependency drug courts. These components may improve communication, coordination and collaboration between the CWS and AOD systems, however, empirical information on the association between these collaborative components and treatment outcomes for parents involved in the CWS is lacking. More information is needed to link the use of collaborative practice approaches between the CWS and the AOD system to certain critical outcomes for substance abusing parents in the CWS, such as access to treatment, treatment participation and retention, and overall treatment success.

Although more empirical research is needed on the interventions identified in this review, it is clear that addressing the problem of substance abuse among parents involved in the child welfare system will likely require a multifaceted approach that integrates the best available individual-level interventions with system-level collaborative approaches. This review has synthesized the available evidence on a number of potentially useful interventions. County agencies may benefit from identifying areas of need in their own localities and choosing from among the various interventions identified in this review. In light of such a limited amount of research, evaluations of these local efforts would help to assess their effectiveness. Ultimately, an approach that integrates individual-level interventions and system-level approaches, along with careful follow-up evaluations, may shed even more light on the types of interventions that are most effective with this vulnerable population.

REFERENCES

Abbott, A. A. (1994). A feminist approach to substance abuse treatment and service delivery. *Social Work and Health Care, 19*(3-4), 67-93.

Ashley, O. S., Marsden, M. E., & Brady, T. M. (2003). Effectiveness of substance abuse treatment programming for women: A review. *The American Journal of Drug and Alcohol Abuse, 29*(1), 19-53.

Baker, P. L., & Carson, A. (1999). "I take care of my kids." Mothering practices of substance-abusing women. *Gender and Society, 13*(3), 347-363.

Bander, K. W., Stilwell, N. A., Fein, E., & Bishop, G. (1983). Relationship of patient characteristics to program attendance by women alcoholics. *Journal of Studies on Alcohol, 44*(2), 318-327.

Bartholomew, N. G., Rowan-Szal, G. A., Chatham, L. R., & Simpson, D. D. (1994). Effectiveness of a specialized intervention for women in a methadone program. *Journal of Psychoactive Drugs, 26*(3), 249-255.

Bauman, P. S., & Levine, S. A. (1986). The development of children of drug addicts. *The International Journal of the Addictions, 21*(8), 849-863.

Bellis, M. D., Broussard, E. R., Herring, D. J., Wexler, S., Moritz, G., & Benitez, J. G. (2001). Psychiatric co-morbidity in caregivers and children involved in maltreatment: A pilot research study with policy implications. *Child Abuse & Neglect 25,* 923-944.

Berkowitz, G., Brindis, C., & Peterson, S. (1998). Substance use and social outcomes among participants in perinatal alcohol and drug treatment. *Women's Health: Research on Gender, Behavior and Policy, 4*(3), 231-254.

Black, M. M., Nair, P., Kight, C., Wachtel, R., Roby, P., & Schuler, M. (1994). Parenting and early development among children on drug-abusing women: Effects of home intervention. *Pediatrics, 94*(4), 440-448.

Burns, K., Chethik, L, Burns, W. J., & Clark, R. (1991). Dyadic disturbances in cocaine-abusing mothers and their infants. *Journal of Clinical Psychology, 47*(2), 316-319.

Carroll, K. M., Change, G., Behr, H., Clinton, B., & Kosten, T. R. (1995). Improving treatment outcome in pregnant methadone-maintained women: Results from a randomized controlled trial. *The American Journal on Addictions, 4*(1), 56-59.

Chaffin, M., Kelleher, K., & Hollenberg, J. (1996). Onset of physical abuse and neglect: Psychiatric, substance abuse, and social risk factors from prospective community data. *Child Abuse and Neglect, 20*(3), 191-203.

Chang, G., Carroll, K. M., Behr, H. M., & Kosten, T. R., (1992). Improving treatment outcome in pregnant opiate-dependent women. *Journal of Substance Abuse Treatment, 9,* 327-330.

Chavkin, W., Paone, D., Friedman, P., & Wilets, I. (1993). Reframing the debate: Toward effective treatment for inner city drug-abusing mothers. *Bulletin of the New York Academy of Medicine, 70,* 50-68.

Clark, H. W. (2001). Residential substance abuse treatment for pregnant and postpartum women and their children: Treatment and policy implications. *Child Welfare, 80*(2), 179-198.

Conners, N.A., Bradley, R. H., Whiteside Mansell, L., Liu, J. Y., Roberts, T. J., Burgdorf, K., & Herrell, J. M. (2004). Children of mothers with serious substance abuse problems: An accumulation of risks. *The American Journal of Drug and Alcohol Abuse, 30*(1), 85-100.

Conners, N. A., Bradley, R. H., Whiteside-Mansell, L., & Crone, C. C. (2001). A comprehensive substance abuse treatment program for women and their children: An initial evaluation. *Journal of Substance Abuse Treatment 21*, 67-75.

Copeland, J., Hall, W., Didcott, P., Biggs, V. (1993). A comparison of a specialist women's alcohol and other drug treatment service with two traditional mixed sex services: Client characteristics and treatment outcome. *Drug and Alcohol Dependence, 32*, 81-92.

deZwart, W. (1991). Treatment of women alcoholics, clinical and epidemiological data. *Alcoholism, 27*(1-2), 17-31.

Dore, M., & Doris, J. M. (1998). Preventing child placement in substance-abusing families: Research informed practice. *Child Welfare 77*(4), 407-426.

Egelko, S., Galanter, M., Dermatis, H., DeMaio, C. (1998). Evaluation of a multisystems model for treating perinatal cocaine addiction. *Journal of Substance Abuse Treatment, 15*(3), 251-259.

El-Bassel, N., Gilbert, L., Schilling, R. & Wada, T. (2000). Drug abuse and partner violence among women in methadone treatment. *Journal of Family Violence, 15*(3), 209-228.

Elk, R., Mangus, L., Rhoades, H., Andres, R., & Grabowski, J. (1998). Cessation of cocaine use during pregnancy: Effects of contingency management interventions on maintaining abstinence and complying with prenatal care. *Addictive Behaviors, 23*(1), 57-64.

Elk, R., Mangus, L. G., LaSoya, R. J., Rhoades, H. M., Andres, R. L., & Grabowski, J. (1997). Behavioral interventions: Effective and adaptable for the treatment of pregnant cocaine-dependent women. *Journal of Drug Issues, 27*(3), 625-658.

Ernst, C. C., Grant, T., Streissguth, A. P., & Sampson, P. D. (1999). Intervention with high-risk alcohol and drug-abusing mothers: II Three-year findings from the Seattle Model of Paraprofessional Advocacy. *Journal of Community Psychology, 27*(1), 19-38.

Famularo, F., Kinscherff, R., & Fenton, T. (1992). Parental substance abuse and the nature of child maltreatment. *Child Abuse and Neglect, 16*, 475-483.

Feig, L. (1998). Understanding the problem: The gap between substance abuse programs and child welfare services. In R. L. Hampton, V. Senatore, & T. P. Gullotta (Eds.). *Substance abuse, family violence, and child welfare: Bridging perspectives* (pgs. 62-95). Thousand Oaks CA: Sage.

Grant, T., Ernst, C. C., Pagalilauan, G., & Streissguth, A. (2003). Post-program follow-up effects of paraprofessional intervention with high-risk women who abused alcohol and drugs during pregnancy. *Journal of Community Psychology, 31*(3), 211-222.

Grella, C. E. (1999). Women in residential drug treatment: Differences by program type and pregnancy. *Journal of Health Care for the Poor and Underserved, 10*(2), 216-229.

Grella, C. E. (1997). Services for perinatal women with substance abuse and mental health disorders: The unmet need. *Journal of Psychoactive Drugs, 29*(1), 67-78.

Harrell, A., & Goodman, A. (1999). *Review of specialized family drug courts: Key issues in handling child abuse and neglect cases.* Washington DC: Urban Institute.

Hien, D., & Honeyman, T. (2000). A closer look at the drug-abuse maternal aggression link. *Journal of Interpersonal Violence, 15*(5), 503-522.

Hiller, M. L., Rowan-Szal, G. A., Bartholomew, N. G., & Simpson, D. D. (1996). Effectiveness of a specialized women's intervention in a residential treatment program. *Substance Use and Misuse, 31*(6), 771-783.

Hohman, M. M., Shillington, A. M., & Grigg Baxter, H. (2003). A comparison of pregnant women presenting for alcohol and other drug treatment by CPS status. *Child Abuse and Neglect, 27*, 303-317.

Hughes, P. H. Coletti, S. D., Neri, R. L., Urmann, C. F., Stahl, S., Sicilian, D. M., Anthony, J. C. (1995). Retaining cocaine-abusing women in a therapeutic community: The effect of a child live-in program. *American Journal of Public Health, 85*(8), 1149-1152.

Hunter, T. N. (2003). Child welfare and alcohol and other drug treatment (AOD): Bridging the gap to comprehensive services. *Journal of Family Social Work, 7*(4), 63-73.

Kearney, M. H., Murphy, S., & Rosenbaum, M. (1994). Mothering on crack cocaine: A grounded theory analysis. *Social Science and Medicine, 38*(2), 351-361.

Kelleher, K., Chaffin, M., Hollenberg, J., & Fischer, E. (1984). Alcohol and drug disorders among physically abusive and neglectful parents in a community-based sample. *American Journal of Public Health, 84*(10), 1586-1590.

Kelley, S. J. (1998). Stress and coping behaviors of substance-abusing mothers. *Journal of the Society of Pediatric Nurses, 3*(1) 103-111.

Killeen, T., & Brady, K. T. (2000). Parental stress and child behavioral outcomes following substance abuse residential treatment: Follow-up at 6 and 12 months. *Journal of Substance Abuse Treatment, 19*, 23-29.

Klein, D., Crim, D., & Zahnd, E. (1997). Perspectives of pregnant substance-using women: Findings from the California Perinatal Needs Assessment. *Journal of Psychoactive Drugs, 29*(1), 55-66.

Knight, D. K., Hood, P. E., Logan, S. M., & Chatham, L. R. (1999). Residential treatment for women with dependent children: One agency's approach. *Journal of Psychoactive Drugs, 31*(4), 339-351.

Ladwig, G. B., & Andersen, M. D. (1989). Substance abuse in women: Relationship between chemical dependency of women and past reports of physical and/or sexual abuse. *The International Journal of the Addictions, 24*(8), 739-754.

Laken, M. P., & Ager, J. W. (1996). Effects of case management on retention in prenatal substance abuse treatment. *American Journal of Drug and Alcohol Abuse, 22*(3), 439-449.

Marsh, J. C., D'Aunno, T. A., & Smith, B. D. (2000). Increasing access and providing social services to improve drug abuse treatment for women with children. *Addiction 95*(8), 1237-1247.

McAlpine, C., Marshall, C. C., Harper Doran, N. (2001). Combining child welfare and substance abuse services: A blended model of intervention. *Child Welfare, 80*(2), 129-149.

McComish, J. F., Greenberg, R., Kent-Bryant, J., Chruscial, H. L., Ager, J., Hines, F., & Ransom, S. B. (1999). Evaluation of a grief group for women in residential substance abuse treatment. *Substance Abuse, 20*(1), 45-58.

McMahon, T. J., & Luthar, S. S. (1998). Bridging the gap for children as their parents enter substance abuse treatment. In R. L. Hampton, V. Senatore, & T. P. Gullotta (Eds.). *Substance abuse, family violence, and child welfare: Bridging perspectives* (pgs. 143-187). Thousand Oaks CA: Sage.

McNichol, T., & Tash, C. (2001). Parental substance abuse and the development of children in family foster care. *Child Welfare, 80*(2), 239-256.

Merikangas, K. R., Stolar, M., Stevens, D. E., Goulet, J., Preisig, M. A., Fenston, B., Zhang, H., O'Malley, S. S., & Rounsaville, B. J. (1998). Familial transmission of substance use disorders. *Archives of General Psychiatry, 55*, 973-979.

Metsch, L. R., Wolfe, H. P., Fewell, R., McCoy, C. B., Elwood, W. N., Wohler-Torres, B., Petersen-Baston, P., Haskins, H. V. (2001). Treating substance-using women and their children in public housing: Preliminary evaluation findings. *Child Welfare, 80*(2), 199-220.

Miller, B. A., Downs, W. R., & Gondoli, D. M. (1989). Spousal violence among alcoholic women as compared to a random household sample of women. *Journal of Studies on Alcohol, 30*(6), 533-540.

Miller, B. A., Downs, W. R., Gondoli, D. M., & Keil, A. (1987). The role of childhood sexual abuse in the development of alcoholism in women. *Violence and Victims, 2*(3), 157-171.

Miller, B. A., Smyth, N. J., & Mudar, P. J. (1997). Mothers' alcohol and other drug problems and their punitiveness toward their children. *Journal of Studies on Alcohol*, 632-642.

Mullins, S. M., Suarez, M., Ondersma, S. J., Page, M. C. (2004). The impact of motivational interviewing on substance abuse treatment retention: A randomized control trial; of women involved with child welfare. *Journal of Substance Abuse Treatment, 27*, 51-58.

Murphy, J. M., Jellinek, M., Quinn, D., Smith, G., Poitrast, F. G., & Goshko, M. (1991). Substance abuse and serious child mistreatment: Prevalence, risk and outcome in a court sample. *Child Abuse and Neglect, 15*, 197-211.

O'Neill, K., Baker, A., Cooke, M., Collins, E., Heather, N., & Wodak, A. (1996). Evaluation of a cognitive-behavioral intervention for pregnant injecting drug users at risk of HIV infection. *Addiction, 91*(8), 1115-1125.

Porowski, A. W., & Burgdorf, & Herrell, J. M. (2004). Effectiveness and sustainability of residential substance abuse treatment programs for pregnant and parenting women. *Evaluation and Program Planning, 27*, 191-198.

Potocky, M., & McDonald, T. P. (1996). Evaluating the effectiveness of family preservation services for the families of drug-exposed infants: A pilot study. *Research on Social Work Practice, 6*(4), 524-535.

Reed, B. G. (1987). Developing women-sensitive drug dependence treatment services: Why so difficult? *Journal of Psychoactive Drugs, 19*(2), 151-164.

Roberts, A. C., Nishimoto, R. H. (1996). Predicting treatment retention of women dependent on cocaine. *American Journal of Drug and Alcohol Abuse, 22*(3), 313-334.

Rosett, H. L., Weiner, L., Zuckerman, B., McKinlay, S., & Edelin, K. C. (1980). Reduction of alcohol consumption during pregnancy with benefits to the newborn. *Alcoholism: Clinical and Experimental Research, 4*(2), 178-184.

Saunders, E. J. (1993). A new model of residential care for substance-abusing women and their children. *Adult Residential Care Journal, 7*(2), 104-117.

Schinka, J. A., Hughes, P. H., Coletti, S. D., Hamilton, N. L., Renard, C. G., Urmann, C. F., & Neri, R. L. (1999). Changes in personality characteristics in women treated in a therapeutic community. *Journal of Substance Abuse Treatment, 16*(2), 137-142.

Schuler, M. E., Nair, P., Black, M. M., & Kettinger, L. (2000). Mother-infant interaction: Effects of a home intervention and ongoing maternal drug use. *Journal of Clinical Child Psychology, 29*(3), 424-431.

Semidei, J., Radel, L. F., & Nolan, C, (2001). Substance abuse and child welfare: Clear linkages and promising responses. *Child Welfare, 80*(2), 109-127.

Shillington, A. M., Hohman, M., & Jones, L. (2001). Women in substance abuse treatment: Are those involved in the child welfare system different? *Journal of Social Work Practice in the Addictions, 1*(4), 25-46.

Smith, B. D. (2003). How parental drug use and drug treatment compliance relate to family reunification. *Child Welfare, 82*(3), 335-365.

Smith, B. D., & Marsh, J. C. (2002). Client-service matching in substance abuse treatment for women with children. *Journal of Substance Abuse Treatment, 22,* 161-168.

Stevens, S. J. & Arbiter, N. (1995). A therapeutic community for substance-abusing pregnant women and women with children: Process and outcome. *Journal of Psychoactive Drugs, 27*(1), 49-56.

Stevens, S., Arbiter, N., & Glider, P. (1989). Women residents: Expanding their role to increase treatment effectiveness. *The International Journal of the Addictions, 24*(5), 425-434.

Stranz, I. H., & Welch, S. P. (1995). Postpartum women in outpatient drug abuse treatment: Correlated of retention/completion. *Journal of Psychoactive drugs, 27*(4), 357-373.

Sowers, K. M., Ellis, R. A., Washington, T. A., & Currant, M. (2002). Optimizing treatment effects for substance-abusing women with children: An evaluation of the Susan B. Anthony Center. *Research on Social Work Practice, 12*(1), 143-158.

Substance Abuse and Mental Health Administration (1996) *Results from the 1996 National Household Survey on Drug Abuse.* Online, retrieved July 8, 2005 from: http://oas.samhsa.gov/nhsda/PE1996/HTTOC.htm.

Substance Abuse and Mental Health Administration (1997). *Substance use among women in the United States.* Rockville MD: Author.

Substance Abuse and Mental Health Administration (2003). *Results from the 2003 National Survey on Drug Use and Health: National Findings.* Online, retrieved July 8, 2005 from: http://www.oas.samhsa.gov/nhsda/2k3nsduh/2k3Results.htm#ch3

Svikis, D., McCaul, M., Feng, T., Stuart, M., Fox, M., & Stokes, E. (1998). Drug dependence during pregnancy: Effect of an on-site support group. *Journal of Reproductive Health, 43,* 799-805.

Sweeney, P. J., Schwartz, R. M., & Mattis, N. G. (2000). The effect of integrating substance abuse treatment with prenatal care on birth outcome. *Journal of Perinatology, 4,* 219-224.

Testa, M. F., Ryan, J. P., Louderman, D., Sullivan, J. A., Gillespie, S., Gianforte, R., Preuter, J., & Quasius, D. (2003). *Illinois AODA IV-E Waiver Demonstration: Interim evaluation report.* Online, retrieved July 5, 2005 from: http://cfrcwww.social. uiuc.edu/pubreports/MainPubs.htm

United States General Accounting Office (1998). *Foster Care: Agencies face challenges securing stable homes for children of substance abusers.* HEHS-98-182. Washington, D.C.: Government Printing Office.

U. S. Department of Health and Human Services, Children's Bureau. (1997). *National study of protective, preventive and reunification services delivered to children and their families.* Washington DC: U. S. Government Printing Office.

U.S. Department of Health and Human Services (1999). *Blending perspectives and building common ground: A report to congress on substance abuse and child protection.* Washington DC: Author.

Volpicelli, J. R., Markman, I., Monterosso, J., Filing, J., & O'Brien, C. P. (2000). Psychosocially enhanced treatment for cocaine-dependent mothers: Evidence of efficacy. *Journal of Substance Abuse Treatment, 18,* 41-49.

Wasserman, D. R., & Leventhal, J. M. (1993). Maltreatment of children born to cocaine-dependent women. *AJDC, 147,* 1324-1328.

Werner, E. E. (1986). Resilient offspring of alcoholics: A longitudinal study from birth to age 18. *Journal of Studies on Alcohol, 47*(1), 34-40.

Wexler, H. K., Cuadrado, M. & Stevens, S. J. (1998). Residential treatment for women: Behavioral and psychological outcomes. In S. J., Stevens, and H. K. Wexler (Eds.). *Women and substance abuse: Gender transparency* (pp, 213-233). Binghamton NY: Hawthorne Medical Press.

Whitesdale-Mansell, L., Crone, C. C., & Conners, N. A. (1998). The development and evaluation of an alcohol and drug prevention and treatment program for women and children. *Journal of Substance Abuse Treatment, 16*(3), 265-275.

Williams-Petersen, M.G. Myers, B. J., McFarland Degen, H., Knisley, J. S., Elswick, R. K., & Schnoll, S. S. (1994). Drug-using and nonusing women: Potential for child abuse, child-rearing attitudes, social support, and attention for expected baby. *The International Journal of the Addictions, 29*(11), 1631-1643.

Wobie, K., Eyler, F. D., Conlon, M., Clarke, L., & Behnke, M. (1997). Women and children in residential treatment: Outcomes for mothers and their infants. *Journal of Drug Issues, 27*(3), 585-606.

Young, N. K., & Gardner, S. L. (2002). *Navigating the pathways: Lessons and promising practices in linking alcohol and drug services with child welfare.* SAMHSA Publication No. SMA-02-3639. Rockville, MD: Center for Substance Abuse Treatment, Substance Abuse and Mental Health Services Administration.

Young, N. K., Gardner S. L., & Dennis, K. (1998). Responding to alcohol and other drug problems in child welfare: Weaving together practice and policy. Washington DC: Child Welfare League of America.

Assessing Parent Education Programs
for Families Involved
with Child Welfare Services:
Evidence and Implications

Michelle A. Johnson, PhD
Susan Stone, PhD
Christine Lou, MSW
Jennifer Ling, MSW
Jennette Claassen, MSW
Michael J. Austin, PhD

SUMMARY. Parent education programs may be offered or mandated at various stages of the child welfare services continuum. However, little is known regarding their efficacy in addressing the parenting problems that bring families to the attention of child welfare services. This article synthesizes outcome data generated from 58 parenting programs with families determined to be at-risk of child maltreatment and/or abusive or neglectful. It places parent education programs within the broader context of research on effective parenting as well as the leading etiological

---

Michelle A. Johnson is Research Director, Department of Social Welfare at UCLA, Los Angeles, CA. Susan Stone is Assistant Professor, Christine Lou is BASSC Doctoral Research Assistant, Jennifer Ling is Doctoral Research Assistant, Jennette Claassen is BASSC Research Assistant, Michael J. Austin is BASSC Staff Director; all are affiliated with the School of Social Welfare, University of California, Berkley, Berkeley, CA 94720.

models of child maltreatment to assess the evaluations of these programs with regard to methodological rigor as well as theoretical salience. Practical and theoretical implications are presented along with recommendations for future research.

KEYWORDS. Parent education, child welfare, parenting programs, parent skills, child maltreatment, child abuse, child neglect

INTRODUCTION

With over 500,000 children currently in out-of-home care and more than a million families receiving child welfare services to maintain the safety and well-being of their children in their homes (NCCAN, 2003), it is apparent that large numbers of parents engage in behaviors that are determined to be harmful to their children. As a function of their involvement with the child welfare services system, it has been estimated that approximately 850,000 families in the U.S. participate in voluntary or court-mandated parent education programs each year (Barth et al., 2005). Parent education programs, whether explicit or implicit, assume an underlying theory of action; that is, intervening with parents directly can improve (a) parenting skills and capacities, (b) certain child outcomes, and, ultimately, (c) can reduce the future risk of maltreatment. Therefore, training for biological parents may be provided at various stages of the child welfare services continuum: as a preventative measure to strengthen and preserve at-risk families or as a response to prevent the recurrence of child maltreatment either in intact families or in families where children have been placed in out-of-home care.

Despite the widespread development and implementation of parenting programs for families that come to the attention of the child welfare services system, little is known about their effectiveness in preventing child maltreatment. The primary focus of this report is to synthesize outcome data generated from parenting programs with families determined to be (a) at-risk of child maltreatment and/or (b) abusive or neglectful. By placing these findings within the broader context of research on effective parenting as well as parenting among maltreating families, our goal is to create a template onto which we map both what are thought to be key intervention elements of parenting programs as well as the key outcomes that have been measured. This report is divided into four sections. We first describe what is understood to be effective parenting in order to frame the context of parenting for families that come to the attention of the child welfare services system. The framework and methods of the review are presented second, followed by major findings and implications for practice.

EFFECTIVE PARENTING

The knowledge, skills, and behaviors that are associated with effective parenting have been defined over time by normative standards regarding the parenting role. Three major bodies of research inform our current understanding of effective parenting: (a) studies examining the effects of parenting styles on child outcomes (see Baumrind, 1978; Dornbusch et al., 1987; Steinberg, Elmen, & Mounts, 1989; Steinberg, Lamborn, Dornbusch, & Darling, 1992; Pettit et al., 2001); (b) studies examining parental affective and behavioral characteristics associated with positive parenting (see Holden, 1983; Gardner, 1987; Pettit & Bates, 1989; Dix, 1991; Grusec & Goodrow, 1994; Rusell & Russell, 1996; Russell, 1997; Hoghughi & Speight, 1998; DeKlyen, Speltz, & Greenberg, 1998; Gardner, Sonuga-Barke, & Sayal, 1999; Gardner, Ward, Burton, & Wilson, 2003); and (c) studies examining contextual factors and parenting strategies associated with family resilience (see Belsky, 1984; Jarrett, 1999; Taylor, Spencer, & Baldwin, 2000; Murry et al., 2001; Walsh, 2002; Hess, Papas, & Black, 2002; Conger & Conger, 2002; Kotchick & Forehand, 2002; Orthner, Jones-Sanpei, & Williamson, 2004; Armstrong, Birnie-Lefcovitch, & Ungar, 2005).

Parenting Styles

Classic studies of parenting styles form the foundation of the early modern research regarding parenting effect on child socialization and academic achievement (see Baumrind, 1967, 1971, 1978). These studies distinguish parental styles on the three domains of parental responsiveness/warmth, psychological autonomy, and behavioral control/demand, and associate parenting success with the extent to which these elements are present in the parent-child relationship: (a) *authoritarian* parents exhibit higher levels of control/demand, and lower levels of parental warmth and autonomy, and tend to raise children who are relatively discontent, withdrawn, and distrustful; (b) *permissive* parents exhibit lower levels of control/demand, and higher levels of warmth and autonomy, and tend to raise relatively less socially responsible and less independent children; and (c) *authoritative* parents exhibit higher levels of control/demand, autonomy, and warmth, and tend to raise children who are socially responsible and independent. Thus, an "authoritative" parenting style can be characterized as the benchmark for successful parenting, and subsequent studies suggest that this style of parenting is related to increased child academic success and psychosocial maturity (Dornbusch et al., 1987; Steinberg, Elmen, & Mounts, 1989; Steinberg, Lamborn, Dornbusch, & Darling, 1992).

Parental Characteristics

In addition to refining categories of parental styles, latter research also identifies "proactive" behavioral and affective parenting characteristics associated with positive parenting and reduced occurrence of child misbehavior and conduct problems. Specifically, it suggests that the following parental techniques have beneficial impacts on promoting healthy parent-child relationships and preventing and/or reducing occurrences of undesirable child outcomes or behaviors: (a) engaging in "pre-emptive" positive involvement with the child, such as joint play or conversation Holden, 1983; Gardner, 1987; Pettit & Bates, 1989; Dix, 1991; Gardner, Sonuga-Barke, & Sayal, 1999; Gardner, Ward, Burton, & Wilson, 2003); (b) demonstrating warmth/affection to the child, such as expressing sensitivity and empathy, responding positively, and showing respect and encouragement Russell & Russell, 1996; Russell, 1997; DeKlyen, Speltz, & Greenberg, 1998); and (c) employing specific parental interaction strategies, such as reasoning, negotiation, and compromise, use of humor, and use of incentives (Grusec & Goodrow, 1994; Gardner, Sonuga-Barke, & Sayal, 1999; Kaplan & Owens, 2004). Hoghughi and Speight (1998) summarize these components of "good parenting" as the provision of love, care and commitment; control/consistent limit setting; and facilitation of development.

Parenting Context and Resilience

Contextual and environmental factors often impact parental ability to implement these proactive strategies and develop positive parental characteristics. Belsky's research on the process model of competent parenting recognizes multiple and layered parenting domains, and identifies three general sources of influence on parental functioning: (a) personal psychological resources of parents, (b) characteristics of the child, and (c) contextual sources of stress and support, specifically, marital relationships, social networks, and employment status (Belsky, 1984). While parenting research has generally focused on the first component of Belsky's model (i.e., personal parental characteristics and behaviors) within primarily middle-class, white, and intact family samples, research has increasingly recognized and examined contextual influences on parenting competence, particularly within minority samples and samples of lower socioeconomic status. Family resilience research suggests that the following factors have protective influences on families in conflict or at risk for deleterious child outcomes: (a) positive child characteristics and behaviors, such as child warmth/affection and an "easy" temperament (Russell, 1997; Hess, Papas, & Black, 2002; Kaplan & Owens; 2004); (b) positive family belief systems, such as making meaning of adversity, positive outlook, and transcendence and spirituality (Walsh, 2002; Kaplan & Owens, 2004); (c) flexible, cohesive, and connected family organizational patterns (Hess, Papas, & Black, 2002; Walsh, 2002); (d) clear family communication patterns that are open to emotional sharing and promote collaborative problem-solving (Conger & Conger, 2002; Walsh, 2002; Kaplan & Owens; 2004; Orthner, Jones-Sanpei, & Williamson, 2004); (e) positive marital quality(Bronstein, Clauson, Stoll, & Abrams, 1993; Russell, 1997; Conger & Conger 2002); and (f) access to social and economic resources, such as supportive social networks and good housing (Taylor, Spencer, & Baldwin, 2000; Murry et al., 2001; Walsh, 2002; Kaplan & Owens; 2004; Orthner, Jones-Sanpei, & Williamson, 2004).

Implicit assumptions based on "effective parenting" about the appropriate use and expression of parental control, degree of parent and child interaction, and level of parental warmth and affection structure the goals of many parenting programs. However, parental characteristics associated with child maltreatment such as poverty, depression, substance abuse, single parenthood, poor problem-solving skills and social isolation are also those that have been found to predict attrition and poorer outcomes in parent training programs (Dore & Lee, 1999). Furthermore, evidence is accumulating to suggest that demographically similar maltreating parents and non-maltreating caretakers differ in important ways, such as having higher levels of anger, stronger beliefs in corporal punishment, less empathy, more role reversal, and higher levels of psychopathology (e.g., Mennen & Trickett, 2006). Therefore, to be effective, parenting programs geared to maltreating parents have the special challenge of addressing the underlying etiology of child maltreatment that not only shapes parenting but also informs program engagement and retention.

ETIOLOGICAL MODELS OF CHILD MALTREATMENT

While there is general consensus that child maltreatment results from a complex interplay between child, caregiver and family characteristics, as well as particular socio-contextual factors (e.g., see Azar, Povilaitis, Lauretti, & Pouquette, 1998; Belsky, 1980; Cichetti & Toth, 2005; Garbarino & Eckenrode, 1997; Gelles, 1985), models of maltreatment differ in terms of the relative emphasis each place on specific aspects of the ecology and the mechanisms by which specific characteristics and conditions combine to raise the likelihood of maltreatment. Despite these differences, aspects of the caregiving environment, such as parenting beliefs, behaviors, and the quality of parent-child interactions and relationships, consistently emerge as key etiological factors in child maltreatment and, indeed, are thought to be critical levers for intervention (Azar, Nix & Makin-Byrd, 2005; Azar et al., 1998). Emergent literature on so-called "risky families" lends additional support to the salience of poorly functioning caregiving environments. Characterized by high levels of aggression and conflict as well as cold and unsupportive relationships, these caregiving environments place children at substantial risk for poor health and mental health outcomes (Repetti, Taylor, & Seeman, 2002). Finally, a robust line of research suggests that social contextual conditions (e.g., low SES, lack of job opportunities, stressors) exert their influence on maltreatment through their effects on parent distress and parenting practices (Conger, Ge Elder, Lorenz, & Simons, 1994; Duncan, Brooks-Gunn & Klebanov, 1994; McLoyd, 1998). In other words, while child maltreatment has multiple determinants at multiple ecological levels, the caregiving environment constitutes an important pathway between caregivers' personal and social characteristics and child outcomes.

PARENTING ISSUES AMONG MALTREATING FAMILIES

Theoretical and empirical work suggests that there are five core domains of parenting difficulty vithin maltreating families. These include deficiencies in (a) social cognitive processing, (b) impulse control, (c) parenting skills, (d) social skills, and (e) stress management (Azar, et al., 2005; Azar, et al., 1998). These domains, which are briefly described below, are thought to generalize across most maltreatment types; that is, similar sets of parenting problems apply in situations of physical abuse, emotional abuse, neglect, and, to a lesser extent, sexual abuse.

Social-Cognitive Processing

Social cognitive processing describes pathways between parenting schemas, parent attributions of children and child behavior, and ultimately parental responses to children (Azar et al., 2005). Problematic schemas include parental perceptions of low levels of control and efficacy as well as inaccurate or incomplete understanding of their children's developmental needs and incorrect parental attributions of children. For example, caregivers at risk for maltreatment often hold hostile attribution biases (that is, attribute hostile intent to the behavior of children) as well as expectations that children, as opposed to parents, will provide comfort and care.

Impulse Control

The domain of impulse control corresponds with parents' responses to children. Impulsive parenting responses occur quickly and without adequate reflection on the purposes and potential consequences of the response. The management of anger may be particularly salient to this domain (Pinkston & Smith, 1998).

PARENTING SKILLS

This third domain relates to parents' actual skills in terms of the day-to-day care of children as well as parent management techniques, monitoring, and discipline of children. Specifically, maltreating parents often possess a limited repertoire of parenting skills and strategies; these limited strategies are often harsh, coercive and inconsistent.

Social and Stress Management Skills

Finally, maltreating parents show deficits in complex social skills, including limited and poor communication with others, over-reliance on negative control and coercive strategies, poor ability to read social cues, and overall insensitivity and unresponsiveness to others' needs. In addition, maltreating parents exhibit elevated levels of emotional arousal in response to stress as well as ineffective coping strategies.

CHARACTERISTICS AND CONTEXTS OF MALTREATING PARENTS

While research suggests a common set of parenting issues among maltreating families, a great deal of heterogeneity exists within this population. Key sources of variation within parents and their contexts that influence caregiving capacities also represent dimensions on which parenting programs may intervene. Factors such as a parents' own childrearing history, the presence of psychopathology (particularly depressive symptomotology and substance abuse), parent age, and cognitive ability increase the risk for maltreatment (Cicchetti & Toth, 2005; Toth, Maughan, Manly, Spagnola, & Cichetti, 2002). In addition, abusive family environments often include high levels of marital and relational discord, including domestic violence, low levels of relational intimacy and satisfaction, and high levels of anger, disruption and conflict (Repetti, Taylor & Seeman, 2002). High levels of social isolation resulting from weak and unsupportive social networks also characterize maltreating families. Maltreating families are disproportionately represented among the lowest economic strata of society, placing these families at increased risk of financial hardship, loose attachment to the labor force, and chronic stressors. Poverty directly influences levels of parental distress, which, in turn, influences the warmth and consistency of their parenting (Conger, Ge Elder, Lorenz, & Simons, 1994; Duncan, Brooks-Gunn & Klebanov, 1994; McLoyd, 1998). Finally, attributes of children such as their age, gender, temperament, and health and mental health characteristics also influence maltreatment risk.

In short, these sources of heterogeneity within maltreating families suggest an important set of factors that may influence the caregiving environment or that may moderate the influence of the caregiving environment on children's outcomes. In addition, recent conceptual work suggests that the presence of many of these factors relate to parent engagement and adherence to treatment.

GOALS OF THE REVIEW

The appropriate match between participant and parenting education program is of heightened concern for parents involved in the child welfare system given that program attendance and completion often represent the criteria against which child placement and reunification decisions are made in legal proceedings (e.g., Barth et al., 2005; Budd, 2001). Shortened timeframes for the termination of parental rights in child maltreatment cases also make the provision of appropriate and effective services imperative. To identify parenting programs that hold promise for parents that come to the attention of the child welfare services system, this review assesses the impacts of parent education programs on the incidence or recurrence of child maltreatment, where assessed, as well as a number of outcomes that are measured at the caregiver environment level. We review parenting programs aimed at parents who have been determined to be at risk of child maltreatment and/or abusive and neglectful and evaluate them in terms of (a) the extent to which they conceptually address particular needs in the caregiving environment thought to be salient in this population, and (b) methodological rigor.

In contrast to "effective parenting," minimal parenting competency is generally considered the "floor" of acceptable parenting that is sufficient to protect the safety and well-being of a child when he or she comes to the attention of child welfare services. However, not only are standards for evaluating parental fitness not well defined or agreed upon, there is a lack of appropriate measures of parenting adequacy (Budd, 2001). Therefore, another goal of the review was to determine how child welfare service practitioners assess the strengths and limitations of the parental caregiving environment to support decisions in initial referral to specific parenting programs.

METHODOLOGY

Search Strategy

This review used pre-determined search terms and search sources to identify research literature within a given topic. This method of searching can reduce the potential for bias in the selection of materials. Using specified search terms, we searched numerous social science and academic databases available through the University of California library. In addition, we conducted overall internet searches and also searched the Websites of research institutes and organizations specializing in systematic reviews, conference proceedings databases, dissertation databases, internet databases (see Appendix A for details of the search protocol). The references in reviews and primary studies were scanned to identify additional articles. The references reviewed were limited to those printed in the English language.

The review included evaluations of parenting programs that explicitly targeted the following populations: (a) parents assessed to be at-risk of child maltreatment, (b) parents referred to a parenting program by a child welfare services agency, and (c) parents that had been indicated or substantiated for a report of child abuse or neglect. In addition, evaluations of programs that explicitly targeted parents with characteristics associated with an increased risk of child maltreatment were reviewed, including (a) parents abusing substances, (b) adolescent parents, (c) ethnic minority and low-income parents, and (d) parents residing in institutional settings.

EVALUATION METHODS

An initial step of the review was to assess the theoretical underpinnings of the parenting programs by reviewing the program goals and documenting the outcomes for which the programs demonstrated empirical support. For example, an outcome of interest to child welfare practitioners might be the number of reports of child maltreatment that occur during program participation or for some period following program completion. As mentioned, indirect measures of effectiveness that address the etiology of child maltreatment might include changes in parental stress, the acquisition of parenting skills, or changes in parental beliefs. While pre- and post-test measurement of these outcomes may suggest changes within program participants that can be attributed to the parenting program, factors other than the program itself can also influence outcomes, such as the receipt of additional services (e.g., substance abuse treatment) or changes family structure (e.g., the placement of a child in foster care), which makes the evaluation of the methodological rigor of each study necessary. In short, to attribute the cause of the change to the parenting program, participants must be randomly assigned to a parent education group or to a control group that does not participate in the program and is followed longitudinally to observe change over time. Changes in the parent education group that exceed changes in the control group represent empirical support for the effectiveness of the program.

The conceptual breadth of each study was assessed by mapping the significant outcomes from each study on to Azar et al.'s (Azar et al.,

2005; Azar et al., 1998) five domains of caregiver functioning, including (a) social cognitive processing, (b) impulse control (c) parenting skills, (d) social skills, and (e) stress management. A code template was developed to categorize study outcomes by caregiver functioning domains. Interrater reliability for the code template was ascertained through a reliability check of 10 percent of the studies (n = 7). Raters agreed on the categorization of outcomes by domain in six of the seven studies (86%) leading to further refinement of the code template and the reassignment of some outcomes from the social cognitive processing domain to the parenting skill and impulse control domains.

While there are many approaches to evaluating the methodological rigor of randomized controlled trials (RCT), such as CONSORT guidelines or Campbell Collaboration guidelines, the few RCTs that were generated through the search criteria prevented the application of these approaches. Given the interest in treatment efficacy (that is, the successful outcomes of clinical trials), treatment effectiveness (the outcomes of interventions conducted under the normal conditions of program delivery in the community), as well as the theory underlying intervention designs, we took an inclusive approach to studies of varying methodological rigor would assist child welfare agencies by defining intervention components, identifying assessment and outcome measurement strategies, and assisting in the development of valid research questions for the future.

The research designs of all studies were reviewed for their methodological rigor and categorized. Randomized control trials (Level 1) were considered the most rigorous types of evaluations, followed by Level 2 quasi-experimental designs including (a) control group studies that collected repeated measures on participants that were assigned to at least one treatment group and a no-treatment control group, and (b) comparison group studies that collected repeated measures on participants that were assigned to one or more treatment groups without no-treatment controls. Level 3 studies included single group or single subject designs that collected repeated measures on participants over time. Several descriptive studies that focused on the development or the implementation of a program were reviewed but were not included in the analysis.

Studies were also reviewed to determine how participants were initially identified for program enrollment. Instruments that were used in pre- and post-test measurement were documented and reviewed.

FINDINGS

The overall assessment of the 70 studies of that were reviewed is presented first, followed by detailed results of (a) the outcomes of the 58 parent education programs by target population, and (b) results related to parenting assessment.

Summary of General Findings

Conceptual Breadth

Our results indicate that parenting programs, especially those focused on maltreating populations, assess outcomes in at least one of the theoretically salient caregiving domains, though child protective service outcomes of interest such as child maltreatment recurrence were monitored in only one-third of cases (n = 23; 33%). The weight of outcomes assessed fall into three particular caregiving domains: social-cognitive processing, parenting skills, and stress management (see Table 1). While we might like to know more about how effective programs are in preventing child maltreatment occurrence or recurrence specifically, this finding is encouraging given that the theoretical work reviewed pinpoints social cognitive processing as a central lever for intervention. Outcomes related to parent impulse control and social skills, however, receive less emphasis. It is unclear what drives this particular finding.

While social cognitive processing is considered a key lever for intervention, Azar et al.'s theoretical model suggests that attention to each of the five key domains outlined is critical for intervention with maltreating families. Of the studies reviewed, a majority (n = 47; 67%) of studies included only one theoretical domain (equally distributed among social cognitive processing or parenting skills). Of the remaining 23, fifteen focused on two domains, mostly including social cognitive processing. Finally, eight included three domains, including a combination of social cognitive processing and parenting skills plus an additional domain of either social skills or stress management. In short, these results suggest a picture of a few multi-pronged programs, a set of programs focused on social cognitive processing and parenting skills in combination, and a set of cognitively based and skills based programs, respectively. On the one hand, these findings raise questions about the availability of particular intervention strategies related to the five domains and/or the availability of adequate measures for these outcomes.

TABLE 1. Empirical Support for Theoretical Domains Addressed in Parenting Program Evaluations

Target Populations of Programs	Outcomes by Theoretical Domain*					Total Number of Studies (N)
	SCP	IC	PS	SS	SM	
At-Risk/Indicated for Child Maltreatment	16	1	18	4	13	45
Substance Abusing Parents	5	0	4	2	0	8
Adolescent Parents	4	0	3	1	0	7
Culturally Specific Parenting Programs	4	0	4	0	1	8
Institutional Settings	2	0	1	0	0	2
TOTAL	31	1	30	7	14	70

*SCP = Social Cognitive Processing, IC= Impulse Control, PS=Parenting Skills, SS=Social Skills, SM= Stress Management

Alternatively, multiple domains may appear less salient to program developers. Further research will be needed to clarify this gap.

Methodological Rigor

Of the 70 studies reviewed, 17 (24%) used randomized controlled trials (RCT); 20 (29%) employed quasi-experimental designs (of these four utilized a sophisticated control strategy), and 33 (47%) drew on single group pre-test post-test designs (see Table 2). Indeed, we have evidence of an emerging research base. Of the RCTs focused on child welfare populations, most were preventative (e.g., home visiting models targeting families at risk for maltreatment). It is notable that the modal study in our review was a single group pre-test post-test intervention study. These studies cannot be used to demonstrate the efficacy of a particular intervention. However, they can be used to (a) assess whether a particular intervention is moving in the hypothesized direction and (b) identify families who may differentially drop out.

Outcomes of Parent Education Programs by Target Population

The significant results of parent education programs are presented in Figures 1 through 4. Outcomes are organized by population: (a) parents determined to be at-risk of child maltreatment and/or indicated for child maltreatment (Figure 1), (b) substance abusing parents (Figure 2), (c) adolescent parents (Figure 3), and (d) specific programs for ethnic minority families (Figure 4). Two programs for parents in prison are also

TABLE 2. Study Designs (n = 70)

Study Designs	Target Populations of Programs					Total Number of Studies (N)
	At-Risk/Indicated for Child Maltreatment	Substance Abusing Parents	Adolescent Parents	Culturally Specific Parenting Programs	Institutional Settings	
RCT	10	4	0	3	0	17
Quasi-Experimental	14	2	2	2	0	20
Single Group	21	2	5	3	2	33
TOTAL	45	8	7	8	2	70

described. In each table, the five domains of the caregiving environment and the developmental stage of the index child targeted by the intervention organize programs that reported statistically significant outcomes for each domain. The methodological rigor of each evaluation is bracketed following the referenced citation that appears in the endnote section (for tables only). Fuller descriptions of each of the studies, including intervention components, program goals, research designs, participant demographics, and overall findings of the studies are provided in the full report.

PROGRAMS FOR PARENTS AT-RISK OR INDICATED FOR CHILD MALTREATMENT

Forty-five studies evaluated 37 programs that were designed to address the parenting needs of families determined to be at risk of maltreatment or had maltreated their children (Figure 1). Of the 45 evaluations, nearly half utilized single group designs (n = 21; 47%) followed by quasi-experimental designs (n = 14; 31%) and randomized control trials (n = 10; 22%). Nearly half of the programs (n = 15; 41%) were designed for parents who were pregnant or specifically parenting children of five years of age or younger (including preschool children). Eight (22%) programs targeted at-risk or maltreating parents of children ranging from preschool age through latency age. Two programs specifically targeted parents of adolescents (5%). Twelve of the programs (32%) either tailored their interventions to the specific needs of the family, as in the Bavolek Nurturing Program (Bavolek, 2005), or did not indicate the specific developmental stage of the child for which the parenting program was designed.

FIGURE 1. Programs for Parents at Risk or Indicated for Child Maltreatment

Caregiving Domains	Developmental Stage of Child		
	Prenatal to 5 yrs	Latency through Adolescence	Child's Age Not Specified
Social Cognitive Processing (e.g., increases in age appropriate expectations, empathic understanding of children, changes in role reversal attitudes)	Home Visitation Programs (Chase & Nelson, 2002 [3]; Fraser et al., 2000 [1]; Hawaii's Healthy Start (Duggan et al., 1999 [1]); Early intervention program Wolfe et al., 1988 [2]; Project SafeCare (Bigelow & Lutzker, 2000 [3]; Gershater-Molko et al., 2003 [3])	Triple-P Positive Parenting Matrix (Sanders et al., 2004 [1]); Family Connections Program (DePanfilis, 2005 [1]); Family Interactions Skills Project (MacMillan et al., 1988 [3])	Social Network Intervention Project (Gaudin et al., 1990/1991 [2]); Bavolek Nurturing Program (Cowen, 2001 [3]; Bavolek, 2005 [3]); San Fernando Valley Child Guidance Clinic (Golub et al., 1987 [3]) Active Parenting Program (Carlsen, 1997 [3]); Anger management program (Acton & During, 1992 [3]); RETHINK Method: Anger Management (Fetch et al., 1999 [3])
Impulse Control (e.g., reduced anger levels)			Clinic based program Barth et al., 1983 [3]
Parenting Skills (e.g., improvements related to parental discipline; increased the responsiveness of neglectful parents; improvements in child management skills)	Home Visitation Programs; Hawaii's Healthy Start; Parenting Young Children Huebner, 2002 [2]; Parent/Child Foster Placement (Nayman & Witkin, 1978 [3]; Project SafeCare (Gershater-Molko et al., 2003 [3]; Mandel et al., 1998 [3]; The Incredible Years (Baydar et al., 2003 [1]	Triple-P Positive Parenting Matrix; Webster-Stratton Parenting Program (Hughes & Gottlieb, 2004 [1]; Parent Training Program (Wolfe et al., 1981 [2]	Social Network Intervention Project Bavolek Nurturing Program; Multisystemic Therapy Training (MST) and Parent Training (PT) (Brunk et al., 1987 [1]); Active Parenting Program; Anger management program; RETHINK Method Parenting Daily Diary (Peterson et al., 2003 [3]).
Social Skills (e.g., improved social support; increase in social network size and quality of contacts)	Home Visitation Program (Chase & Nelson, 2002 [3]); Special Social Support Training Project (SSST: Lovell et al., 1992 [3])		Social Network Intervention Project
Stress Management (e.g., reduction in parenting stress; lowered anxiety)	Home Visiting (Fraser et al., 2000 [1]; Hawaii's Healthy Start; Parenting Young Children; Errorless Compliance Training (Ducharme et al., 2001 [3]; Family Growth Center Programs (Whipple, 1999 [2]; STAR (Fox et al.,1991 [3])	Triple-P Positive Parenting Matrix; Parent-Child Interaction Therapy (PCIT; Timmer et al., 2005 [2]); Family Connections Program	Multisystemic Therapy Training (MST) and Parent Training (PT); Anger management program; Parent Training program

Programs for parents of young children. In terms of conceptual breadth, home visiting models that addressed the social cognitive processing domain tended to be the broadest of the fifteen programs for parents of young children by also addressing parenting skills and/or stress management. In many cases the evaluation of these programs were the most methodologically rigorous. However, several of the gains identified were lost at follow-up. In some cases the presence of domestic violence in the home was found to moderate this effect (Eckenrode et al., 2000). Project SafeCare, which was the most comprehensively evaluated program for parents of young children, demonstrated improvements in the ability of parents to identify their children's health symptoms and to seek treatment (Bigelow & Lutzker, 2000; Gershater-Molko et al., 2003). Improvements were also observed in the increased use of planned activities, parent training techniques, positive parent behaviors, and improvements in home safety (Gershater-Molko et al., 2003; Mandel et al., 1998). Families that completed all three training programs were less likely to recidivate (Gershater-Molko et al., 2002), and parents reported high levels of program satisfaction (Taban & Lutzker, 2001).

Other programs achieved positive outcomes in single domains of the caregiving environment, such as the reduction of parental stress (Fox, Fox, & Anderson, 1991; Ducharme et al., 2001; Whipple, 1999), as well as in a combination of two domains, such as reduction in parenting stress and improvement in the home environment (Huebner, 2002). The Incredible Years, which targets parents with preschool-aged children in weekly two-hour sessions from eight to twelve weeks, observed reductions in harsh, negative, inconsistent and ineffective parenting with increases in supportive and positive parenting (Baydar et al., 2003). Significant reductions in incidences of substantiated abusive head injury were also observed in a program that targeted the prevention of Shaken Infant Syndrome (Dias et al., 2005).

Programs for parents of children preschool age through latency. Of the eight programs that targeted at-risk or maltreating parents of children ranging from preschool age through latency age, empirical support for improvements in three caregiving domains was demonstrated by the Triple-P Positive Parenting Matrix based on a randomized control trial (Sanders et al., 2004). This 12-week, clinically based program targeted parents at risk for child maltreatment with children aged 2 to 7 years and appeared to be effective in improving negative parental attributions of child's misbehavior, lowering levels of dysfunctional parenting and lessening parental distress while demonstrating short term gains in child abuse potential and high levels of client satisfaction. The community-based Family Connections Program also demonstrated increases in appropriate parenting attitudes while reducing parenting stress in a randomized control trial. This program was also successful in addressing characteristics that tend to be more common in maltreating parents, including decreasing parent's depressive symptoms and drug use (DePanfilis, 2005).

The remainder of the programs reviewed addressed single domains of the caregiving environment, including reductions in parenting stress along with reductions in abuse risk (Timmer et al., 2005), improvement in parenting skills (Hughes & Gottlieb, 2004), and improvements in parent effectiveness and child management skills (Wolfe et al., 1981). In Wolfe et al.'s study (1981), no reports of child maltreatment recurrence were documented at one-year follow up in a quasi-experimental design.

Whereas home visiting programs appear to be the most promising intervention modality for young children, nurse home visiting was found to be no more effective than standard services for preventing child maltreatment recurrence in a randomized control trial at three-year follow-up (MacMillan et al., 2005), suggesting that families with existing child maltreatment histories may need different services than those offered in early prevention programs. Carlo found experiential learning to demonstrate a significant increase in movement toward family reunification among families whose children had been placed in residential treatment when compared with didactic learning alone in a quasiexperimental design (Carlo, 1993).

Programs for parents of adolescents. The two programs specifically targeted to parents of adolescents, Mission Possible (Riesch et al., 2003) and Parenting Adolescents Wisely (PAW; Kacir & Gordon, 1999) were unable to demonstrate positive changes in the caregiving environment, though PAW did demonstrate a reduction in children's problem behaviors at post-test.

Individualized programs. Of the twelve programs that either tailored their interventions to the specific needs of the family or did not specify the developmental stage of the child as part of the program's target population, there was a great deal of variability in program outcomes. When Multisystemic Therapy Training (MST), an 8-week individual and tailored family treatment based in the home or in the clinic, which focuses on changing family interaction patterns, was compared with Parent Training (Brunk et al., 1987), an 8-week group treatment based in a clinic that focuses on instruction in human development and child management to increase positive parent-child interaction and reduce aversive child behavior, both treatments were found to decrease parental psychiatric symptomology, reduce overall stress and reduce the severity of identified problems. However MST was found to be more effective in restructuring parent-child relations and increasing neglectful parent responsiveness. PT was more effective at reducing identified social problems.

The Social Network Intervention Project (Gaudin, 1990/1991), a case management program monitored by a specialized social worker, demonstrated improvements in three domains of the caregiving environment for neglectful parents, including increases in age appropriate expectations, the empathic understanding of children, and changes in role reversal attitudes. The program also demonstrated improved parenting skills and increases in the social networks of subjects. The Parent Training Program, a 10-session group meeting program with individual work assignments, demonstrated reductions in stress, anxiety, and the frequency of emotionally abusive behavior (Iwaniec, 1997).

Several of the remaining programs reviewed were conceptually strong but lacked the methodological rigor upon which to draw conclusions given their single subject designs. For example, the Bavolek Nurturing Program demonstrated several improvements in social cognitive processing (Cowen, 2001; Bavolek, 2005) and decreased family conflict but was unable to demonstrate sustained change at one-year follow-up (Bavolek, 2005).

Programs for Parents with Substance Abuse Problems

Eight studies that evaluated seven programs addressing the parenting needs of substance using parents were reviewed (Figure 2). Nearly half of these programs were based on Bavolek's Nurturing Parent curriculum (Harm et al., 1998; Moore & Finkelstein, 2001; Saxe, 1997) and most programs tended to focus on the parenting skills and social cognitive processing domains of the caregiving environment. Suchman's Relational Psychotherapy Mother's Group (RPMG; Suchman et al., 2004) and Webster-Stratton's ADVANCE program (Webster-Stratton, 1994) were the most theoretically comprehensive and the most rigorously evaluated. The RPMG program addressed three caregiving domains, including parenting skills, social skills, and social cognitive processing and demonstrated more positive psychosocial adjustment, greater involvement with children and improvements in parent-child relationships and lower levels of risk for child maltreatment among RPMG

FIGURE 2. Parenting Programs for Substance Abusing Parents

Caregiving Domains	Developmental Stage of Child		
	Prenatal to 5 Years	Latency through Adolescence	Child's Age Not Specified
Social Cognitive Processing	Integrated parenting training curriculum (Velez et al., 2004 [3])	ADVANCE Webster - Stratton, 1994 [1]; Relational Psychotherapy Mother's Group (RPMG; Luthar & Suchman, 2000 [1])	Nurturing Program for Families in Substance Abuse (Moore & Finkelstein, 2001); Skillful Parenting Program (Saxe, 1997 [1]); Course in state prison system based on Nurturing Parent curriculum (Harm et al., 1998 [2])
Impulse Control			
Parenting Skills		ADVANCE Relational Psychotherapy Mother's Group (RPMG; Luthar & Suchman [1], 2000; Suchman et al., 2004b [1])	Nurturing Program for Families in Substance Abuse
Social Skills		ADVANCE	
Stress Management			

mothers when compared with participants who received standard drug counseling (Suchman et al., 2004). The ADVANCE program demonstrated improved problem solving, improved communication, and improved family relations and family functioning (Webster-Stratton, 1994). Overall, programs for substance abusing parents were associated with the following outcomes: lower risk levels for child maltreatment (Luthar & Suchman, 2000; Saxe, 1997; Suchman, MaMahon, & Luthar, 2004); improved parenting skills (Moore & Finkelstein, 2001); improved parental knowledge (Velez et al., 2004); enhanced parental competence (Moore & Finkelstein, 2001); more positive parental psychosocial adjustment (Luthar & Suchman, 2000); increased parent-child interaction and improved parent-child affective interactions (Suchman, MaMahon, & Luthar, 2004); and increased parental self-esteem (Saxe, 1997).

Programs for Adolescent Parents

Seven studies evaluated programs that addressed the parenting needs of adolescent parents (Figure 3). Similarly to parent education programs for other populations, most programs for adolescent parents tended to focus on social cognitive processing and parenting skills domains. Specifically, programs were associated with parental improvements in parent knowledge, beliefs, and skills regarding infant growth child development (Britner & Reppucci, 1997; Culp et al., 1998; Dickonson & Cudaback, 1992; Fulton et al., 1991; Weinman et al., 1992), home safety (Culp et al., 1998), parent-child interactions (Britner &

FIGURE 3. Parenting Programs for Adolescent Parents

Caregiving Domains	Developmental Stage of Child		
	Prenatal to 5 Years	Latency through Adolescence	Child's Age Not Specified
Social Cognitive Processing			Project Baby Care (Roberts, Wolman, & Harris-Looby, 2004 [3]); Parent Education/Home Visitation Program (Culp et al., 1998 [3]); Adolescent Parenting Program (Fulton et al., 1991 [3]); Parent Education Program (Weinman, Schreiber, & Robinson, 2002 [3])
Impulse Control			
Parenting Skills	Parenting booklets (Dickinson & Cudaback, 1992 [2])		Parent Education/Home Visitation Program Adolescent Parenting Program
Social Skills			Parent Education/Home Visitation Program
Stress Management			

Reppucci; Fulton et al., 1991), and corporal punishment (Roberts, Wolman, & Harris-Looby, 2004). Other outcomes included a lower incidence of child neglect and abuse (Dickonson & Cudaback, 1992; Flynn, 1999), a lower percentage of low birthweight (Flynn, 1999), and a delay of subsequent pregnancies and increased maternal educational attainment (Britner & Reppucci, 1997).

Programs for Culturally Specific Populations

Culturally specific populations may have different needs and require different approaches in parent education programs; in particular, disciplinary practices and positive parent-child interactions have been identified as areas in which parents from disadvantaged and/or minority backgrounds may deviate from normative standards. Consequently, social cognitive processing and parenting skills in these areas have been the major focus of parent education programs for these populations (Figure 4). Of the three randomized control trials reviewed, two demonstrated no significant effects (Constantino et al., 2001; St. Pierre & Layzer, 1999). However, the Incredible Years BASIC Program (Gross et al., 2003) demonstrated increases in parenting self-efficacy as well as the reduced use of coercive discipline strategies with Latino parents. Other programs demonstrated increases in parental ability to use more positive and diversionary methods and decreases in occurrences of emotional/physical punishment and other aggressive practices in disciplinary strategies (Project SafeCare for Spanish-speaking Parents, Cor-

FIGURE 4. Culturally Specific Parenting Programs

Caregiving Domains	Developmental Stage of Child		
	Prenatal to 5 Years	Latency through Adolescence	Child's Age Not Specified
Social Cognitive Processing	The Incredible Years BASIC Program (Gross et al., 2003 [1])	STEP for Chicana mothers (Villegas, 1977 [2])	Listening to Children (Wolfe & Hirsch, 2003 [2])
Impulse Control			
Parenting Skills	The Incredible Years BASIC Program	MADRE (Herrierias, 1988 [3])	Project Safe Care for Spanish speaking (Cordon et al., 1998 [3])
Social Skills			
Stress Management			Listening to Children

don et al., 1998; MADRE, Herrerias, 1988; STEP for Chicanas, Villegas, 1997). Additionally, the Listening to Children program (Wolfe & Hirsch, 2003) demonstrated improvements in parental attitudes and reductions in parenting-related stress and the Strong Families/Familias Fuertas (McGrogan, 1998) was associated with reductions in child abuse potential. Although home visiting has been widely employed as a parent education modality, it was not found to be an effective means of social service delivery and parenting education for low-income and/or minority families (St. Pierre & Layzer, 1999).

Programs in Institutional Settings

Parents residing in institutional settings such as prisons may share similarities with parents whose children have been placed in out-of-home care in that they are separated from their children and are therefore challenged to improve their parenting in the absence of immediate and ongoing parent-child interaction. Furthermore, children of incarcerated parents often come to the attention of child welfare services given their need for out-of-home placement. To assess the feasibility of institutionally-based programs for child welfare populations, evaluations of the Parent Education Project (Howze Browne, 1989) and the Parent Center Training Program (Harm & Thompson, 1997) were reviewed. These programs demonstrated improved outcomes in multiple domains of caregiving, including social cognitive functioning, parenting skill, and social skills in single group (Howze Browne, 1989) and quasi-experimental group designs (Harm & Thompson, 1997). Each modality used a parenting class format ranging from 15 to 24 weeks, which the Parent Center Training program combined with written communication with children. These preliminary findings suggest that due to low self-esteem and lack of empathy toward their children, incarcerated mothers are at a high risk for maltreatment; however, by working with parents prior to prison release, parenting programs have the potential to ease the transition toward reunification.

PARENTING ASSESSMENT

As part of the structured literature review, a large number of self-report and observational assessment instruments (150) were identified in relationship to their use in either initially assessing or subsequently monitoring program participants. These instruments typically reflect items relevant to the outcomes of child maltreatment prevention and intervention (e.g., developmental screening, risk assessment, and treatment planning); however, consideration must be given in relation to their use when evaluating improvements in parenting outcomes. Podsakoff, MacKenzie, Lee & Podsakoff (2003) summarize four key sources of common method biases, as well as efforts to reduce these biases.Unfortunately, it is not always clear what the direction of potential bias and the variation in their magnitude by discipline. These biases include (1) common rater effects (e.g., social desirability), (2) item characteristic and context effects, and (3) measurement context effects (i.e., similarities in media and method). Of these, common rater and measurement context effects may be particularly important sources of biases.

Because child maltreatment represents deviation from social norms and mores, parents may over-report positive items and underreport negative items in directly administered measures. Of the promising programs, the majority relied upon parental self-report instruments to assess program outcomes; however, many also included at least one observational measure (such as the Home Observation for Measure of the Environment Inventory, which is completed by the social worker) and/or an administrative measure (such as maltreatment rates collected from the child welfare agency). Given that most studies employed pre- and post-test comparisons, significant findings based on self-report measures suggest that the program minimally increased parental awareness of socially acceptable attitudes, behaviors, and practices associated with effective parenting.

Aside from these common rater effects, many studies use similar media (e.g. parent self report or child behavior scales).General strategies to avoid problems from either source can be both procedural and statistical. These include using multiple sources, creating separation (e.g., temporal) of measurement occasions or methods, and creating opportunities for respondent anonymity, as well as latent variable statistical modeling techniques.Within studies reviewed, there was typically some attempt to control for these biases, especially through using multiple reporting sources.

It is not clear if and how these instruments are used by child welfare workers in making referrals to parenting programs. For example, how are the strengths and limitations of family functioning and parenting capacities assessed in terms of the most appropriate referral? While the assessment of parenting competencies (using psychometrically validated instruments) may hold promise for developing the appropriate match between available programs and the needs of prospective participants, more research is needed to identify the relevant criteria for generating this match. This topic is explored in more detail in the next BASSC structured review of family assessment instruments.

DISCUSSION

As this review suggests, significant efforts have been made to demonstrate the efficacy of parent education programs. However, knowledge development in this area has been stymied by the methodological limitations of many of the existing studies reviewed, such as single group designs, small sample sizes, and the infrequent use of alternative conditions that would allow for the selective evaluation of key treatment components. Nonetheless, the majority of studies describe some positive outcomes for participants to suggest that parenting programs may be important mechanisms for changing some aspects of the caregiving environment. However, the linkage between parent education programs and the effective prevention of child maltreatment occurrence or recurrence is less well understood, primarily because studies typically do not monitor these outcomes. Despite these limitations, the evidence base for parent education programs for families involved in child welfare services is growing and we are increasingly able to make recommendations for what we see as promising programs for various stages of a child's development based on the more rigorous research designs (see Figure 5).

Of the programs that we reviewed for parents at-risk or indicated for child maltreatment, home visiting programs appeared to hold the most promise for at-risk parents of young children. Typically, parenting pro-

FIGURE 5. Promising Parent Education Programs

Promising Programs for Parents At Risk or Indicated for Child Maltreatment			
Child's Dev Stage	Program Description	Outcomes	Contact
Prenatal to 3 years	**Home Visitation.** Prevention and early intervention program that typically targets families at-risk of or in early stages for child maltreatment. Program content varies but is typically based in the families' home and seeks to achieve the following objectives: establish a relationship of trust between the professional home visitors and the family, promote maternal-infant attachment, improve parental adoption of health promoting behaviors, promote positive parenting practices, reduce parental stress and improve maternal mood, reduce child abuse potential, and promote the use of community and neighborhood support systems to assist families.	Improved parenting competence[24] and parenting efficacy;[25] Improvement in home environment.[26] Promoted use of non-violent discipline[27] and reduction in parenting stress[28] Fewer child maltreatment reports[29] Decreased injuries from partner violence in the home and linked families with resources;[30] Improved maternal mood adjustment[31]	Ruth A. O'Brien, Ph.D., RN Kempe Prevention Research Ctr. for Family & Child Health 1825 Marion Street Denver, CO 80218 (303) 864-5210 Fax: (303) 864-5236 obrien.ruth@tchden.org **Website:** http://www.strengtheningfamilies.org/html/programs_1999/12_PECNHVP.html
Preschool	**The Incredible Years.** Targets parents with preschool-aged children. The program teaches child-directed play skills, positive discipline strategies, effective parenting skills, strategies for coping with stress, and way to strengthen children's pro-social and social skills. The training is offered either in weekly 2-hr sessions for 8 to 9 or 12 week sessions	Reduction in harsh, negative, inconsistent & ineffective parenting; increase in supportive, positive parenting[1]	Carolyn Webster-Stratton, Ph.D. Director, Parenting Clinic, University of Washington, 1411 Eighth Avenue West, Seattle, WA 98119 Phone and Fax: (206) 285-7565; Toll-Free Phone and Fax: (888) 506-3562 Email: incredibleyears@comcast.net **Website**: www.incredibleyears.com
0-5 years	**Project SafeCare.** Targets parents with children between birth and 5 and have been reported for physical abuse or neglect. In-home service up to 24 weeks designed to improve parenting skills in infant and child health care, home safety and cleanliness, and parent-child interactions to reduce future occurrences of maltreatment.	Improved ability to identify children's health symptoms & seek treatment;[2] Increased use of planned activities & parent training techniques; positive parent behaviors; improvement in home safety;[3] Reductions in home hazards maintained at 4-month follow-up[4] Families who completed all three training components less likely to recidivate. [5] High levels of program satisfaction[6]	John R. Lutzker, Ph.D. Executive Director Marcus Institute 1920 Briarcliff Road, Atlanta, GA 30329 404-419-4000 404-419-4505 (FAX)

Promising Programs for Parents At Risk or Indicated for Child Maltreatment			
Child's Dev Stage	Program Description	Outcomes	Contact
Preschool	**Special Social Support Training Project (SSST).** Targets low-income mothers (age 25-42) with preschool children who are involuntary CPS clients at high risk for child maltreatment. 12-week program is based within a therapeutic nursery school; seeks to strengthen pro-social attitudes and skills needed to build more satisfying relationships with friends, neighbors, and family.	Increase in social network size & quality of contacts; increased satisfaction with social support, increased duration of interactions & % of daily contacts with friends; [7]More daily contact with professional service providers, higher % of daily contact with people in the community; [8]High levels of program satisfaction reported[9]	Madeline L. Lovell, MSW, Ph.D., Director, Social Work Program Department of Society, Justice, & Culture Seattle University 900 Broadway, Seattle WA 98122 206-296-5387; mlovell@seattleu.edu
2-7 years	**Triple-P Positive Parenting Matrix.** Targets parents at risk for child maltreatment. 12-week group-administered program is based in a clinical setting supported with telephone consultation; seeks to reduce parents' negative attributions for children's behavior and reduce risk factors for child maltreatment.	Greater parental self-efficacy; short term improvement on measures of negative parental attributions for child's misbehavior & unrealistic parental expectations; Lower levels of dysfunctional parenting; less relationship conflict; Less parental distress; Short term improvement in potential for child abuse; High levels of consumer satisfaction, lower levels of disruptive child behavior. No significant long-term benefits for children reported[10]	**Website:** http://www.triplep.net/ Email contact@triplep.net Ph: 61 7 3236 1212 Fax: 61 7 3236 1211 Address: Level 3, 424 Upper Roma Street, Brisbane, QLD, 4000, Australia PO Box: 1300 Milton, Qld, 4064, Australia
5-11 years	**Family Connections Program.** Targets at-risk families with children who have no current CPS involvement but exhibit risk for child neglect and abuse. Community-based psychosocial, early intervention seeks to promote the safety and well-being of child and families through family and community services, professional education and training, and research and evaluation.	Increase in appropriate parenting attitudes & satisfaction with parenting; Reduction in parenting stress; Decrease in parent's depressive symptoms, drug use, and child's behavioral problems reported[11]	**Website -** http://www.familyconnections.org/index.htm
4-13 years	**Parent Education vs. Parent Involvement.** Targets parents of emotionally/behaviorally disturbed children removed from the home and placed in residential care. 6-month intervention is based in a residential treatment facility for disturbed children to resocialize parents to more competent parental roles through monitored interaction with their children.	Increase in the movement towards reunification[12]	Paul Carlo, Ph.D, MSW, Director, USC Center on Child Welfare USC School of Social Work University Park Campus Montgomery Ross Fisher Building Los Angeles, CA 90089-0411 nraman@usc.edu

FIGURE 5 (continued)

Promising Programs for Parents At Risk or Indicated for Child Maltreatment			
Child's Dev Stage	**Program Description**	**Outcomes**	**Contact**
Individualized	**Multisystemic Therapy Training (MST) and Parent Training (PT).** Targets abusive and neglectful families. MST is an 8-week individual and tailored family treatment based in home or in clinic, and uses joining, reframing, and prescribed tasks designed to change interaction patterns. PT is an 8-week group treatment based in clinic, and focuses on instructing both parents (when available) in human development and child management techniques to develop parents' capacity to increase positive parent-child interactions and to reduce aversive child behavior.	Improvements in the restructuring of parent-child relations; increased the responsiveness of neglectful parents; Reduced overall stress; Decreased parental psychiatric symptomology; reduction in severity of identified problems; decreased maltreated children's passive compliance[13]	Marshall Swenson, MSW, MBA MST Services, Inc. 710 J. Dodds Boulevard Mount Pleasant, SC 29464 Phone: (843) 856-8226 x11 Fax: (843) 856-8227 Email: marshall.swenson@mstservices.com **Website**: www.mstservices.com or www.mstinstitute.org
Not specified	**Social Network Intervention Project.** Targets neglectful parents with at least 1 child in the home. Case management based program is monitored by a social worker trained in a specialized approach to increasing the social networks of the families, from 2-23 months	Increases in age appropriate expectations, empathic understanding of children, & role reversal attitudes; Improved parenting skills; Increased social networks[14]	James M. Gaudin Jr., Professor The University of Georgia School of Social Work Athens, GA 30602 Phone (706) 542-5454 FAX (706) 542-3282 E-Mail Address: JGAUDIN@UGA.CC.UGA.EDU
Not specified	**Parent Training Program.** Targets emotionally abusive and neglectful parents through weekly sessions covering: 1) developmental counseling, 2) improving parent-child interactions, 3) managing children's and parent's problematic behavior. Program consisted of individual work and a 10 session, 2-hour group meeting.	Reduction in stress and state anxiety; Reduction in frequency of emotionally abuse behavior[15]	Dorota Iwaniec Director of the Institute of Child Care Research, Queen's University of Belfast 5a Lennoxvale, Belfast, BT9 5BY Tel: 028 90 975428 Fax: 028 90 687416 Email: d.iwaniec@qub.ac.uk

Promising Parenting Programs for Substance Abusing Parents			
Child's Dev Stage	Program Description	Outcomes	Estimated Costs
3-8 yrs	**ADVANCE.** Targets families with children who have a history of misconduct and a clinically significantly number of behavioral problems. 26-week program that combines video training with weekly group meetings with a therapist in a clinical setting. Goals are to improve personal self-control, communication skills, problem-solving skills, and strengthen social support and self-care. The ADVANCE program is used in conjunction with a basic parenting program.	Improved problem solving; Improved family relations and family functioning; Improved communication; Improvements in child behavior[16]	Carolyn Webster-Stratton, Ph.D. Director, Parenting Clinic, University of Washington, 1411 Eighth Avenue West, Seattle, WA 98119 Phone and Fax: (206) 285-7565; Toll-Free Phone and Fax: (888) 506-3562 Email: incredibleyears@comcast. net Website: www.incredibleyears.com
<16 yrs	**Relational Psychotherapy Mother's Group (RPMG).** Targets heroin-addicted mothers with children up to 16 years of age. 24-week program is designed to be an "add-on" treatment to methadone maintenance counseling at methadone clinics. This developmentally informed, supportive, nondirective psychotherapy group treatment seeks to address psychosocial vulnerabilities, and facilitating optimal parenting, among at-risk mothers.	More positive psychosocial adjustment;[17] Greater involvement with children;[18] Improvement in parent-child relationship;[19] Improved affective interaction; Lower levels of risk for child maltreatment;[20] At 6 month follow-up post-treatment mothers showed greater improvements in level of opioid use;[21] As maternal interpersonal maladjustment increased, parenting problems improved for RPMG mothers and remained the same or worsened for mothers in standard drug counseling[22]	Suniya S. Luthar, PhD Associate Professor of Psychology and Education, Teachers College, Columbia University Director of Child & Family Research, the APT Foundation, New Haven, CT Email:S/504@Columbia.edu
Promising Culturally Specific Parenting Programs			
Preschool	**The Incredible Years BASIC Program.** Targets parents from minority ethnic backgrounds raising children in low-income, under sourced communities. 12-week program is based in day care centers that seeks to reduce parents' coercive discipline strategies and to decrease child conduct problems in classrooms.	Increases in parenting self-efficacy; Positive effects for parent behavior; parents used more positive and less directive behaviors with toddlers; reduced use of coercive discipline strategies[23]	Carolyn Webster-Stratton, Ph.D. Director, Parenting Clinic, University of Washington, 1411 Eighth Avenue West, Seattle, WA 98119 Phone and Fax: (206) 285-7565; Toll-Free Phone and Fax: (888) 506-3562 Email: incredibleyears@comcast. net **Website:** www.incredibleyears.com

[1] Fraser et al., 2000 [1]
[2] Duggan et al., 1999 [1]
[3] Fraser et al., 2000 [1]
[4] Duggan et al., 1999 [1]

FIGURE 5 (continued)

[5] Fraser et al., 2000 [1]; Duggan et al., 1999 [1]
[6] Eckenrode et al., 2000 [1]
[7] Duggan et al., 1999 [1]
[8] Fraser et al., 2000 [1]
[9] Baydar et al., 2003 [1]
[10] Bigelow & Lutzker, 2000 [3]; Gershater-Molko et al., 2003 [3]
[11] Gershater-Molko et al., 2003 [3]
[12] Mandel et al., 1998 [3]
[13] Gershater-Molko et al., 2002 [1]
[14] Taban & Lutzker, 2001 [2]
[15] Lovell et al., 1992 [3]
[16] Lovell & Richey, 1997 [2]
[17] Lovell & Richey, 1991 [3]
[18] Sanders et al., 2004 [1]
[19] DePanfilis, 2005 [1]
[20] Carlo, 1993 [2]
[21] Brunk et al., 1987 [1]
[22] Gaudin et al., 1990/1991 [2]
[23] Iwaniec, 1997 [2]
[24] Webster- Stratton, 1994 [1]
[25] Luthar & Suchman, 2000 [1]
[26] Luthar & Suchman [1], 2000; Suchman et al., 2004b [1]
[27] Suchman et al., 2004b [1]
[28] Luthar & Suchman, 2000 [1]; Suchman et al., 2004a [1]
[29] Luther & Suchman, 2000 [1]
[30] Suchman et al., 2004a [1]
[31] Gross et al., 2003 [1]

grams represented one component of a larger array of home visiting services. These programs appeared to be the broadest conceptually by addressing multiple domains of the caregiving environment and were also the most rigorously evaluated. However, while effective at post-test, many program gains were lost at follow-up. Several explanations are possible. One suggests that as children develop, their behaviors present parents with new challenges that early intervention education is unlikely to address. Another suggests that while these programs are successful in helping parents to maintain an acceptable level of caregiving during the early years, they may not necessarily be effective in addressing the underlying problems that characterize maltreating families. In either case, it is encouraging that these programs demonstrate short-term improvements in parenting during early childhood when deficits in the caregiving environment may have more detrimental consequences given a young child's vulnerability and dependence. Other literature reviews that have focused specifically on early intervention approaches to the prevention of physical child abuse and neglect have noted that early intervention programs that report positive outcomes employ some form of parenting guidance or education to enhance the parent-infant interaction (e.g., Guterman, 1997), suggesting that direct parenting support is crucial to the success of these programs.

For preschool aged children, The Incredible Years appeared to be effective in reducing harsh, negative, and inconsistent parenting while demonstrating increases in positive parenting (Baydar et al., 2003). The Incredible Years BASIC program was also noteworthy in that it was effective in increasing parenting self-efficacy among parents from ethnic minority backgrounds who were raising children in low-income communities (Gross et al., 2003). The Triple-P Positive Parenting Matrix, with its attributional retraining and anger management focus, demonstrated short-term reductions in potential for child abuse as well as improvements in three domains of the caregiving environment among parents of children 2 to 7 years of age (Sanders et al., 2004). Given the importance of engagement and retention in services for child welfare clients, it was also encouraging to see that this program received high levels of consumer satisfaction.

The Family Connections program (DePanfilis, 2005) and Multisystemic Therapy Training and Parent Training (Brunk et al., 1987) also appear to be promising programs that have demonstrated effectiveness in making changes in certain caregiving domains, such as reducing parenting stress and improving parent-child relations. These programs also reported improvements in specific characteristics that place caregivers at risk of maltreatment, such as reductions in substance use and psychiatric symptomology. Two additional programs that may hold promise for improving the parenting of substance abusing caregivers include the Relational Psychotherapy Mother's Group (RPMG; Luthar & Suchman, 2000; Suchman et al., 2004b) and the ADVANCE program. The RPMG targets heroin-addicted mothers with children up to 16 years of age and is a 24-week "add-on" treatment to methadone maintenance counseling at methadone clinics. ADVANCE targets families with children age 3 to 8 years and is a 26-week program that combines video training with weekly group meetings with a therapist in a clinical setting.

Although evaluations of Project SafeCare were predominately based on single subject designs, this program is promising in that families who completed all three of its training components in child health care, parent-child interaction, and home safety and accident prevention were less likely to recidivate in a randomized control trial. The home safety and cleanliness component of this program is reported to be an efficient and inexpensive method for reducing hazards in the home. At the same time, the project appears to experience a high rate of attrition despite the report of high levels of program satisfaction.

Other approaches that appeared promising in quasi-experimental designs but are in need of more empirical support include the Special Social Support Training Project (Lovell et al.) and Social Network Intervention Project (SNIP; Gaudin, 1990/1991) for neglectful families. Both of these programs demonstrated increased positive influences on the social network size of participants, and in the SNIP, significant changes in parenting skills. Iwaniec's (1997) parent training program achieved significant reductions in emotionally abuse behaviors and Carlo (1993) demonstrated that a combination of parent education and parent involvement in children's residential placement leads to an increased probability of family reunification. These findings, although preliminary, suggest that a number of intervention modalities, either alone or in combination, may be effective in improving child welfare service outcomes.

Previous research has suggested that several factors lead to differential drop-out rates or poorer treatment outcomes. In this review, factors included the presence of domestic violence in the family (Eckenrode et al., 2000); parenting children with more behavioral problems (Fox et al., 1991); participant depression or mental illness (Baydar et al., 2003; Choi et al., 1997); parental poverty and unemployment (Choi et al., 1997); and a participant's African American ethnicity (Timmer et al., 2005). Some factors also appeared to improve retention and program outcomes, including participants that were better educated, older at first pregnancy, and more satisfied with their social support (Hughes & Gottlieb, 2004), as well as participants with fewer risk factors (Landy & Munro, 1996) and participants who were single (Carlsen, 1997). The coupling of the parenting program with other resources was also found to improve parenting outcomes (Chase & Nelson, 2002).

CAVEATS AND CONSIDERATIONS

Though many of the promising programs featured have demonstrated positive changes in parenting, agencies considering the adaptation and/or implementation of these programs should be aware of several caveats (see Figure 6). The conditions under which most research is conducted differs in many ways from the conditions under which programs are delivered in everyday settings. These settings differ in terms of the training and style of the practitioners that implement the

FIGURE 6. Caveats and Considerations in Program Implementation (adapted from Schoenwald & Hoagwood, 2001)

Promising programs replicated in the San Francisco Bay Area may not produce the same results. Sources of variation in program outcomes include:

- Implementation of intervention (e.g. adherence to model, tweaking, modifying components)

- Practitioner characteristics (e.g., training, clinical supervision, type of practitioner)

- Participant characteristics (e.g., developmental stage of child and parent; child welfare referral problems, such as substance use; source of referral, such as judge, social worker, etc.; ethnicity and cultural identification of parents; family context, such as presence of domestic violence; timing of and participation in other services, such as counseling or substance abuse treatment)

- Service delivery characteristics (e.g., physical location of sessions, organizational culture, policies affecting personnel)

- Service system characteristics (e.g., financing methods, interagency working relationships)

program model, the presenting problems of parents and their children, as well as the timing and duration of other services that they may be enrolled in simultaneously. Variation in these characteristics may lead to outcomes that differ from the results presented here. Other factors include the physical location of the sessions, characteristics of the organization responsible for service delivery, as well as other elements of service delivery such as payment and financing. Furthermore, deviations or modifications from the original intervention model will likely lead to outcomes that differ from the results reported here. Therefore, the process of moving a promising program into the practice setting requires decision making about which variables are most relevant, close monitoring of adherence to the program model, and careful measurement and monitoring of outcomes.

RESEARCH RECOMMENDATIONS

While several promising programs were identified, only two programs, home visitation and Project SafeCare (Eckenrode et al., 2000; Gershater-Molko et al., 2002), demonstrated improvement in specific child welfare outcomes with child welfare populations in the most rigorous evaluations. Given the caveats of implementation mentioned in Figure 6, the major message is that more research is necessary to determine the effectiveness of promising programs for child welfare populations in addressing child welfare outcomes of interest.

To build evidence for parenting programs for child welfare we recommend the launch of multi-year research and development projects. Such projects would involve the consensus-based selection of a promising program that ideally has already demonstrated some degree of efficacy in a randomized control trial for implementation in multiple counties or jurisdictions. Such a project would systematically monitor implementation and evaluate program outcomes at multiple time points in relation to child welfare indicators of interest while taking into consideration those parent, child, and programmatic characteristics that typically predict program drop-out for families that come to the attention of the child welfare services system.

PROGRAM IMPLICATIONS

One of the goals of this review was to assist child welfare practitioners in their efforts to identify the most appropriate parenting programs for both contracting as well as referral purposes. There are many issues connected with this goal and they are illustrated in Figure 7 as they relate to contracting decisions. The issues are laid out in the form of a guide for practice that includes key questions that emerged from the literature review. The questions have been categorized into the following sections: (1) program objectives, (2) program content, (3) program implementation, (4) program evaluation, and (5) program costs. Program objectives refer to the relevance of the program for child welfare populations and how these objectives are specified. Along these lines, agencies are encouraged to harness existing information about the characteristics of the families that enter their systems through their administrative databases to better target contracted services. Program content includes the appropriateness of the program for different client populations as well as the elements of the program that are linked to specific outcomes. Program implementation refers to the effectiveness and efficiency of the way the program is managed and how the participants are involved in the program. Program evaluation involves the degree to which the objectives are measured and how they are linked to specified outcomes. Finally, program costs relate to the fees charged for each participant, the cost of related training materials, and the costs associated with follow-up and on-going support.

THEORETICAL IMPLICATIONS

In this review, we opted to conduct two parallel appraisals of the research in the area of parenting programs: (a) critical appraisal of the evidentiary base to assess the extent to which we can infer that a particular parenting program achieves its desired outcomes and to determine the client and setting characteristics to which outcomes are generalizable, and (b) critical appraisal of the conceptual base to assess the extent to which program outcomes are matched to theoretical accounts of maltreating parents and the extent to which theoretical accounts match the realities of child welfare populations and practices. Based on these assessments we identified implications for child welfare agencies to consider for future research and for contracting for parenting education programs. We also identified several implications for theory. Broadly speaking, these questions relate to an overall theme of what we would term "ecological validity." In other words, to what extent are program outcomes matched to theoretical accounts of maltreating parents? To what extent do theoretical accounts match the realities of child welfare populations and practices?

Although links do exist between theory and outcomes, these linkages lack depth and breadth. As mentioned, Azar's theoretical model suggests that attention to each of the five key domains outlined is critical in intervention with maltreating families. Of the studies reviewed, a majority of studies included only one theoretical domain (equally distributed among social cognitive processing or parenting skills). Of the remaining 24, fifteen focused on two domains, mostly including social cognitive processing. Finally, eight included three domains, including a combination of social cognitive processing and parenting skills plus an additional domain of either social skills or stress management. In short, these results suggest a picture of a few multi-pronged programs, a set of programs focused on social cognitive processing and parenting skills in combination, and a set of cognitively based and skills based programs, respectively.

This distribution and patterning of program outcomes across theoretical domains raises several areas of discussion points and implications. A first area of discussion centers on the relationship between program breadth and outcomes. Combining results from our empirical and theoretical appraisals, it appears that more theoretically deep interventions were associated with more positive outcomes. What is less clear is whether this relates to program intensity or whether it reflects strong alignment with key causal mechanisms associated with parenting within maltreating families.

A second area of discussion relates to the question of the specificity of intervention effects. Clearly, the caregiving domains specified in Azar's framework overlap considerably and, as noted above, Azar's own writings clearly implicate the social-cognitive processing domain as central. From the perspective of intervention, this raises the question of whether a single treatment domain or, alternatively, particular combinations of domains appear especially powerful. This is important to consider from the perspective of theory refinement. But it is also has important implications for intervention. From the perspective of child welfare organizations, the more complex the program, the more difficult it is to implement.

A third set of discussion points center around the utility of theoretically-based programs in general. There is always a complex set of trade-offs involved in linking theoretical knowledge to interventions. By definition, theories are abstractions. One set of trade-offs is involved in the process of operationalizing this set of interactions. This raises issues as to the success of the operationalization process. Did we adequately capture the theory in this respect? There is also a second trade-off. Theories are not meant to accurately represent real situations or persons. In short, is there evidence that there is a good enough match between the realities faced by child welfare workers and parents and the general propositions of the theory. In other words, is the Azar framework applicable to practice?

FIGURE 7. Contracting for Parenting Programs (adapted from Mathews & Hudson, 2001)

Relevance of Program Objectives	• Target population? (development stage/problems of parents and/or children) • Behaviors to be affected? (described in measurable terms) • Types of situations? (circumstances or conditions in which the behaviors are to be modified or strengthened?) • Measurement? (standards/criteria for assessing new behaviors) • Frequency of measurement? (specific points in time when measurements will be taken) • Outcome measures? (specific outcomes against which performance of new behaviors will be assessed)
Program Content	• How many of the core parenting issues will be addressed? (social cognitive processing, impulse control, parenting skills, social skills, and stress management?) • How has this content been validated with prior evaluation? (what prior outcomes does the program demonstrate?) • How age-appropriate (children) and adult-learning acceptable are the training methods (experiential, safety hazards, etc.?)
Program Implementation	• To what extent does the advertised program match the actual delivery of the program? (Does content of program match what is described in the materials? Can program demonstrate adherence to original treatment model, if relevant?) • How are parents involved in the program? (attendance, task completion, etc.?) • How are factors related to program drop-out managed? (How are issues related to substance abuse, depression, domestic violence, etc. managed?) • To what extent does the program reflect a manageable capacity to serve clients (how many clients will the program serve per year?)
Program Evaluation	• How are the performance goals for each parent assessed in relationship to the program objectives? (Do the outcomes match up with the program objectives?) • How is the management of program drop out evaluated? (How will the program communicate drop out issues with the child welfare worker?) • How is participant satisfaction monitored throughout the implementation of the program? (Are satisfaction assessments made anonymously or are they completed in the presence of the program managers?) • How is the communication with the child welfare agency (participant progress and participation) assessed?
Program Costs	• What are the costs associated with sending one person through the program? • What are the costs of the training materials and instructor training associated with the program if we were to train our own staff to operate the program? • How do the costs associated with various programs compare with one another? • Are the differences in costs related to differences in outcomes?

A fourth set of discussion points center around the utility of the Azar framework in general. Does the Azar framework appear to adequately cover the sources of parenting issues among maltreating families? Finally, current conceptualizations of child maltreatment draw heavily upon the ecological paradigm. In these models, parenting is one of many factors that place families at risk for maltreatment. Drawing upon these more generalized models of child maltreatment, we might not expect that intervention exclusively focused on parent beliefs and practices would necessarily have a large impact on maltreatment-related outcomes at either the family or child level. While there is an accumulating body of research that maltreating parents have distinct parenting characteristics, we know less about how other key risk factors specifically related to parenting.

REFERENCES

Acton, R. G., & During, S. M. (1992). Preliminary results of aggression for management training for aggressive parents. *Journal of Interpersonal Violence, 7*(3), 410-417.

Adams, J. (2001). Impact of parent training on family functioning. Child *& Family Behavior Therapy, 23*(1), 29-42.

Armstrong, M. I., Birnie-Lefcovitch, S., & Ungar, M. T. (2005). Pathways between social support, family well beings, quality of parenting, and child resilience: What we know. *Journal of Child and Family Studies, 14*(2), 269-281.

Azar, S. T., Povilaitis, T.Y., Lauretti, A.F., & Pouquette, C.L. (1998). The current status of etiological theories in intrafamilial child maltreatment. In J. R. Lutzker (Ed.), *Handbook of Child Abuse Research and Treatment.* (pp. 3-30). New York: Plenum Press.

Azar, S. T., Nix, R.L., & Makin-Byrd, K. N. (2005). Parenting schemas and the process of change. *Journal of Marital and Family Therapy, 31*(1), 45-58.

Barlow, J., & Coren, E. (2001). Parent training programmes for improving maternal psychosocial health. Retrieved 10 September, 2005, from ebn.bmjjournals.com

Barth, R. P., Blythe, B. J., Schinke, S. P., & Schilling, R. F. I. (1983). Self-control training with maltreating parents. *Child Welfare, 62*(4), 313-324.

Barth, R. P., Landsverk, J., Chamberlain, P., Reid, J. B., Rolls, J. A., Hurlburt, M. S. et al. (2005). Parent-training programs in child welfare services: Planning for a more evidence-based approach to serving biological parents. *Research on Social Work Practice, 15*(5), 353-371.

Baumrind, D., & Black, A. E. (1967). Socialization practices associated with dimensions of competence in preschool boys and girls. *Child Development, 38*(2), 291-327.

Baumrind, D. (1971). Harmonious parents and their preschool children. *Developmental Psychology, 4*, 99-102.

Baumrind, D. (1978). Parental disciplinary patterns and social competence in children. *Youth and Society, 9*(3), 239-276.

Bavolek, S. (2005). The nurturing parenting programs. Retrieved May 2005, 2005, from www.nurturingparenting.com/research_validation/index.htm

Baydar, N., Reid, M. J., & Webster-Stratton, C. (2003). The role of mental health factors and program engagement in the effectiveness of a preventative parenting program for head start mothers. *Child Development, 74*(5), 1433-1453.

Belsky, J. (1980). Child maltreatment: An ecological integration. *American Psychologist, 35*(4), 320-335.

Belsky, J. (1984). The determinants of parenting: A process model. *Child Development, 55,* 83-96.

Bigelow, K., & Lutzker, J. (2000). Training parents reported for or at risk for child abuse and neglect to identify and treat their children's Illness. *Journal of Family Violence, 15*(4), 311-330.

Brems, C., Baldwin, M., & Baxter, S. (1993). Empirical evaluation of a self psychologically oriented parent education program. *Family Relations, 42*(1), 26-30.

Britner, P., & Reppucci, D. (1997). Prevention of child maltreatment: Evaluation of a parent education program for teen mothers. *Journal of Child and Family Studies, 6*(2), 165-175.

Browne, D. C. H. (1989). Incarcerated mothers and parenting. *Journal of Family Violence, 4*(5), 211-221.

Brunk, M., Henggeler, S. W., & Whelan, J. P. (1987). Comparison of multisystemic therapy and parent training in the brief treatment of child abuse and neglect. *Journal of Consulting and Clinical Psychology, 55*(2), 171-178.

Carlo, P. (1993). Parent education vs. parent involvement: Which type of efforts work best to reunify families? *Journal of Social Service Research, 17*(1/2), 135-151.

Carlsen, L., & Lightfield, E. (1997). Analysis of the effects of a parenting program upon attitudes and behaviors of abusive parents mandated to participate. *Dissertation Abstracts International, 58*(1), 305-306.

Choi, N. G., Berger, J. L., & Flynn, N. (1997). Effectiveness of a parent-aide services program. Families in Society: *The Journal of Contemporary Human Service*s, September-October, 529-548.

Cicchetti, D. T., S.L. (2005). Child Maltreatment. *Annual Review of Psychology, 1*(1), 409-438.

Conger, R. D., Ge, X., Elder, G.H., Lorenz, F.O., & Simons, R.L. (1994). Economic stress, coercive family process, and developmental problems of adolescents. *Child Development, 65*(2), 541-561.

Conger, R. D., & Conger, K. J. (2002). Resilience in Midwestern families: Selected findings from the first decade of a prospective, longitudinal study. *Journal of Marriage and Family, 64*(2), 361-373.

Constantino, J., Hashemi, N., Solis, E., Alon, T., Haley, S., McClure, S. et al. (2001). Supplementation of urban home visitation with a series of group meetings for parents and infants: Results of a "real-world" randomized, control trial. *Child Abuse & Neglect, 25*(12), 1571-1581.

Cordon, I. M., Lutzker, J. R., Bigelow, K. M., & Doctor, R. M. (1998). Evaluating Spanish protocols for teaching bonding, home safety, and health care skills to a mother reported for child abuse. *Journal of Behavior Therapy and Experimental Psychiatry, 29*(1), 41-54.

Cowen, P. S. (2001). Effectiveness of a parent education intervention for at-risk families. *Journal of the Society of Pediatric Nurses, 6*(2), 73-82.

Culp, A. M., Blankemeyer, M., & Passmark, L. (1998). Parent education home visitation program: Adolescent and nonadolescent mother comparison after six months of intervention. *Infant Mental Health Journal, 19*(2), 111-123.

DeKlyen, M., Speltz, M L., & Greenberg, M. T. (1998). Fathering and early onset conduct problems: Positive and negative parenting, father-son attachment, and the marital context. *Clinical Child and Family Psychology Review, 1*(1), 3-21.

Depanfilis, D. (2005). Demonstrated effective programs: Family connections, 2005, from http://nccanch.acf.hhs.gov/topics/prevention/emerging/report/emergingb.cfm# fam

Dias, M. S., Smith, K., deGuehery, K., Mazur, P., Li, V., & Shaffer, M. (2005). Preventing abusive head trauma among infants and young children: A hospital-based, parent education program. *Pediatrics, 115*(4), e470-477.

Dickinson, N. S., & Cudaback, D. (1992). Parent Education for adolescent mothers. *The Journal of Primary Prevention, 13*(1), 23-35.

Dinkmeyer, D., & McKay, G. D. (1989). *The Parent's Handbook–Systematic Training for Effective Parenting*. Circle Pines, MN: American Guidance Service.

Dix, T. (1991). The affective organization of parenting: Adaptive and maladaptive processes. *Psychological Bulletin, 110*(1), 3-25.

Dornbusch, S. M., Ritter, P. L., Leiderman, H., Roberts, D. F., & Fraleigh, M. J. (1987). The relation of parenting style to adolescent school performance. *Child Development, 58*(5), Special Issue on Schools and Development), 1244-1257.

Ducharme, J. M., Atkinson, L., & Poulton, L. (2001). Errorless compliance training with physically abusive mothers: A single-case approach. *Child Abuse & Neglect, 25*(6), 855-868.

Duggan, A., McFarlane, E., Windham, A., Rohde, C., Salkever, D., Fuddy, L. et al. (1999). Evaluation of Hawaii's Healthy Start Program. *The Future of Children, 9*(1), 66-90.

Duncan, G. J., Brooks-Gunn, J. & Klebanov, P.K. (1994). Economic deprivation and early childhood development. *Child Development, 65*(2), 296-318.

Eckenrode, J., Ganzel, B., Henderson, C. R., Jr., Smith, E., Olds, D., Powers, J. et al. (2000). Preventing child abuse and neglect with a program of nurse home visitation: The limiting effects of domestic violence. *JAMA: Journal of the American Medical Association, 284*(11), 1430-1431.

Fetsch, R. J., Schultz, C. J., & Wahler, J. J. (1999). A preliminary evaluation of the Colorado rethink parenting and anger management program. *Child Abuse & Neglect, 23*(4), 353-360.

Flynn, L. The adolescent parenting program: improving outcomes through mentorship. *Public Health Nursing, 16*(3), 182-189.

Forgatch, M. S., & DeGarmo, D. S. (1999). Parenting through change: An effective prevention program for single mothers. *Journal of Consulting and Clinical Psychology, 67*(5), 711-724.

Fox, R., Fox, T. A., & Anderson, R. (1991). Measuring the effectiveness of the star parenting program with parents of young children. *Psychological Reports, 68*(1), 35-40.

Fraser, J. A., Armstrong, K. L., Morris, J. P., & Dadds, M. R. (2000). Home visiting intervention for vulnerable families with newborns: Follow-up results of a randomized controlled trial. *Child Abuse & Neglect, 24*(11), 1399-1429.

Fricker-Elhai, A., Ruggiero, K., & Smith, D. (2005). Parent-child interaction therapy with two maltreated siblings in foster care. *Clinical Case Studies, 4*(1), 13-39.

Fulton, A., Murphy, K. R., & Anderson, S. L. (1991). Increasing adolescent mothers' knowledge of child development: an intervention program. *Adolescence, 26*(101), 73-81.

Garbarino, J., & Eckenrode, J. (1997). *Understanding Abusive Families: An Ecological Approach to Theory and Practice.* San Francisco: Jossey-Bass.

Gardner, F. E. M. (1987). Positive interaction between mothers and conduct-problem children: Is there training for harmony as well as fighting? *Journal of Abnormal Child Psychology, 15*(2), 283-293.

Gardner, F. E. M., Sonuga-Barke., E. J. S., & Sayal, K. (1999). Parents anticipating misbehavior: An observational study of strategies parents use to prevent conflict with behavior problem children. *Journal of Child Psychology and Psychiatry, 40*(8), 1185-1196.

Gardner, F. E. M., Ward, S., Burton, J., & Wilson, C. (2003). The role of mother-child joint play in the early development of children's conduct problems: A longitudinal observational study. *Social Development, 12*(3), 361-378.

Gaudin, J. M., Wodarski, J. S., Arkinson, M. K., & Avery, L. S. (1990/1991). Remedying child neglect: Effectiveness of social network interventions. *The Journal of Applied Social Sciences, 15*(1), 97-123.

Gelles, R. J. (1985). Family Violence. *Annual Review of Sociology, 11*, 347-367.

Gershater-Malko, R. M., Lutzker, J. R., & Wesch, D. (2002). Using recidivism data to evaluate project safecare: teaching bonding, safety, and health care skills to parent. *Child Maltreatment, 7*(3), 277-285.

Gershater-Malko, R. M., Lutzker, J. R., & Wesch, D. (2003). Project SafeCare: Improving health, safety, and parenting skills in families reported for, and at risk for child maltreatment. *Journal of Family Violence, 18*(8), 377-385.

Golub, J., Espinosa, M., Damon, L., & Card, J. (1987). A videotape parent education program for abusive parents. *Child Abuse & Neglect, 11*(2), 255-265.

Gray, J., Spurway, P., & McClatchey, M. (2001). Lay therapy intervention with families at risk for parenting difficulties: The Kempe Community Caring program. *Child Abuse & Neglect, 25*(5), 641-655.

Gross, D., Fogg, L., Webster-Stratton, C., Garvey, C., Julion, W., & Grady, J. (2003). Parent training of toddlers in day care in low-income urban communities. *Journal of Consulting and Clinical Psychology, 71*(2), 261-278.

Grusec, J. E., & Goodnow, J. J. (1994). Impact of parental discipline methods on the child's internalization of values: A reconceptualization of current points of view. *Developmental Psychology, 30*(1), 4-19.

Guterman, N. B. (1997). Early prevention of physical child abuse and neglect: existing evidence and future directions. *Child Maltreatment, 2*(1), 12-34.

Harm, N. J., & Thompson, P. J. (1997). Evaluating the effectiveness of parent education for incarcerated mothers. *Journal of Offender Rehabilitation, 24*(3/4), 135-152.

Harm, N. J., Thompson, P. J., & Chambers, H. (1998). The effectiveness of parent education for substance abusing women offenders. *Alcoholism Treatment Quarterly, 16*(3), 63-77.

Hebert, M., Lavoie, F., & Parent, N. (2002). An assessment of outcomes following parents' participation in a child abuse prevention program. *Violence and Victims, 17*(3), 355-372.

Herrerías, C. (1988). Prevention of child abuse and neglect in the Hispanic community: The MADRE parent education program. *Journal of Primary Prevention, 9*(1&2), 104-119.

Hess, C. R., Papas, M. A., & Black, M. M. (2002). Resilience among African Americian adoelescent mothers: Predictors of positive parenting in early infancy. *Journal of Pediatric Psychology, 27*(7), 619-629.

Hoghughi, M., & Speight, A. N. P. (1998). Good enough parenting for all children - a strategy for a healthier society. *Archives of Disease in Childhood, 78*(4), 293-296.

Holden, G. W. (1983). Avoiding conflict: Mothers as tacticians in the supermarket. *Child Development, 54*(1), 233-240.

Huebner, C. E. (2002). Evaluation of a clinic-based parent education program to reduce the risk of infant and toddler maltreatment. *Public Health Nursing, 19*(5), 377-389.

Hughes, J. R., & Gottlieb, L. N. (2004). The effects of the Webster-Stratton parenting program on maltreating families: Fostering strengths. *Child Abuse & Neglect, 28*(10), 1081-1097.

Iwaniec, D. (1997). Evaluating parent training for emotionally abusive and neglectful parents: Comparing individual versus individual and group intervention. *Research on Social Work Practice, 7*(3), 329-349.

Jarrett, R. L. (1999). Successful parenting in high-risk neighborhoods. *The Future of Children, 9*(2), 45-50.

Joyce, M. R. (1995). Emotional relief for parents: Is rational-emotive parent education effective? *Journal of Rational-Emotive & Cognitive-Behavior Therapy, 13*(1), 55-75.

Kacir, C. D., & Gordon, D. A. (1999). Parenting adolescents wisely: The effectiveness of an interactive videodisk parent training program in appalachia. *Child & Family Behavior Therapy, 21*(4), 1-22.

Koger, D., Jodi, S., & Contreras, D. (2003). *The influence of a home visitation, parent education program on parenting behaviors: Are changes substantiated over time?* Paper presented at the The 65th National Council on Family Relations Annual Conference, Vancouver, BC Canada.

Kotchick, B. A., & Forehand, R. (2002). Putting parenting in perspective: A discussion of the contextual factors that shape parenting practices. *Journal of Child and Family Studies, 11*(3), 255-269.

Landy, S., & Munro, S. (1998). Shared parenting: Assessing the success of a foster parent program aimed at family reunification. *Child Abuse & Neglect, 22*(4), 305-318.

Lovell, M. L., Reid, K., & Richey, C. A. (1992). Social support training for abusive mothers. *Social Work with Groups, 15*(2-3), 95-107.

Lovell, M. L., & Richey, C. (1991). Implementing agency-based social-support skill training. *Families in Society: The Journal of Contemporary Human Service, 72*(9), 563-572.

Lovell, M. L., & Richey, C. A. (1997). The impact of social support skill training on daily interactions among parents at risk for child maltreatment. *Children and Youth Services Review, 19*(4), 221-251.

Luthar, S., & Suchman, N. (2000). Relational psychotherapy mothers' group: A developmentally informed intervention for at-risk mothers. *Development and Psychopathology, 12*(2), 235-253.

Lutzker, J. R., Bigelow, K. M., Doctor, R. M., & Kessler, M. L. (1998). Safety, health care, and bonding within an ecobehavioral approach to treating and preventing child abuse and neglect. *Journal of Family Violence, 13*(2), 163-185.

MacMillan, H. L., & Thomas, B. H. (1993). Public health nurse home visitation for the tertiary prevention of child maltreatment: Results of a pilot study. *Canadian Journal of Psychiatry, 38*(6), 436-442.

MacMillan, H. L., Thomas, B. H., Jamieson, E., Walsh, C., Boyle, M., Shannon, H. et al. (2005). Effectiveness of home visitation by public-health nurses in prevention of the recurrence of child physical abuse and neglect: A randomised controlled trial. *The Lancet, 365*(9473), 1786-1793.

MacMillan, V. M., Guevremont, D. C., & Hansen, D. J. (1988). Problem-solving training with a multiply distressed abusive and neglectful mother: Effects on social insularity, negative affect, and stress. *Journal of Family Violence, 3*(4), 313-326.

Mandel, U., Bigelow, K., M. & Lutzker, J. R. (1998). Using video to reduce home safety hazards with parents reported for child abuse and neglect. *Journal of Family Violence, 13*(2), 147-162.

Matthews, J. M., & Hudson, A. M. (2001). Guidelines for evaluating parent training programs. *Family Relations, 50*(1), 77-86.

McCabe, K., Yeh, M., Garland, A. F., Lau, A. S., & Chavez, G. (2005). The GANA program: A tailoring approach to adapting parent child interaction therapy for Mexican Americans. *Education & Treatment of Children, 28*(2), 111-129.

McGrogan, K. L. (1998). *The development and pilot test in a community center of a Latino parenting group for limited-literacy, Spanish-speaking families with children at risk.* New Jersey: Rutgers, State University of New Jersey.

McInnis-Dittrich, K. (1996). Violence prevention: An ecological adaptation of systematic training for effective parenting. *Families in Society: The Journal of Contemporary Human Services, 77*(7), 414-422.

McLoyd, V. C. (1998). Socioeconomic disadvantage and child development. *American Psychologist, 53*(2), 185-204.

Mennen, F. E., & Trickett, P. (2006). *Parenting Attitudes, Family Environments, and Psychopathology in Maltreating and Non Maltreating Urban Parents.* Presented at the 10th Annual Conference of the Society for Social Work and Research, January 12-15, 2006, San Antonio, TX.

Moore, J., & Finkelstein, N. (2001). Parenting services for families affected by substance abuse. *Child Welfare, 80*(2), 221-238.

Murry, V. M., Bynum, M. S., Brody, G. H., Willert, A., & Stephens, D. (2001). African American single mothers and children in context: A review of studies on risk and resilience. *Clinical Child and Family Psychology Review, 4*(2), 133-155

Naughton, A., & Heath, A. (2001). Developing an early intervention programme to prevent child maltreatment. *Child Abuse Review, 10*(2), 85-96.

Nayman, L., & Witkin, S. (1978). Parent-child foster placement: An alternate approach in child abuse and neglect. *Child Welfare, 57*(4), 249-258.

National Clearinghouse on Child Abuse and Neglect Information (NCCAN). (2003). *Foster Care National Statistics.* Washington, DC: U.S. Department of Health and Human Services.

Openshaw, K. D., Mills, T., A., Adams, G. R., & Durso, D. D. (1992). Conflict resolution in parent-adolescent dyads: The influence of social skills training. *Journal of Adolescent Research, 7*(4), 457-468.

Orthner, D. K., Jones-Sanpei, H., & Williamson, S. (2004). The resilience and strengths of low-income families. *Family Relations, 53*(2), 159-167.

Pehrson, K. L., & Robinson, C. C. (1990). Parent education: Does it make a difference. *Child Study Journal, 20*(4), 221-236.

Peterson, L., Termblay, G., Ewigman, B., & Popkey, C. (2002). The parental daily diary. *Behavior Modification, 26*(5), 627-647.

Peterson, L., Tremblay, G., Ewigman, B., & Saldana, L. (2003). Multilevel selected primary prevention of child maltreatment. *Journal of Consulting and Clinical Psychology, 71*(3), 601-612.

Pettit, G. S., & Bates, J. E. (1989). Family interaction patterns and children's behavior problems from infancy to 4 years. *Developmental Psychology, 25*(3), 413-420.

Pettit, G. S., Laird, R. D., Dodge, K. A., Bates, J. E., Criss, M. M. (2001). Antecedents and behavior-problem outcomes of parental monitoring and psychological control in early adolescence. *Child Development, 72*(2), 583-598.

Pinkston, E., & Smith, M. D. (1998). Contributions of parent training to child welfare: Early history and current thoughts. In J. R. Lutzker (Ed.), *Handbook of Child Abuse Research and Treatment: Issues in Clinical Child Psychology* (pp. 377-399). New York: Plenum Press.

Price, A., & Wichterman, L. (2003). Shared family care: Fostering the whole family to promote safety and stability. *Journal of Family Social Work, 7*(2), 35-54.

Repetti, R. L., Taylor, S.E., & Seeman, T.E. (2002). Risky families: Family social environments and the mental and physical health of offspring. *Psychological Bulletin, 128*(2), 330-366.

Riesch, S.K., Henriques, J., & Chanchong, W. (2003). Effects of communication skills training on parents and young adolescents from extreme family types. *Journal of Child and Adolescent Psychiatric Nursing, 16*(4), 162-175.

Riley, D., Meinhardt, G., Nelson, C., Salisbury, M., & Winnett, T. (1991). How effective are age-paced newsletters for new parents–A replication and extension of earlier studies. *Family Relations, 40*(3), 247-253.

Roberts, C., Wolman, C., & Harris-Looby, J. (2004/05). Project Baby Care: A parental training program for students with emotional and behavioral disorders (EBD). *Issues in Education, 81*, 101-103.

Russell, A., & Russell, G. (1996). Positive parenting and boys' and girls' misbehaviour during a home observation. *International Journal of Behavioral Development, 19*(2), 291-308.

Russell, A. (1997). Individual and family factors contributing to mothers' and fathers' positive parenting. *International Journal of Behavioral Development, 21*(1), 111-132.

Sanders, M. R., Pidgeon, A. M., Gravestock, F., Connors, M. D., Brown, S., & Young, R. W. (2004). Does parental attributional retraining and anger management enhance the effects of the Triple P-Positive Parenting Program with parents at risk of child maltreatment? *Behavior Therapy, 35*(3), 513-535.

Saxe, H. B. (1997). The impact of the Los Angeles unified school district's skillful parenting program on the prevention of child abuse and neglect on parents with alcohol or drug-related histories. *Dissertation Abstracts International Section A: Humanities & Social Sciences, 58*(6-A), 2074.

Schoenwald, S. K., & Hoagwood, K. (2001). Effectiveness, transportability, and dissemination of interventions: What matters when? *Psychiatric Services, 52*(9), 1190-1197.

St. Pierre, R., & Layzer, J. (1999). Using home visits for multiple purposes: The comprehensive child development program. *The Future of Children, 9*(1), 134-151.

Steinberg, L., Elmen, J. D., & Mounts, N. S. (1989). Authoritative parenting, psychosocial maturity, and academic success among adolescents. *Child Development, 60*(6), 1424-1436.

Steinberg, L., Lamoborn, S. D., Dornbusch, S. M., & Darling, N. (1992). Impact of parenting practices on adolescent achievement: Authoritative parenting, school involvement, and encouragement to succeed. *Child Development, 63*(5), 1266-1281.

Suchman, N., Mayes, L., Conti, J., Slade, A., & Rounsaville, B. (2004). Rethinking parenting interventions for drug-dependent mothers: From behavior management to fostering emotional bonds. *Journal of Substance Abuse Treatment, 27*(3), 179-185.

Suchman, N.E., McMahon, T.J., & Luthar, S.S. (2004). Interpersonal maladjustment as predictor of mothers' response to a relational parenting intervention. *Journal of Substance Abuse Treatment, 27*(2), 135-143.

Taban, N., & Lutzker, J. R. (2001). Consumer evaluation of an ecobehavioral program for prevention and intervention of child maltreatment. *Journal of Family Violence, 16*(3), 323-330.

Taylor, J., Spencer, N., & Baldwin, N. (2000). Social, economic, and political context of parenting. *Archives of Disease in Childhood, 82*(2), 113-117.

Taylor, K. D., & Beauchamp, C. (1988). Hospital-based primary prevention strategy in child abuse: A multi-level needs assessment. *Child Abuse & Neglect, 12*(3), 343-354.

Timmer, S., Urquiza, A. J., Zebell, N. M., & McGrath, J. M. (2005). Parent-child interaction therapy: Application to maltreatment parent-child dyads. *Child Abuse & Neglect, 29*(7), 825-842.

Toth, S. L., Maughan, A., Manly, J.T., Spagnola, M., & Cichetti, D. (2002). The relative efficacy of two interventions in altering maltreated preschool children's representational models: Implications for attachment theory. *Development and Psychopathology, 14*(4), 877-908.

Velez, M., Jansson, L., Montoya, I., Schweitzer, W., Archie, G., & Svikis, D. (2004). Parenting knowledge among substance abusing women in treatment. *Journal of Substance Abuse Treatment, 27*(3), 215-222.

Villegas, A. V. (1997). *The efficacy of systematic training for effective parenting with Chicana mothers.* Arizona State University: UMI Dissertation Services HQ 755.7 V544.

Walsh, F. (2002). A family resilience framework: Innovative practice applications. *Family Relations, 51*(2), 130-137.

Webster-Stratton, C. (1994). Advancing videotape parent training: A comparison study. *Journal of Consulting and Clinical Psychology, 62*(3), 583-593.

Weinman, M.L., Schreiber, N.B., & Robinson, M. (1992). Adolescent mothers: Were there any gains in a parent education program? *Family & Community Health, 15*(3), 1-10.

Whipple, E. E. (1999). Reaching families with preschoolers at risk of physical child abuse: What works? *Families in Society: The Journal of Contemporary Human Services, 80*(2), 148-160.

Wolfe, D.A., Edwards, B., Manion, I., & Koverola, C. (1988). Early intervention for parents at risk of child abuse and neglect: A preliminary investigation. *Journal of Consulting and Clinical Psychology, 56*(1), 40-47.

Wolfe, D.A., Sandler, J., & Kaufman, K. (1981). A competency-based parent training program for child abusers. *Journal of Consulting and Clinical Psychology, 49*(5), 633-640.

Wolfe, R. B., & Hirsch, B. J. (2003). Outcomes of a parent education program based on reevaluation counseling. *Journal of Child and Family Studies, 12*(1), 61-76.

APPENDIX A. BASSC Search Protocol

Search Terms

parent training, parent skills, parent education, child welfare, child mal-treatment, abuse, neglect, outcome, intervention, and evaluation

Databases

Academic databases for books and articles
Pathfinder or Melvyl
ArticleFirst
Current Contents Database
ERIC
Expanded Academic ASAP
Family and Society Studies Worldwide
PAIS International
PsychInfo
Social Science Citation Index
Social Services Abstracts
Social Work Abstracts
Sociological Abstracts

Systematic Reviews

Cochrane Collaboration
Campbell Collaboration

Reference lists from primary & review articles

Research Institutes

Mathmatica
Urban Institute
RAND
GAO
National Academy of Sciences
Chapin Hall
CASRC (San Diego)

Brookings Institute

Manpower Demonstration Research Corporation
Annie E. Casey Foundation

Conference proceedings

PapersFirst (UCB Database)
Proceedings (UCB Database)

Dissertation Abstracts

DigitalDissertations (UCB database)

Professional Evaluation Listserves

Child Maltreatment

Internet

Google
Dogpile

Experts / personal contacts

Exclusion/Inclusion Criteria

Exclusion Criteria:

Articles describing parenting interventions focused primarily on children's behavioral outcomes
Articles describing parenting interventions for improving children's educational outcomes, court based programs for parenting in the context of divorce and custody, programs focused on parenting children with special needs
Articles describing interventions or program approaches with no data
Studies that provided only descriptive data with no outcome data
Studies that reported preliminary results for which a subsequent evaluation provided full results
Studies that provided no description of the intervention

Inclusion Criteria:

Experimental randomized controlled trials
Quasi-experimental designs: pre and post tests/ no control group, control group that is not randomized, comparing groups that differed in the dosage of treatment they received.
Single group designs

PART II

EVIDENCE FOR MANAGEMENT PRACTICE

Evidence-Based Practice in the Social Services: Implications for Organizational Change

Michelle Johnson, PhD
Michael J. Austin, PhD

SUMMARY. Evidence-based practice integrates individual practitioner expertise with the best available evidence while also considering the values and expectations of clients. Research can be categorized into two broad areas: primary (experiments, clinical trials, and surveys) and secondary research (overviews of major studies, practice guidelines, and decision and economic analyses). One of the major challenges to incorporating research evidence into organizational life is the absence of an evidence-based organizational culture within human service agencies. This article identifies multiple strategies and case examples for creating such an organizational culture. Three major implications emerge from this analysis: (a) agency- university partnerships to identify the data to support evidence-based practice, (b) staff training (in the agencies and

Michelle Johnson is a Doctoral Research Assistant and Michael J. Austin is Professor, School of Social Welfare, University of California, Berkeley.

This article was originally published in *Administration in Social Work*, Vol. 30 (3) 2006. © 2006 by The Haworth Press, Inc on campuses) that features problem-based learning approaches to support the introduction and utilization of evidence-based practice, and (c) the modification of agency cultures to support and sustain evidence-based practice.

KEYWORDS. Evidence-based practice, social services, organizational change

INTRODUCTION

The use of research evidence to guide practice and develop policies in the human services has become increasingly important given the limited resources and the pressures to document service outcomes. These pressures have emerged from increased scrutiny of public expenditures and the call for information about the impact of interventions on the reduction or elimination of social problems. The most significant progress in the testing and evaluation of interventions has been made in the field of health care. For example, in the United Kingdom (U.K.) National Health Service, all doctors, nurses, pharmacists, and other health professionals now have a contractual duty to provide clinical care based on the best available research evidence. The establishment of the Cochrane Collaboration, a worldwide network designed to prepare, maintain, and disseminate high-quality systematic reviews of research on the outcomes and the effects of health care interventions began in the early 1990s (Bero & Rennie, 1995). In 1999, the Cochrane model was replicated in the fields of social science, social welfare and education with the launch of the Campbell Collaboration. Meanwhile, empirically-based governmental initiatives such as the Child and Family Service (CFS) Reviews have emerged in the U.S. to ensure that state child welfare agency practice is in conformity with federal child welfare requirements and national standards through the use of qualitative and quantitative information sources.

What has become clear, however, is that the reliance on the random diffusion of a growing volume of research information to health and human service professionals is unlikely to adequately inform staff or improve client services. For example, Kirk and Penska (1992) found that of 276 randomly selected U.S. MSW-trained social workers, 92 percent reported reading at least one professional article a month. However, the extent to which practitioners implement research findings in practice is unclear. Conventional continuing education activities, such as conferences and courses that focus largely on the transfer of knowledge, appear to have little impact on the behavior of health professionals. The circulation of guidelines without an implementation strategy is also unlikely to result in changes in practice (Bero et al., 1998; Gira, Kessler, & Poertner, 2003).

For research evidence to impact practice and policy, scholars have identified at least five requirements: (a) agreement on the nature of evidence, (b) a strategic approach to the creation of evidence and the development of a cumulative knowledge base, (c) effective research dissemination approaches combined with effective strategies for accessing knowledge, (d) initiatives to increase the use of evidence in both policy and practice, and (e) a variety of action steps at the organizational level (Davies & Nutley, 2001; Kitson, Harvey, & McCormack, 1998). The purpose of this analysis is to consider evidence-based practice in the context of complex human service organizations. We begin by exploring the nature of the evidence base and issues related to the translation of research findings into agency practice. We then review key findings from studies that have examined issues related to the integration of evidence at the organizational level and provide recommendations for future work in this area.

WHAT IS EVIDENCE-BASED PRACTICE?

The concept of evidence-based practice (EBP) was first developed by a Canadian medical group at McMaster University. The group defined EBP as a process that includes "the conscientious, explicit, and judicious use of current best evidence in making decisions about the care of individuals" (Sackett, Richardson, Rosenberg, & Haynes, 1997). The process itself involves the following steps: (a) becoming motivated to apply evidence-based practice, (b) converting information needs into a well-formulated answerable question, (c) achieving maximum efficiency by tracking down the best evidence with which to answer the question (which may come from the clinical examination, the diagnostic laboratory, the published literature or other sources), (d) critically appraising the evidence for its validity and applicability to clinical practice, (e) applying the results of this evidence appraisal to policy/practice, (f), evaluating performance, and (g) teaching others to do the same (Sackett et al., 1997; Greenhalgh, 2001). According to Gambrill (1999), a notable feature of EBP process is the attention that is given to the values and expectations of clients and to their active involvement in decision-making processes. Evidence-based social work practice involves clients as informed participants by searching for practice-related research findings related to important decisions and sharing the results of such a search with clients. If no evidence can be found to support a service decision, the client needs to be informed and practitioners need to describe their rationale for making recommendations to clients.

Sackett and his colleagues (1997) suggest that the problem-based EBP approach to learning can increase the ability of practitioners to help clients by providing opportunities to access newly generated evidence, update practitioner knowledge to improve performance (which is often subject to deterioration), and overcome some of the deficiencies that are present in traditional continuing education programs.

WHAT IS THE BEST EVIDENCE?

There are differing opinions about what information is considered appropriate for implementing evidence-based practice. In general, research evidence can be divided into two broad categories: primary and secondary research. Primary research includes: (a) experiments, where an intervention is tested in artificial and controlled surroundings, (b) clinical trials, where an intervention is offered to a group of participants that are then followed up to see what happens to them, and (c) surveys, where something is measured in a group of participants. Secondary research includes: (a) overviews or summaries of primary studies, which may be conducted systematically according to rigorous and predefined methods (such as procedures used in the Cochrane Collaboration) or may integrate numerical data from more than one study as in the case of meta-analyses; (b) guidelines that are used to draw conclusions from primary studies about how practitioners should behave; (c) decision analyses that use the results of primary studies to generate probability trees for use in making choices about clinical management or resource allocation, and (d) economic analyses that use the results of primary studies to find out whether a particular course of action is a good use of resources. Traditionally, the import and relevance of evidence has been arrayed hierarchically with systematic reviews considered to be the best evidence and case reviews considered to be the least rigorous as noted in Figure 1.

The hallmark of EBP is the systematic and rigorous appraisals of research related to relevant practice questions. The primary focus is on the validity of assessment measures and the effectiveness of interventions. For example, systematic reviews prepared for the Cochrane Collaboration require reviewers to clearly state decision-making rules for each stage of the process with respect to how studies were identified and the

FIGURE 1. Hierarchy of Evidence from a Research Perspective*

Research Design	Description
Systematic reviews and meta-analyses	Secondary research papers where all primary studies on a particular topic have been critically appraised using rigorous criteria
Randomised controlled trials with (a) definitive results (i.e., confidence intervals which do not overlap the threshold clinically significant effect), and (b) non-definitive results (i.e., a point estimate which suggests a clinically significant effect but with confidence intervals overlapping the threshold for this effect)	Participants are randomly allocated by a process equivalent to the flip of a coin to either one intervention or another. Both groups are followed up for a specified time period and analyzed in terms of specific outcomes defined at the outset of the study.
Cohort studies	Two or more groups of individuals are selected on the basis of differences in their exposure to a particular agent and followed up to see how many in each group develop a particular condition or other outcome
Case-control studies	Participants with a particular condition are identified and "matched" with control cases. Data are then collected on past exposure to a possible causal agent for the condition. Case-control studies are generally concerned with the etiology of a condition rather than treatment.
Cross-sectional surveys	A sample of participants are interviewed, examined, or otherwise studied to gain answers to a specific question. Data are collected at a single time-point but may refer retrospectively to experiences in the past.
Case reports	A case report describes the history of a single participant in the form of a story. Case reports are often run together to from a case series in which the histories of more than one participant with a particular condition are described to illustrate an aspect of the condition, the treatment, or their adverse reaction to treatment.

* Adapted from Guyatt, G. H., Sackett, D. L., Sinclair J. C., Hayward, R., Cook, D. J., Cook, R., J. (1995). Users' guides to the medical literature. IX. A method for grading health care recommendations. *Journal of the American Medical Association, 174*, 1800-1804.

criteria they used to assess the methodology used, the quality of the findings and the ways in which the data were extracted, combined and analyzed (Oxman & Guyatt, 1993).

The development of systematic reviews for the human services is still in its infancy but is growing largely due to the efforts of the Campbell Collaboration, a sibling of the Cochrane organization for research reviews in the social and behavioral sectors, criminology, and education. The inaugural meeting of the Campbell Collaboration was held in February 2000 at the University of Pennsylvania and attended by 85 participants representing thirteen countries that reflected the international interest and momentum. Today the Campbell Collaboration houses over 12,000 randomized and possibly randomized trials in education, social work and welfare, and criminal justice. It provides free access to reviews and review-related documents in these content areas.

However, in considering the traditional hierarchy of evidence, some scholars note that evaluating the potential contribution of a particular study requires considerably more effort than simply examining its basic design. For example, a methodologically flawed meta-analysis would rarely be placed above a large, well-designed cohort study. Further, many important secondary types of research, such as guidelines, economic and decision analyses, qualitative studies, and evaluations of risk assessment, which are of particular salience for child and family services are not included in this hierarchy of research methodologies. As a general rule, the type of evidence needed will depend, to a large extent, on the type of questions asked. Figure 2 illustrates the broad topic categories and preferred study designs for addressing questions that emerge in child and family services. For example, the randomized controlled trial is preferred for the determination of treatment effectiveness, whereas a cross-sectional survey may be sufficient to demonstrate the validity and reliability of an assessment instrument.

Up to this point, the focus has been on the hierarchy of research methods used to generate evidence. However, there is another way of viewing evidence; namely, the multiple sources of knowledge that are available to practitioners who seek to engage in evidence-based practice. Based on the work of the Social Care Institute for Excellence in London, Pawson et al. (2003) have identified five types of knowledge that could relate to evidence-based practice. As defined in Figure 3, the first domain includes evidence supplied by users or consumers of social services as well as the family members, volunteers, and others who assist service users and are considered to be paraprofessionals (e.g., foster parents, home health aides, volunteers, etc.). This domain of knowledge is

FIGURE 2. Topic Categories and Preferred Study Designs*

Topic	Purpose	Study Design
Treatment Effectiveness	Testing the efficacy of treatments, procedures, client education, or other interventions	Preferred study design is the randomized controlled trial
Diagnosis/Assessment	Demonstrating whether a new test or assessment is valid (can we trust it?) and reliable (would we get the same results every time?)	Preferred study design is the cross-sectional survey in which both the new test and the gold standard test are performed
Screening/Prevention	Demonstrating the value of tests that can be applied to large populations and that pick up disease at a presymptomatic stage	Preferred study design is cross-sectional survey
Prognosis	Determining what is likely to happen to someone whose disease is picked up at an early stage (e.g., risk assessment)	Preferred study design is the longitudinal cohort study
Causation	Determining whether a putative harmful agent is related to the development of a condition	Preferred study design is cohort or case-control study, depending on how rare the disease is, but case reports may also provide crucial information

* Adapted from Greenhalgh, T. (2001). *How to Read a Paper: The Basics of Evidence Based Medicine.* (2ⁿᵈ ed.). London: BMJ Books.

rarely captured and reported in the practice literature but represents another perspective on Gambrill's (1999) notion of client involvement. If this domain is placed on a hierarchy of knowledge, some would suggest that this represents the highest level in assessing the outcomes of services.

The next domain in Figure 3 refers to practitioner knowledge, often poorly researched except in the form of practice guidelines. Practitioner knowledge can be viewed from the perspectives of both line staff and management staff. The next level in the hierarchy involves organizational knowledge, sometimes codified in policy and procedure manuals and often reflected in administrative data. Similar to organizational knowledge, policy knowledge is captured in both the policy development stage (white papers and legislative testimony) and the policy implementation stage (outcome and process studies). And finally, research as noted earlier in Figure 1 comprises the generally accepted method of compiling knowledge related to service users and providers as well as organizational and policy specialists. Based on these research and practice hierarchies, it is instructive to consider how the translation of other empirically-based materials might improve social services.

FIGURE 3. Hierarchy of Knowledge from a Practice Perspective*

Service User and Care Provider Knowledge As active participants in the use or provision of services, service users possess often unspoken and undervalued knowledge gained from the use of and reflection on various interventions. Similarly, paraprofessional providers of care (e.g., foster parents, home health assistants, volunteers, etc.) have unspoken and undervalued knowledge gained from the provision of various interventions.
Professional Practitioner Knowledge *Line staff:* Practitioners possess tacit knowledge, often shared informally with colleagues, that is based on their repeated experiences in dealing with clients of similar backgrounds and problems. Similarly, practitioners have acquired knowledge how organizations function to facilitate or inhibit service delivery, how policy changes impact service delivery, and how community (neighborhood) factors influence service provision. This knowledge tends to be acquired one practitioner at a time and specific to service settings and may be difficult to articulate and aggregate. *Management staff:* Practitioners at the supervisory, middle management, or senior management levels have acquired knowledge about client populations, staff experiences, internal organizational dynamics, and external inter-agency dynamics that also tends to be acquired one practitioner at a time and may be difficult to articulate and aggregate.
Organizational Knowledge Often assembled in the form of policies and procedures manuals, organizational knowledge also includes administrative data gathered on a regular basis to account for the number of clients served, the outcomes of service, and the costs associated with service provision. The aggregation of this data is captured in quarterly or annual reports to funding sources (government, foundations, and donors) and to the community at large.
Policy Knowledge Often assembled in the form of legislative reports, concept papers, grand jury investigations, court decisions, technical reports, and monographs from research institutes, this form of knowledge focuses on what is known that could inform policy development or what has been learned from policy implementation that can inform administrative practice as well as future policy development.
Research Knowledge Often derived from empirical studies utilizing an array of quantitative and qualitative research methodologies, this knowledge is displayed in research reports, service evaluations, and service instrumentation (see hierarchy of research methodologies noted in Figure 1). It is also possible for research knowledge acquisition to focus on one or more of the previous categories noted above (user/carer, practitioner, organizational, and policy)

*Adapted from Pawson, R, Boaz, A. Grayson, L., Long, A. & Barnes, C. (2003). *Types and Quality of Knowledge in Social Care*. London, UK: Social Care Institute for Excellence.

Best Practices and Guidelines

The mushrooming guidelines industry owes its success, in part, to the growing "accountability culture" that is now being set in statute in many countries and within many fields. Officially produced or sanctioned guidelines, defined as "systematically developed statements to assist practitioner decisions about appropriate care for specific clinical circumstances" (Greenhalgh, 2001, p. 140) are used to achieve several objectives in the provision of clinical care. Practice guidelines are designed to make standards explicit and accessible, simplify clinical decision making, and improve cost effectiveness. Practice guidelines are also used to assess professional performance, to externally control practitioners, to delineate divisions of labor, and to educate patients and professionals about best practices. Despite these benefits, there are drawbacks to the use of guidelines and best practice statements when they reflect "expert opinion" that may have, in fact, formalized unsound practices. For example, Bartels et al. (2002) cautioned that in interdisciplinary fields, the consensus of experts may inadvertently incorporate disciplinary biases. Similarly, practice guidelines developed at national or regional levels may not reflect local needs, ownership by local practitioners, or differences in demographic or clinical factors. The wholesale implementation of practice guidelines may have the effect of inhibiting innovation and preventing individualized approaches to treatment. Furthermore, by reducing practice variation, guidelines may standardize "average" rather than best practice. The drawbacks include legal and political dimensions. For example, judicial decisions could use practice guidelines to determine competent practice or shift the balance of power between different professional groups (e.g., between clinicians and administrators or purchasers and providers).

Gibbs (2003) recommends the use of guidelines that can be easily interpreted as disconfirming and confirming evidence based on thorough search procedures and objective standards for evaluating evidence. For example, Saunders, Berliner, and Hanson (2003) note that recently released guidelines for the mental health assessment and treatment of child abuse victims and their families were developed by an advisory committee of clinicians, researchers, educators, and administrators for the U.S. Office for Victims of Crime. They evaluated the treatment protocols based on their theoretical grounding, anecdotal clinical evidence, acceptance among practitioners in the child abuse field, potential for causing harm, and empirical support for utility with victims of abuse. The manual advises readers that treatment protocols with the highest levels of empirical and clinical support should be considered "first choice" interventions. Appendix A provides an example of a guideline considered "well-supported and efficacious."

Groups that have researched the effectiveness of guidelines conclude that the most effective guidelines have been: (a) developed locally by the people who are going to use them, (b) introduced as part of a specific educational intervention, and (c) implemented via a client specific prompt that appears at the time of the consultation (Greenhalgh, 2001). While local adoption and ownership is crucial to the success of a guideline or best practice program, local practitioners also need to draw upon the range of resources available from national and international databases related to evidence-based practice.

While there are many approaches to the development and implementation of practice guidelines, the research partnership between the Children and Family Research Center of the University of Illinois at Urbana-Champaign and the Illinois Department of Children and Family Services demonstrates an important collaborative effort. Through this partnership, the Department of Children and Family Services (Research Practice Integration Committee) selects and prioritizes Center-funded research projects for use in agency practice. The Center develops the research questions, methodology, and findings; this is followed by a joint agency-university effort to identify the implications for practice. Members of the partnership draft clinical procedures linked to caseworker behaviors. After a process of discussion and refinement among the partners, the clinical procedures and caseworker behaviors are reviewed and approved by the Department's Best Practices Committee before they are integrated into departmental policies and training programs. The resulting practice guides are shared with staff and illustrated in Appendix B. Emerging and Promising Practices

The documentation of emerging and promising practices related to innovative programs and interventions can provide practitioners and policy makers with ideas that may be transferable to other settings. For example, in 2001 the Office on Child Abuse and Neglect (OCAN) initiated a project on the *Emerging Practices in the Prevention of Child Abuse and Neglect* to feature and share the designs and outcomes of effective and innovative programs for the prevention of child maltreatment. For example, new or creative ideas and strategies for preventing child abuse and neglect are illustrated in a program called "Hui Makuakane" (Appendix C). As a first-time effort, OCAN recommended the development of a more precise definition of the universe of prevention programs and the specification of standards to maximize objectivity, standardization, and interrater reliability. In another example of federal leadership, the U.S. Children's Bureau has began publishing promising child welfare approaches identified during their reviews of statewide Child and Family Services, such as Delaware's Child Welfare Staff Training and Retention Initiatives (Appendix D).

TRANSLATING THE EVIDENCE TO POLICY AND PRACTICE

Despite advances in research and dissemination efforts, a substantial body of literature documents the failure of conventional educational approaches to promote the transfer of various types of research evidence into practice and policy. Rosenheck (2001) notes that the recent evaluations of new mental health treatments is a sequential two-part process that begins with: (a) efficacy research conducted in highly controlled research settings, and (b) followed by effectiveness research in which interventions are evaluated in settings that more closely approximate the "real world." However, the fit between the intervention or guideline and the context of service delivery is not always taken into consideration (Hoagwood et al., 2001). This dimension of "fit" is referred to as "transportability" or "translational" research that focuses on whether validated interventions produce desired outcomes under different conditions (Schoenwald & Hoagwood, 2001). For example, a randomized controlled trial of an intervention that has been validated in an efficacy study may not be effective when implemented with a different population or in a different agency setting. Therefore, some aspects of the intervention, the population, and the setting may need to be modified for use in "real world" service settings.

Researchers in the field of child mental health have made an important contribution to transportability research by developing frameworks for validating interventions in different settings (Schoenwald & Hoagwood, 2001). The questions that they have applied to transportability research include: "What is the intervention?", "Who can and will conduct the intervention in question, under what circumstances, and to what effect?", and "Which aspects of the protocols, practice guidelines, and practice settings require modification?". At each step in the research and intervention development process, decisions are made about the variables that are considered the most relevant. The following dimensions and variables have been used to compare conditions in research and practice settings (adapted from Schoenwald & Hoagwood, 2001):

1. Intervention characteristics (focus of treatment, model complexity, implementation specifications)
2. Practitioner characteristics (training, clinical supervision, types of practitioner such as social worker, physician, parent, etc.)
3. Client characteristics (age, gender, ethnicity and cultural identification, family context, referral source)

4. Service delivery characteristics (frequency, duration, source of payment)
5. Organizational characteristics (structure, hierarchy, procedures, organizational culture and climate, size, mission and mandates)
6. Service system characteristics (financing methods, legal mandates, interagency working relationships)

Given that organizational factors can be the most significant obstacles or enhancers of evidenced-based practices, there has been call for "dissemination research" that would bring more attention to the role of organizational life (Rosenheck, 2001). For example, in an implementation study of family psycho-education programs in Maine and Illinois, Rosenheck (2001) found that the external organizational factors (e.g., statewide advocacy and coalition building) were the most important predictor of successful implementation. While developing best practices guidelines, disseminating evidence, and sponsoring research-oriented workshops and conferences are important, one of the major challenges to implementing EBP involves the building of an evidence-based organizational culture inside and outside social service agencies.

ORGANIZATIONAL ISSUES

Several studies have documented the barriers to the implementation of research findings at the individual practice level, particularly in the field of health care (see Bero et al., 1998; Gira et al., 2003). However, less is known about the experiences of organizations that have attempted to develop an organizational culture that supports evidence-based practice and policy. The barriers identified by Hampshire Social Services (1999) in Appendix E include the organizational culture, practice environment, and educational environment. The solutions that they identified are noted in Figure 4 According to Hodson (2003), EBP is an innovation that requires: (a) ideological and cultural change (by winning over the hearts and minds of practitioners to the value of evidence and the importance of using it when making decisions), (b) technical change (changing the content or mode of service delivery in response to evidence about the effectiveness of interventions), and (c) organizational change (changing the organization and management to support EBP).

Based on interviews with staff responsible for promoting the development of EBP in the U.K., Hodson (2003) found that a combination of "micro" and "macro" approaches is more likely to achieve lasting

FIGURE 4. Organizational Barriers and Solutions*

Barrier		Solution Suggested
Organizational Culture	Little history, culture or expectation that evidence is routinely and systematically used to underpin practice	Creating the right culture and expectation through reinforcement of expectations and setting specific objectives for individuals
	A belief that achieving evidence-based ways of working is entirely a central departmental responsibility, rather than a joint responsibility with individuals locally,	Reflect evidence in operational practice with the approval, encouragement, and guidance of managers; reflect evidence in training, strategy, and policy
	Risk aversion mitigates against taking action in response to new ideas	
Practice Environment	Workload and time pressures of staff mitigate against discovering relevant evidence or generating it through evaluating initiatives or practice	
	Poor systems to establish and share best practice across the department	Encourage formal evaluation of practice and sharing of best practice results
Educational Environment	Skepticism about how transferable or generalizable evidence is, which mitigates against adoption of new ideas	within and across areas; establish networks, collate materials in the library; assess research deficits; develop a research agenda
	Evidence is not available in easily digestible formats which allow simple translations into policy and practice	Raise awareness about available materials, foster skill development in utilizing these resources through training, set up "reading clubs" and learning sets to help digest and disseminate evidence; utilize trainers

* Hampshire Social Services *Notes on Our Strategy* (1999)

change; "micro" approaches refer to altering the attitudes, ways of working and behaviors of individual practitioners and "macro" approaches relate to the "top-down" strategy to redesign key systems (such as the system for dissemination of evidence or the system for developing policy). Organizational approaches, which may include micro and macro strategies, focus on the context within which practitioners and systems operate. This approach removes impediments to new ways of working by redesigning embedded routines and practices as well as established cultures and behaviors. It also supplies the supportive structures that are necessary to sustain EBP processes (Hodson, 2003).

Evidence for Micro Approaches

Research reviews on micro approaches have focused on the effectiveness of various dissemination and implementation strategies in the field of health care (see Figure 5). In their review of twelve meta-analy-

FIGURE 5. Micro Strategies to Promote Professional Behavioral Change

Bero et al. (1998)	Gira, Kessler, & Poertner (2004)				
	Strong	**Moderate**	**Weak to Moderate**	**Weak**	**Not Evaluated**
Consistently Effective	Reminders (computerized)	Interactive Educational Meetings[1]	Educational Outreach Visits		Reminders (manual)
	Multifaceted Interventions[2]		Audit and Feedback[3]		
Mixed Effects				Local Opinion Leaders[4]	Local Consensus Process[5]
				Educational Materials[6]	Patient Mediated Interventions[7]
					Didactic Educational Meetings (lectures)
Not Evaluated		Use of Computers[8]			

[1] Participation of health care providers in workshops that include discussion or practice
[2] A combination that includes two or more of the following: audit and feedback, reminders, local consensus process, marketing
[3] Any summary of clinical performance
[4] Use of providers nominated by their colleagues as 'educationally influential'
[5] Inclusion of participating providers in discussion to ensure that they agreed that the chosen clinical problems were important and the approach to managing the problem was appropriate
[6] Distribution of published or printed recommendations for clinical care, including clinical practice guidelines, audio-visual materials and electronic publications
[7] Any intervention aimed at changing the performance of health care providers where specific information was sought from or given to patients
[8] For use in accessing clinical data, guidelines, and protocols; making clinical decisions; and in interactive patient education, therapy, and treatment adherence

ses of multiple strategies, Gira et al. (2004) found that certain types of continuing education and computer utilization demonstrated moderate to strong effects, whereas educational outreach visits and audits showed weaker outcomes. For example, the use of printed educational materials, local opinion leaders, and continuous quality improvement were found to be among the weakest interventions. However, a combination of approaches for changing practitioner behaviors was found to be effective and consistent with other studies. Bero et al.(1998) categorized efforts to promote changes in the behaviors of practitioners as either consistently effective, having mixed effects, or having little or no effect. While their review of eighteen systematic analyses found that passive dissemination of information was generally ineffective, interactive approaches such as educational outreach visits and educational meetings were found to be more effective. More intensive efforts to alter practice are more successful when coordinated with active dissemination and implementation strategies to enhance the utilization of research findings. The central issues for dissemination strategies appear to be the characteristics of the message, the recognition of external barriers to change, and the practitioner's level of preparedness for engaging in change.

Evidence for Macro Approaches

In contrast to the large number of studies on efforts to change individual behaviors, the research on macro approaches to changing organizational cultures related to EBP is limited by the small number qualitative studies (Barratt, 2003; Hodson, 2003). For example, Barratt (2003) found that few individuals within organizations in the United Kingdom held common views about the nature of evidence along and little consensus on how evidence could be effectively utilized. In addition, there was little clarity about the types of mechanisms needed to promote and sustain an evidence-based organizational culture. However, Barratt (2003) found considerable consensus on the need for organizations to share a common understanding of what constitutes "best evidence" by fostering continuous dialogue about the nature and relevance of evidence. Such dialogue was needed before practitioners could be expected to effectively manage the dissemination, implementation and adoption processes at either the management or line levels. In addition, there was a high level of agreement that responsibility and accountability for EBP should be devolved down through an agency. The active leadership of top management using coordinated strategy groups is needed to support the continuous use of evidence-base practice throughout the organization. At the same time, there was equally strong agreement that accessing evidence and reflecting upon its relevance should be an integral part of everyone's job with time allocated during the work week to read and reflect.

Hodson's (2003) found that the major barriers to the implementation of EBP were: (a) lack of time to fulfill the EBP role, (b) isolation within their agencies in terms of driving EBP initiatives, (c) lack of resources, and (d) a lack of a sound knowledge base of relevant evidence. The major strategies to address these barriers included a willingness to address organizational issues, specific EBP leadership competencies, and leadership support in the form of regional meetings and seminars to maintain momentum. Some of these strategies can be handled internally in the agency while others (e.g., developing or enhancing EBP competencies, discussion facilitation, and accessing networking opportunities) may require external assistance or training.

In addition, Hodson (2003) identified the following competencies related for introducting EBP into an agency: (a) setting agency directions and expectations for staff, (b) increasing staff competence, supporting and enabling critical thinking about practice, (c) using evidence to improve services, (d) generating and sharing evidence, and (e) creating strategic partnerships through networking and personal skills. In addition, the modeling of appropriate EBP behaviors included: (a) a demonstrated commitment to one's own personal development (i.e., "still learning" rather than "burnt out"), (b) demonstrating a belief that research evidence can be used to advance practice, (c) seeing the connection between research and practice whereby EBP is part of everyday work, and (d) demonstrating awareness of key issues and being sufficiently well-read to identify research evidence relevant to key issues.

EVIDENCE ON ORGANIZATIONAL APPROACHES

Based on work with more than 900 Veteran's Affairs programs, Rosenheck (2001) identified four major organizational factors for consideration in the implementation of evidence-based intervention. The first is the development of decision-making coalitions at the top and/or bottom of the organization. He noted that if the impetus comes from the higher ranks of the organization, the initiative has a higher potential for widespread impact. At the same time, if the impetus comes from line staff, it is more likely to succeed because consensus is easier to achieve with fewer stakeholders. His second factor is the degree to which the new initiative is consistent with current organizational goals and objectives. The third factor is the verification and dissemination of implementation results and the fourth factor involves the development of "learning subcultures."

In a similar manner, Sheldon and Chilvers (2000) identified the following organizational strategies for supporting the provision of evidence-based social services: (a) regularly scheduled staff training programs that make reference to research (on the nature and development of social problems as well as what is known about the effectiveness of different approaches designed to address them, (b) staff supervision that regularly draws upon research to inform decisions about cases and projects, (c) staff meetings that regularly include references to research on what has been tried elsewhere, regionally, nationally and internationally, (d) support facilities to assist staff in efforts to keep abreast of relevant research, (e) a workforce that would take personal responsibility for acquainting itself with the empirical evidence on service effectiveness, and (f) a range of collaborative arrangements between social services departments and local and regional research institutes and universities. Both top-down and bottom-up strategies are noted in Figure 6.

FUTURE DIRECTIONS

In the context of limited resources and accountability pressures, agencies need innovative strategies to harness information for the benefit of the individuals and communities that they serve. Based on the literature reviewed, evidence-based practice appears to operate best within an organizational context that supports practitioners at each stage of the EBP process, which is noted in Figure 7. Future directions suggest that agency-university partnerships, staff training, and the modification of agency cultures may be an effective place for organizations to begin considering EBP.

Agency-university partnerships can be used to identify the data that will support evidence-based practice. Key questions that need to be addressed are: (a) how will human service agencies develop the research questions needed to guide the systematic search of the literature? (b) how will research questions be addressed by researchers?, and (c) how will results be shared and incorporated into practice?.

Staff training, within human service agencies and on university campuses, that feature problem-based learning approaches are in the best position to support the introduction and utilization of evidence-based

FIGURE 6. Creating and Sustaining an Evidence-Based Organizational Culture in Social Service Agencies*

1. Team or unit level strategies:

    *   Develop and disseminate an in-house newsletter on relevant research
    *   Form and support monthly journal clubs to discuss an article or book of relevance to practice and to encourage knowledge sharing among practitioners
    *   Include research on the agenda of supervisory meetings, unit meetings, and departmental meetings

FIGURE 6 (continued)

- Involve students in agency field placements to search for, summarize, and share relevant research
- Create a library in every supervisor's office of relevant research articles, reports, and books
- Help staff access existing databases (Cochrane and Campbell Collaboratives) (cont'd)

2. Department or agency level strategies:

- Develop an organizational environment that recognizes the importance of research in making decisions at all levels of the organization
- Identify champions for evidence-based practice (chief information officer, knowledge manager, etc.)
- Demonstrate ownership of evidence-based practice by senior and middle management (may require special orientation sessions)
- Provide resources for evidence-based practice (internet access, training, library materials, etc.)
- Establish a steering committee responsible for implementing evidence-based practice
- Support the design, implementation, and utilization of service evaluations
- Create a climate of continuous learning and improvement (learning organization)
- Promote evidence-based training and evidence-based decision-making
- Develop system of email alerts of recent, relevant articles
- Create a policy on supervision that includes evidence-based practice
- Consider mandatory in-service training on evidence-based practice and lobbying for similar content in local pre-service university programs
- Promote protected reading time for staff to review relevant research
- Structure student placements around evidence-based practice

3. University/institute research development and dissemination strategies:

- Provide clear, uncomplicated, user-friendly presentations of research findings
- Conduct research relevant to the service mission of the organization
- Develop research and evaluation partnerships between agencies and universities/institutes
- Utilize multiple methods of dissemination
- Build dissemination into all research projects
- Engage practitioners in research topic identification and development

4. Implications for senior management

- Develop and circulate a policy statement that clearly identifies the value-added qualities of evidence-based practice including:
  - An approach to assessing service effectiveness
  - A way of finding promising practices for adaptation/incorporation
  - Provide evidence to support decision-making at the line and management levels

- An approach to making decisions about the effectiveness of contracted services

- Develop an orientation program whereby senior staff become thoroughly acquainted with evidence-based practice and begin to redesign the organizational culture to make it possible to install this new approach to service delivery

- Identify a champion from the rank of either senior management or middle management to serve as the agency's chief information officer (knowledge manager) to guide this organizational change (based on a well-defined job description or work portfolio)

- Identify a university/institute partner to conduct systematic reviews of existing evidence by involving agency staff in:
  o selecting the areas for review,
  o reviewing the results of the reviews and recommendations,
  o designing the strategies for incorporating new knowledge into ongoing practice and evaluating the outcomes
  o coordinating all agency efforts to promote evidence-based practice through the agency's chief information officer or knowledge manager.

* Adapted from Center for Evidence-based Social Services (2004). Becoming an evidence-based organization: Applying, adapting, and acting on evidence – Module 4. *The Evidence Guide: Using Research and Evaluation in Social Care and Allied Professions.* Exeter, UK: University of Exeter

FIGURE 7. Steps Involved in Implementing Evidence-Based Practice (Sackett et al., 1997)

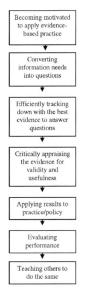

practice. Major questions might include the following: To what extent are practice guidelines needed and how can they be incorporated in staff training programs? How can training become more "problem-based" in order to apply evidence-based research? How can the transfer of learning be efficiently/effectively assessed?

Finally, the modification of agency cultures may be necessary to support and sustain evidence-based practice. The modification of an agency's culture needs to include strategies that address the reality that practitioners generally do not consult the research literature to guide practice decision-making due to an overwhelming volume of information, lack knowledge about searching techniques, lack of time, and lack access to information and libraries (Bunyan & Lutz, 1991). In essence, what does management need to do to build and sustain the supports for evidence-based practice? What do supervisors need to do to assist line staff in the process of adopting evidence-based practice? And what adjustments do line staff members need to make to incorporate evidence-based practice into their daily routines?

CONCLUSION

Evidence-based practice seeks to integrate the expertise of individual practitioners with the best available evidence within the context of the values and expectations of clients. While the development of evidence that is based on randomized controlled trials in the human services is still in its infancy, other types of knowledge hold promise for improving practice. This knowledge is increasingly available within agencies as well as at state, regional, and federal levels. The strategies related to agency-university partnerships, problem-based learning in training programs, and the transformation of agencies into learning organizations hold much promise for building evidence-based organizational cultures within the human services.

REFERENCES

Barratt, M. (2003). Organizational support for evidence-based practice within child and family social work: A collaborative study. *Child and Family Social Work, 8,* 143-150.

Bartels, S. J., Dums, A. R., Oxman, T. E., Schneider, L. S., Arean, P. A., Alexopoulos, G. S. et al. (2002). Evidence-based practices in geriatric mental health care. *Psychiatric Services, 53*(11), 1419-1431.

Bero, L., & Rennie, D. (1995). The Cochrane Collaboration. Preparing, maintaining, and disseminating systematic reviews of the effects of health care. *Journal of the American Medical Association, 274*(24), 1935-1938.

Bero, L. et al. (1998). Getting research findings into practice: An overview of systematic reviews of interventions to promote the implementation of research findings. *British Medical Journal, 317*, 465-468.

Bunyan, L. E., & Lutz, E. M. (1991). Marketing the hospital library to nurses. *Bulletin of the Medical Library Association, 79*(2), 223-225.

Caliber Associates. (2003). *Emerging practice in the prevention of child abuse and neglect.* Washington, DC: US Department of Health and Human Services. Available at http://www.calib.com/nccanch/prevention/emerging/index.cfm

Center for Evidence-based Social Services (2004). Becoming an evidence-based organization: Applying, adapting, and acting on evidence - Module 4. *The Evidence Guide: Using research and evaluation in social care and allied professions.* Exeter, UK: University of Exeter

Davies, H. & Nutley, S. (2002). Evidence-based policy and practice: Moving from rhetoric to reality, *Discussion Paper 2. Scotland: St Andrews University, Research Unit for Research Utilization.* www.st-andrews.ac.uk/~ruru/RURU%20publications%20list.htm

Chalmers, I., Sackett, D., & Silagy, C. (1997). The Cochrane collaboration. In A. Maynard & I. Chalmers (Eds.), *Non-random reflections on health services research: On the 25th anniversary of Archie Cochrane's effectiveness and efficiency.* (pp. 231-249). London: BMJ.

Gambrill, E. (1999). Evidence-based practice: An alternative to authority-based practice. *Families in Society: The Journal of Contemporary Human Services, 80*(4), 341.

Gibbs, L. E. (2003). *Evidence-based practice for the helping professions: A practical guide with integrated multimedia.* Pacific Grove, CA: Brooks Cole.

Gira, E. C., Kessler, M. L., & Poertner, J. (2004). Influencing social workers to use research evidence in practice: Lessons from medicine and the allied health professions. *Research on Social Work Practice, 14*(2), 68-79.

Greenhalgh, T. (2001). *How to read a paper: The basics of evidence based medicine. (2nd ed.).* London: BMJ Books.

Guyatt, G. H., Sackett, D. L., Sinclair J. C., Hayward, R., Cook, D. J., & Cook, R. J. (1995). Users' guides to the medical literature. IX. A method for grading health care recommendations. *Journal of the American Medical Association, 174*, 1800-1804.

Hampshire Social Services (1999). *Evidence-based practice in Hampshire Social Services: Notes on our strategy.* Hampshire, UK: Hampshire Social Services.

Hoagwood, K., Burns, B. J., Kiser, L., Ringeisen, H., & Schoenwald, S. K. (2001). Evidence-based practice in child and adolescent mental health services. *Psychiatric Services, 52*(9), 1179-1189.

Hodson, R. (2003). *Leading the drive for evidence based practice in services for children and families: Summary report of a study conducted for research in practice.* UK: Research in Practice. Available at *http://www.rip.org.uk/devmats/leadership. html*

Kirk, S. A., & Penska, C. E. (1992). Research utilization in MSW education: A decade of progress? In A. J. Grasso, & I. Epstein (Eds.). *Research utilization in the social services: Innovations for practice and administration.* New York: Haworth.

Kitson, A., Harvey, G., & McCormack, B. (1998). Enabling the implementation of evidence-based practice: A conceptual framework. *Quality in Health Care, 7,* 149-158.

Oxman, A. D., & Guyatt, G. H. (1995). The science of reviewing research. In K. S. Warren & F. Mosteller (Eds.), *Doing more good than harm: The evaluation of health care interventions.* New York: New York Academy of Sciences.

Pawson, R, Boaz, A. Grayson, L., Long, A. & Barnes, C. (2003). *Types and quality of knowledge in social care.* London, UK: Social Care Institute for Excellence.

Poertner, J. (2000). *Parents' expectations of caseworkers: Research integration practice guide.* Urbana, IL: Children and Family Research Center. Available at http://cfrcwww.social.uiuc.edu/respract/respracproc1.htm

Rosenheck, R. A. (2001). Organizational process: A missing link between research and practice. *Psychiatric Services, 52*(12), 1607-1612.

Sackett, D. L., Straus, S. E., Richardson, W. S., Rosenberg, W., & Haynes, R. B. (1997). *Evidence-based medicine: How to practice and teach EBM (2nd ed.).* Edinburgh: Churchill-Livingstone.

Saunders, B.E., Berliner, L., & Hanson, R.F. (Eds.). (2003). *Child Physical and Sexual Abuse: Guidelines for Treatment (Final Report: January 15, 2003).* Charleston, SC: National Crime Victims Research and Treatment Center. Available at http://www.musc.edu/cvc/guide1.htm

Schoenwald, S. K., & Hoagwood, K. (2001). Effectiveness, transportability, and dissemination of interventions: What matters when? *Psychiatric Services, 52*(9), 1190-1197.

Sheldon, B., & Chilvers, R. (2000). *Evidence-based social care: A study of prospects and problems.* Lyme Regis: Russell House Publishing.

United States Department of Health and Human Services (USDHHS), Children's Bureau. (2000). Child and Family Services Review Procedures Manual. Washington, DC: US Department of Health and Human Services. Available at *http://www. acf.hhs.gov/programs/cb/publications/procman/index.htm.*

APPENDIX A. Trauma-focused Cognitive-Behavioral Therapy (CBT) (Adapted from a summary by Judy Cohen, M.D. and Esther Deblinger, PhD)

Brief Description:

> Trauma-focused cognitive behavioral therapy, an intervention based on learning and cognitive theories, is designed to reduce children's negative emotional and behavioral responses and correct maladaptive beliefs and attributions related to the abusive experiences. It also aims to provide support and skills to help non-offending parents cope effectively with their own emotional distress and optimally respond to their children. See references for theory and rationale.

Treatment Components (12-18 sessions):

1. Psychoeducation about child abuse, typical reactions, safety skills and healthy sexuality
2. Gradual exposure techniques including verbal, written and/or symbolic recounting (i.e., utilizing dolls, puppets, etc.) of abusive event(s).
3. Cognitive reframing consisting of exploration and correction of inaccurate attributions about the cause of, responsibility for, and results of the abusive experience(s).
4. Stress management techniques such as focused breathing and muscle relaxation exercise, thought stopping, though replacement, and cognitive therapy interventions.
5. Parental participation in parallel or conjoint treatment including psychoeducation, gradual exposure, anxiety management and correction of cognitive distortions.
6. Parental instruction in child behavior management strategies.
7. Family work to enhance communication and create opportunities for therapeutic discussion regarding the abuse.

Treatment Manuals or Protocol Descriptions:

Deblinger, E., & Heflin, A.H. (1996). *Treatment for sexually abused children and their non-offending parents: A cognitive-behavioral approach.* Thousand Oaks, CA: Sage.

Cohen, J.A., Mannarino, A.P. (1993). A treatment model for sexually abused preschoolers. *Journal of Interpersonal Violence, 8,* 115-131.

APPENDIX A (continued)

Treatment Outcome Study References:

Berliner, L. & Saunders, B.E. (1996). Treating fear and anxiety in sexually abused children: Results of a controlled 2-year follow-up study. *Child Maltreatment, 1*(4), 294-309.

Celano, M., Hazzard, A., Webb, C., McCall, C. (1996). Treatment of traumagenic beliefs among sexually abused girls and their mothers: An evaluation study. *Journal of Abnormal Child Psychology,* 24, 1-16.

Cohen, J.A., & Mannarino, A.P. (1996). A treatment outcome study for sexually abused pre-school children: Initial findings. *Journal of the American Academy of Child and Adolescent Psychiatry,* 35, 42-50.

Cohen, J.A., & Mannarino, A.P. (1997). A treatment study of sexually abused preschool children: Outcome during a one year follow-up. *Journal of the Academy of Child and Adolescent Psychiatry,* 36(9), 1228-1235.

Cohen, J.A., & Mannarino, A.P. (1998). Interventions for sexually abused children: Initial treatment findings. *Child Maltreatment,* 3, 17-26.

Deblinger, E., McLeer, S. V. & Henry, D. (1990). Cognitive behavioral treatment for sexually abused children suffering post-traumatic stress: Preliminary findings. *Journal of the American Academy of Child and Adolescent Psychiatry,* 19, 747- 752.

Deblinger, E., Lippmann, J., & Steer, R. (1996) Sexually abused children suffering posttraumatic stress symptoms: Initial treatment outcome findings. *Child Maltreatment,* 1, 310- 321.

Stauffer, L. & Deblinger, E. (1996). Cognitive behavioral groups for nonoffending mothers and their young sexually abused children: a preliminary treatment outcome study. *Child Maltreatment,* 1(1), 65-76.

Deblinger, E., Steer, R.A., & Lippmann, J. (1999). Two year follow-up study of cognitive behavioral therapy for sexually abused children suffering post-traumatic stress symptoms. *Child Abuse & Neglect,* 23(12), 1371-1378.

APPENDIX B

To bridge research and practice, the Children and Family Research Center and the Illinois Department of Family Services have designed a client satisfaction inventory to highlight 24 caseworker behaviors iden-

tified as important to parents, describe the clinical implications of the behaviors, and identify specific casework interventions that can be implemented to address each issue. An example of Caseworker Behavior 1 is presented here.

Caseworker Behavior 1: My caseworker encourages me to discuss times when things were better in my family.

Clinical Implications: Encouraging clients to discuss times when things were better in their family offers them the opportunity to identify and acknowledge family strengths and resources. Through recognition of sequences of positive patterns, families can begin to make conscious use of their strengths and resources to work toward a desired future.

Casework Interventions:
1. Ask the clients to discuss the positive patterns they observe in themselves and their families.
2. Tell clients about the positive patterns observed in the clients and/ or their families.
3. Ask the clients how they will know when things are better.
4. Discuss with the clients what changes DCFS is wanting to see to ensure their child's safety.

These activities can be done periodically throughout the life of the case.

Source: *Parents' Expectations of Caseworkers: An Abbreviated Summary (Adapted from John Poertner, Dennette M. Derezotes, Ellyce Roitman, Casandra Woolfolk, Jo Anne Smith, Children and Family Research Center, School Social Work, University of Illinois at Urbana-Champaign)*

APPENDIX C
The Hui Makuakane Program developed a program to engage fathers in home visitation programs and increased the involvement and participation of fathers in family home visits. The program description, as it appeared in OCAN's Emerging Practices in the Prevention of Child Abuse and Neglect, is presented here.

Hui Makuakane aims to recognize and support the role of fathers in the family through the following services goals:

APPENDIX C (continued)

1. Increase fathers' understanding of how their babies grow and what to expect as they grow
2. Increase fathers' knowledge of the kinds of activities they can do with their children to help them grow and develop
3. Increase the amount of time fathers spend with their children in play and in fulfilling their day-to-day needs (e.g., changing diapers, feeding)
4. Teach fathers how to set limits and enforce them using positive disciplinary techniques
5. Help fathers feel good about themselves as parents and to have loving, nurturing relationships with their children
6. Help fathers set personal goals and make progress toward those goals

The program engages fathers in the following activities in order to increase their participation in the services for the entire family: group activities, home visits, career development, job help, support in crisis, referral to other community resources, and outreach to fathers in correctional facilities. Home visits by Father Facilitators for all fathers enrolled in the program are the primary service provided by Hui Makuakane. Father Facilitators provide personal help with answering fathers' questions about their children and learning new and fun activities to do with their children including:

1. Infant massage instruction is provided during home visits as a way to increase positive parent-child interaction
2. Help fathers establish and reach vocational and educational goals
3. Making referrals to other community resources to help fathers meet their goals
4. Providing fathers with 24-hour access to Father Facilitators via cell phones in case of a crisis
5. Group outings are available for the entire family, for just fathers in the program, for just fathers and children, or for just fathers and their partners

APPENDIX D

Promising Approach: Delaware's Child Welfare Staff Training and Retention Initiatives

I. Identifying Information

Agency Sponsor: Delaware Department of Services to Children, Youth and Families

Target Population: Child welfare caseworkers and supervisors

Required/Funding Source: personnel budget.

Length of Operation: 1997 to present

Personnel procedures: Educational requirements for prospective child welfare caseworkers include a bachelor's degree in a field closely related to child welfare.

II. Description of Promising Approach

Staff retention is one of the challenges facing child welfare agencies, which typically experience significant staff turnover in short periods of time. The Delaware Department of Services to Children, Youth, and Their Families has put in place procedures for stabilizing their workforce, building on a legislative initiative enacted in response to several child fatalities.

The Child Abuse Prevention Act of 1997 established systems designed to improve the training and retention of State child welfare caseworkers, using an "overhire" process that supports new staff development. Through these changes and other new procedures, the department is hiring faster, providing more staff training, and improving staff management.

APPENDIX E

The barriers identified by Hampshire Social Services (1999) in the U.K. (organizational culture, practice environment, and educational environment) represent common challenges and some of the solutions are noted in Figure 4.

APPENDIX E (continued)

Introduction

The requirement for Social Services Departments to use empirical evidence in developing policy and practice is becoming increasingly important with the growing focus on best value and performance results in terms of effectiveness. Evidence-based practice is defined as " the conscientious, explicit and judicious use of current best evidence in making decisions about the welfare of service users." (adapted from Sackett et al., BMJ 1996; 312; 71-72)

Evidence is based on the results of soundly based effectiveness research published in refereed journals. However, evidence can also include unpublished work by practitioners if it is methodologically sound and transferable. Professional experience about "what works" built up over many years of practice may also constitute evidence and must not be ignored. The key imperative is for "judicious use" of the "best evidence" available from the full range of sources.

Reliance only on "practice wisdom" means that we do not challenge what we are doing. When we intervene in the lives of others, we should do so with the best evidence available about the likely outcomes of that intervention. The goal is to get the Social Service organization into a position where:

- there is both an expectation and a desire to know what evidence says about how best to approach interventions,
- there is ready access to and awareness of best available evidence,
- where evidence is not available, steps are taken to plug this gap,
- staff are able to understand and interpret evidence in order to inform policy development, training and practice decisions,
- service delivery reflects what the evidence is saying about best practice,
- the results of policy and practice decisions are routinely evaluated to gauge outcomes,
- evaluation results are disseminated in order to add to the body of available evidence.

APPENDIX E (continued)

There are multiple barriers to implementing evidence-based practice in the social services and they include some of the following:

- little history, culture or expectation that evidence is routinely and systematically used to underpin practice,
- a belief that achieving evidence-based ways of working is entirely a departmental (central) responsibility, rather than a joint responsibility with individuals locally,
- workload and time pressures of staff mitigate against discovering relevant evidence (or generating it through evaluating initiatives/practice),
- evidence is not available in easily digestible formats which allow simple translation into policy and practice,
- poor systems to establish and share best practice across the department,
- skepticism about how transferable or generalizable evidence is (this is likely to be a combination of a "not invented here" syndrome, concerns about the validity of "old" research and a lack of skills to appraise evidential material) which together mitigate against adoption of new ideas,
- risk aversion also mitigates against taking" action in response to new ideas.

Any strategy to promote evidence-based practice across the department needs to explicitly and directly address these factors.

The organizational resources and opportunities available to promote evidence-based practice include the achievement of evidence-based practice within the department requires that a very broad range of issues are effectively addressed, including: departmental culture, processes (and responsibilities) for the development and improvement of practice, staff skills, information systems and workload management.

The ultimate aim is to ensure the practice of front-1ine staff in every client group and area is evidence-based and therefore maximizes positive outcomes for our service users. The key groups of staff that the strategy will need to impact are therefore:

- *front-line practitioners:* who will need to routinely challenge and review their practice in the light of best evidence, and if required, amend their ways of working,

APPENDIX E (continued)

- *operational managers:* who will need to set the expectation of routine review of practice, facilitate and encourage this process, allowing innovative or new ways of working to be adopted, and play a key role in sharing best practice with colleagues,
- *HQ commissioning staff:* who will need to ensure that current and future strategies, policies and procedures to which practitioners turn for guidance and direction, are founded on available evidence about what works and what is best practice in service delivery,
- *trainers:* who will need to ensure that current and future training material reflects available evidence about effective practices and best approaches, and that the training agenda material focuses on the development of appropriate skills in the staff to understand, use and generate evidence.

In addition, existing frameworks will need to be harnessed to explore more evidence-based ways of working such as the following:

- meetings of individual teams, of unit / team managers, and of service managers to discuss research and its application in each client group,
- performance development (appraisal) and supervision could be used to set specific staff practice objectives related to the explicit use of evidence,
- the care management process could be used more explicitly to review current practice, plan evidence-based interventions for individual users and record the outcomes,
- technology (such as Hantsnet, WWW) is a readily available resource which could also be exploited further.

Creating the right organizational culture

The challenge is to create a culture that promotes the basics of performance management (assessing how well we currently do things, questioning practice in an attempt to continuously improve, and measuring our achievements in so doing). The routine use of evidence to underpin practice then becomes a natural corollary.

This requires a strong commitment to this way of working (rather than "practice wisdom") because this change might be seen as threatening by some staff. Managers clearly have a crucial role to play in setting clear expectations about the use of evidence in underpinning interventions or strategies. Managers need to use the practices mentioned above (team meetings, performance development and supervision of care management practice, performance agreements) to (a) reinforce these expectations, (b) set specific objectives for individuals and (b) value, acknowledge and encourage achievements.

The notion of "champions" is also a useful way of promoting culture change. This will be achieved by creating a network of staff (through workshops, training events and projects) who are interested in developing evidence-based ways of working. The primary implementation components include:

- providing mechanisms to help staff access "digestible" evidence-based literature,
- developing skills of all staff to generate and exploit evidence through training programs
- reflecting evidence in operational practice (supporting the risk-taking of trying out new ways of working through individual supervision and care management processes,
- reflecting evidence in training, strategy and policy (the training calendar needs to reflect the topics on which there is clear evidence that suggest future changes in practice),
- developing a research agenda (directing more of the available research towards systematic reviews of current evidence so available resources can then be targeted to meet these needs).

Source: Evidence-based practice in Hampshire Social Services (England): An abbreviation of the 1999 organizational strategy.

Implementing Evidence-Based Practice in Human Service Organizations: Preliminary Lessons from the Frontlines

Michael J. Austin, PhD
Jennette Claassen, MSW

SUMMARY. Evidence-based practice (EBP) involves the integration of the expertise of individual practitioners with the best available evidence within the context of values and expectations of clients. Little is known about the implementation of evidence-based practice in the human services. This article is based on a comprehensive search of the literature related to the organizational factors needed to introduce EBP into a human service agency, tools for assessing organizational readiness for EBP, and lessons learned from the current implementation efforts. Three approaches to implementing EBP are investigated: the micro (increasing worker skills), macro (strengthening systems and structures), and the combination (focusing on both aspects). Conclusions and recommendations are drawn from the literature review and framed in the form of a tool for assessing organizational readiness for EBP implementation.

Michael J. Austin is Professor and Jennette Claassen is Research Assistant, School of Social Welfare, University of California, Berkeley.

KEYWORDS. Evidence-based practice, human services, frontline lessons, organizations

INTRODUCTION

Evidence-based practice (EBP) involves the integration of the expertise of individual practitioners with the best available evidence within the context of values and expectations of clients (Sackett, Richardson, Rosenberg, & Haynes, 1997; Gambrill, 1999). The principles and practices of EBP are drawn from the health care field and only recently have become a part of the social service arena. As the social service and mental health fields move towards embracing EBP, most of the literature seeks to promote the adoption of evidence-based practices, rather than actually engaging in and evaluate the use of evidence-based practice (Mullen, Schlonsky, Bledsoe, & Bellamy, 2005). As a result, there are very few evaluations that examine the elements needed to successfully incorporate evidence-based practice into agency operations.

There is recognition in the literature that implementing EBP is a complex and difficult task. Organizational environments and individual capacities need to be considered in designing implementation efforts (Gerrish & Clayton, 2004; Proctor, 2004). The complexity of implementing EBP includes: 1) motivating and facilitating practitioners to gain interest and trust in utilizing research (Proctor, 2004; Mullen & Bacon, 2000), 2) increasing the capacity of staff and agencies to utilize the information available (Barratt, 2003), and 3) mobilizing resources to experiment and sustain EBP practices (Mullen & Bacon, 2000; Barratt, 2003).

Since EBP represents a change in the life of an organization, it is important to include in this analysis the research on implementing organizational change as well as findings on the dissemination and utilization of research. The focus of this review of research is on the different approaches to implementing EBP and the implications for human service organizations.

ORGANIZING CHANGE AND RESEARCH UTILIZATION

Since EBP is a new approach to practice, it is important to view it in the context of organizational change. The successful introduction and sustainability of an innovation into the life of an organization requires an understanding of: (1) the process of change including its barriers and incentives, (2) the culture of an organization, and (3) the strategies for effective dissemination and utilization.

While it is widely recognized that organizational change is a complex process, there is little consensus about the strategies that can ensure successful change. However, there is growing consensus about the following key elements in understanding and managing change: (1) type of change (Damanpour, 1988; Frey, 1990; Pearlmutter, 1998), (2) degree of change (Pearlmutter, 1998; Damanpour, 1988; Proehl, 2001), (3) facilitators and inhibitors of change (Arad, Hanson, & Schneider, 1997; Frambach & Schillewaert, 2002), (4) staff receptivity and resistance to change (Diamond, 1996; Jaskyte & Dressler, 2005), and (5) organizational readiness for change (Robbins Collins, Liaupsin, Illback, & Call, 2003; Hodges & Hernandez, 1999; Lehman, Greener, & Simpson, 2002). Each of these element is explored in greater detail in Austin and Claassen (2006).

An essential component of organizational change strategies is the culture of the organization. Organizational culture and its impact on organizational change process has receive limited attention in the research literature. The focus on organizational culture as an ingredient in organizational change includes the following elements: (1) understanding organizational culture in terms of basic assumptions, values and beliefs, and symbolic artifacts that exist within the organization (Schein, 1985), (2) identifying the types of organizational cultures such as informal culture, role culture, and results-driven culture (Handy, 1995; Cameron & Quinn, 1999), and (3) developing strategies for managing organizational culture in relationship to the roles of leaders (Khademian, 2002).

Another aspect of organizational change related to EBP involves the dissemination and utilization of research. There are at least four critical elements needed to bridge the gap between research and practice and they include: (1) the *source* of the research information is credible and competent, (2) the *content* of the message is focused on practical application, (3) the *method* of transfer includes multiple, reliable delivery approaches, and (4) the *audience* is consulted prior to dissemination (Barwick, Blydell, Stasiulis, Ferguson, Blase, & Fixsen, 2005). In addition, there is a complex interaction between the individual, the organization, the research, and communication in dissemination and utilization processes (Rogers, 1995). Despite this complexity, the most promising dissemination strategies include the utilization of the following combination of experts: persons specifically trained to disseminate information, local opinion leaders who are trusted community professionals, and evaluators who can audit the process and provide feedback mechanisms (Oxman, Thomson, Davis, & Haynes, 1995). These issues are explored in more detail in Lemon and Austin (2006).

In essence, the introduction of EBP requires special attention to the processes of organizational change, the understanding of organizational culture, and the specialized expertise to promote the successful dissemination and utilization of research. With this view in mind, the focus of this analysis shifts to documented case studies that describe the implementation of EBP in human service organizations.

INTRODUCING AND IMPLEMENTING EVIDENCE-BASED PRACTICE

EBP as Change

Since evidence-based social service practice is a relatively new concept in the U.S., most of the literature focuses on assessing its appropriateness and feasibility. However, much can be learned from colleagues in the United Kingdom who have more experience in searching for the most effective methods for implementing and sustaining EBP (Sheldon, & Chilvers, 2000; Pawson, Boaz, Grayson, Long, & Barnes, 2003; Nutley, Walter, Percy-Smith, McNeish, & Frost, 2004; Smith, 2004). While there is growing agreement that EBP represents a significant change in social service practice (Lawler & Bilson, 2004; Proctor, 2004, Nutley & Davies, 2000), it is also clear that EBP requires special attention to the following types of barriers and facilitators of change: (a) ideological and cultural change related to creating "buy-in" to the value of evidence and the importance of using it in decision-making, (b) technical change that may require changes in the content or mode of service delivery in response to evidence on the effective interventions, and (c) organizational change affecting all levels of staff (Hodson, 2003, Nutley & Davies, 2000).

Creating an EBP Culture

Preliminary evidence suggests that the implementation of EBP is more likely to be successful if it is introduced into a supportive organizational culture that is reflected at all levels from front-line staff to top management (Barwick et al., 2005; Lawler & Bilson, 2004). Barwick et al. (2005) found that a supportive EBP culture includes: (a) clarity of mission and goals among staff, (b) staff cohesiveness and autonomy, (c) openness of communication and openness to change, (d) low levels of job stress, (e) careful attention given to staff selection, training, coaching, and (f) the use of continuous quality improvement feedback systems. The major components of organizational culture that are supportive of EBP include: (1) *leadership* provided by change managers or champions, (2) the *involvement* of stakeholders at all levels and phases of implementation, (3) the development of a cohesive *team*, (4) the availability of organizational *resources*, and (5) readiness to become a *learning organization*. Each of these five areas is explored in this section.

Leadership: Effective managerial leadership that demonstrates open and honest communication can significantly influence the change process and create an environment open to learning (Barwick et al., 2005; Proctor, 2004). Barwick et al. (2005) found that, "only strong leadership can build an organizational culture supportive of change, establish aims for improvement, and mobilize resources to meet those aims" (p.101). In addition, agency leaders can set the tone for developing a culture that is supportive of innovation, risk-taking, and the continuous identification and evaluation of the most effective interventions.

While any staff member can assume a leadership role or champion an idea, the development of an evidence-based culture is heavily dependent on middle and top management. A study of 36 social service agency managers indicated that the responsibility and accountability for evidence-based practice should be devolved down through an agency but with a critical role for the director to "lead from the front" (Barratt, 2003). While identifying evidence and reflecting on its relevance for practice should be part of everyone's job, managers need to be mindful of the competing pressures on staff. For example, expecting staff to take the lead in locating and evaluating evidence is rarely feasible given the workload demands placed upon social service staff.

Involvement of Stakeholders: The process of introducing and sustaining EBP requires the involvement of stakeholders at all levels of the organization. (Barwick et al., 2005). Bringing together different parts of the organization, including multiple disciplines and levels of staff, to modify the current knowledge of staff creates an opportunity to develop new and promising practices (Wenger, McDermott, & Synder, 2002). The group of stakeholders needs to include individuals who are ready for change and can help inspire and motivate others. The involvement of the broadest array of staff can help to create "buy-in" where these future implementers understand the advantages of the EBP and the relevance of valid and reliable evidence related to practice (Barwick et al., 2005). This "buy-in" can alleviate potential staff resistance and create a trusting environment where critical analysis can thrive.

Teamwork: Helping practitioners develop the capacity to evaluate evidence and modify practice requires teamwork (Lawler & Bilson, 2004, Barratt, 2003). Teamwork provides an important opportunity to reflect, question, and discuss practice in general. The process of change for practitioners might involve questioning their basic assumptions about practice, which can cause considerable discomfort. Implementing EBP can involve challenging long-held assumptions and altering patterns of behavior. The ability to reflect and change as members of a team can provide staff members with support and can ease their fears. The use of teams needs to be well-planned and managed. While teams can be a catalyst for change when given appropriate leadership and direction; if poorly led, they can lead to substantial resistant to change (Barratt, 2003).

Organizational Resources: In the Barwick et al. (2005) survey of mental health staff, there appeared to be adequate levels facilities, training, and equipment. Clinical staff and executive directors had a favorable view of the adequacy of office space, staff turnover was not a problem, and there was an appropriate amount of staff training. Access to computers and the internet, a commonly cited barrier of EBP, was not a problem as 95% of the clinical and executive staff have a computer in their personal workspace. In contrast, Sheldon and Chilvers (2002) found that over one third of clinical staff reported having no access to library facilitates, journals, or appropriate research material.

In addition to physical resources, it is also important to assess human resources. The attitudes and desires of staff to change has been linked to four key areas: (1) professional growth, (2) confidence in own skills, (3) willingness to persuade coworkers, and (4) ability to adapt to a changing environment. Several surveys noted that practitioners perceive few opportunities for personal and professional growth in their organizations (Mullen & Bacon, 2000; Barwick et al., 2005; Sheldon & Chilvers, 2002). Barwick et al. (2005) found that 42% of clinical staff report that they do not regularly (monthly) read about new techniques or treatments on a monthly basis. Similar results were found by Mullen and Bacon (2000) who noted that social workers do not use research methods or findings to inform their practice. Contrary to perceiving few opportunities for professional growth, Barwick et al. (2005) found that more than two-thirds of the clinical staff and executive directors in their study had a high level of confidence in their own clinical skills which, in turn, facilitated the implementation of EBP. Barwick et al. (2005) also found that both clinicians and management perceived themselves as willing to try new ideas or to adapt quickly to changing situations (only 20% admitted to feeling too cautious or slow to make changes).

Readiness to Become a Learning Organization: Prior to introducing a new idea or change into an existing organization, it is important to assess the readiness for change, from an organizational, individual, and system level. While there are several instruments for assessing organizational readiness for change, Lehman, Greener, and Bilson (2002) Organizational Readiness for Change (ORC) instrument was found to be particularly helpful in assessing individual and organizational readiness (Barwick et al., 2005). The instrument focuses on motivation and personality attributes of program leaders and staff, institutional resources, staff attributes, and organizational climate. The three factors identified by the instrument are: (1) what is important for change to occur, (2) what is necessary but not always sufficient for change to occur, and (3) what change is appropriate in the current situation. The motivational dimensions are divided into individual and organization factors and include the following three areas: (1) program need for improvement (assessing program's current strengths and weaknesses); (2) training needs assessment; and (3) pressure for change from the internal or external environments. The institutional resources section is divided into five areas: (1) office, (2) staffing, (3) training resources, (4) computer access, and (5) electronic communication. The third section focuses on staff attributes and includes: (1) growth, (2) efficacy (3) influence, and (4) adaptability. The last section is the largest and evaluates organizational climate as indicated by: (1) clarity of mission and goals, (2) staff cohesion, (3) staff autonomy, (4) openness of communication, (5) stress, and (6) openness to change. The ORC was originally developed for drug abuse treatment agencies; in 2003, it was redesigned for use in social service agencies.

A second useful framework for understanding an organization and individual readiness for implementation of EBP is the use of the "four A's"–acquire, assess, apply, and adapt (CHSRF, 2001). By using the "four A's" concept, an organization is able to explore the capacity of staff to implement and adopt research information and identify barriers prior to implementation. The four A's explores the ability of an individual and organization to find research they need, assess whether the research is reliable, adapt the information to suit its needs, and implement the research within their context. Utilizing the "four A's", Barwick et al. (2005) designed a staff survey to identify organizational processes that needed strengthening prior to the implementation of EBP as well as to develop a baseline of information on which to evaluate future progress.

In assessing staff readiness to implement EBP, the most important area was staff's capacity to understand research methods. The capacity of staff to seek out, understand, and utilize research findings is limited (Mullen & Bacon, 2000; Barwick et al., 2005; Tozer & Bournemouth, 1999). Social workers rely on a combination of their own experience and the experiences of consultants and supervisors for their practice-based decision-making rather than use research findings or research methods in their practice (Mullen & Bacon, 2002). In addition, a substantial gap exists between self-perceived knowledge of research and their ability to use it (Sheldon & Chilvers, 2002). For example, while a large percentage of clinical staff responded positively to reading published research, very few could actually identify or describe a study and reflected only a minimal understanding of basic research methods. These findings related to a reliance on experience and limited understanding of research methods suggest that an overview of research methods need to be incorporated in plans for introducing EBP.

Promoting a Learning Organization: The ability of an organization to successfully implement EBP requires an organizational culture that values and encourages learning. Such cultures promote the freedom of staff to work autonomously and make changes, share information openly, are flexible and adaptable, encourage and reward risk-taking and creativity, and accept mistakes (Jaskyte & Dressler, 2005). Efforts to create a learning organization require staff to be engaged in the learning process (Stevens and Gist, 1997), given opportunity to apply new knowledge or ideas, be motivated to increase their own knowledge (Noe & Schmitt, 1986), and work in an environment that supports feedback, coaching, and recognition (Huczybski & Lewis, 1980; Mathieu, Tannenbaum & Salas, 1996). The development of an organizational learning culture involves a "cultural overhaul" including making employee growth and development a priority, adopting a "development" philosophy, helping staff overcome fear through supportive relationships, adding rewards or incentives to application of learning, and establishing open lines of communication for staff to share thoughts and ideas (Danielson & Wiggenhorn, 2003).

DIFFERENT APPROACHES TO IMPLEMENTING EVIDENCE-BASED PRACTICE

Three approaches appear in the literature that utilize different strategies to address the challenges of implementing EBP. Each approach focuses on a different aspect of the change process: individual, systems, and context (Hodson, 2003). The micro approach focuses extensively on individual learning, the systems approach works from macro, "top-down" perspective, and the combination approach is a blend of the micro and macro approaches.

The micro approach to implementation of EBP involves the teaching of practice skills needed to appropriately utilize evidence (Hodson, 2003; Mullen, Bellamy, Bledsoe, 2004). This approach seeks to enhance motivation to engage in lifelong learning by providing the necessary learning and application skills. Practitioners are introduced to the process of problem formulation, evidence search tools, evidence appraisal skills, information integration skills, and the implementation process (Gibbs & Gambrill, 2002). This approach is generally found in pre-service university education programs. However, this approach has also been utilized successfully as part of agency in-service training (Newhouse, Dearhold, Poe, Pugh, & White, 2005; Thurston & King, 2004). The micro approach views the implementation of EBP as a long-term organizational process designed to slowly alter the attitudes, practices, and behaviors of individual practitioners (Hodson, 2003).

In contrast, the macro approach seeks to achieve planned change through the "top down" redesign of key organizational systems (Hodson, 2003). Top-level decision-makers identify evidence-based, empirically supported practices and develop tools for practitioners to use in adopting the new practices. Dissemination and utilization strategies (including guidelines, toolkits, intervention-specific training, and consultants) are employed to change practice through the adoption of a predetermined, specific intervention (Gira, Kessler, & Poertner, 2004). While this approach is frequently used in agencies, there is little empirical evidence related to assessing the outcomes of the macro approach. The largest example of this approach is the National Implementing Evidence-Based Practice Project (Torrey, Lynde, & Gorman, 2005) that promotes the adoption of six evidence-based practices for assisting mentally ill adults by using implementation guides designed at the national level but implemented at the local level.

The combination approach utilizes components of the micro and macro approaches in order to create structures and systems that support the sustainability of evidence-based practice. This approach involves the redesign of existing routines and practices in an effort to establish new cultures and behaviors (Hodson, 2003). Instead of viewing the introduction of EBP as a one-time activity, the combination approach combines the increase in the research knowledge, skills, and attitude of staff with the organizational processes and procedures required to incorporate evidence-based approaches into the daily routine. This approach is relatively new and faces significant challenges. Several projects have been started but the outcomes of the efforts have yet to be reported, with the exception of a three-year longitudinal project in a mental health organization (Dickenson, Duffy, & Champion, 2004).

Findings Related to the Micro Approach

Two hospitals employed similar strategies for providing clinical nurses with the structure and tools necessary to acquire EBP knowledge, skills, and to incorporate EBP into their working environments. Both interventions focused on teaching professional staff to become critical thinkers, increase their skill levels, and become comfortable with evidence-based practices (Newhouse et al., 2005; Thurston & King, 2004).

The first hospital utilized the Johns Hopkins Nursing EBP Model (Figure 1) and Guidelines (Figure 2) focusing on a mentored educational experience. The framework in Figure 1 includes internal and external environments within a triangle of practice, education, and research which seeks to combine the expertise of the practitioner and patient, available research, expert opinions, and other accessible evidence. The guidelines provide a step-by-step approach to move from practice questions, to evidence, and finally to the translation to the practice setting. The pilot study was implemented on a large scale throughout the hospital using five education sessions (one-to two hours) over a period of eight weeks. Those identified as leaders, change agents, and potential champions of EBP were trained first with subsequent trainings for the remaining staff. The nurses were given paid time away from day-to-day responsibilities to participate in the education sessions. Mentors provided the nurses with support during the educational sessions to assist with the following areas: (1) problem identification, (2) literature searches, (3) rating of evidence, and (4) creation of recommendations for practice. The nursing units, with support from the mentors, identified questions using an evidence-based approach. For example, two question identified were: (1) "For patients experiencing pain who have a history of substance abuse, what are the best nursing interventions to manage the pain?" and (2) "Should a hyperthermia blanket be used for patients experiencing fever?" Similar examples could be generated in the social services (e.g., "what does research tell us about the most effective ways to recruit foster parents?").

FIGURE 1. The Johns Hopkins Nursing Evidence-Based Practice Model

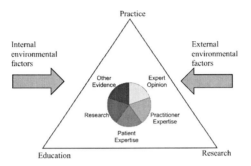

FIGURE 2. Guidelines for Implementation of Evidence-Based Practice Model

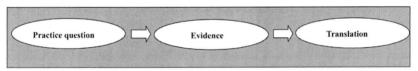

Practice question
 Step 1: Identify EBP question
 Step 2: Define Scope of practice question
 Step 3: Assign responsibility for leadership
 Step 4: Recruit multidisciplinary team
 Step 5: Schedule team conference

Evidence
 Step 6: Conduct internal and external search for evidence
 Step 7: Critique all types of evidence
 Step 8: Summarize evidence
 Step 9: Rate strength of evidence
 Step 10: Develop recommendations for change in processes of care or systems on the basis of strength of evidence

Translation
 Step 11: Determine appropriateness and feasibility of translating recommendations into specific practice setting
 Step 12: Create action plan
 Step 13: Implement change
 Step 14: Evaluate outcomes
 Step 15: Report results of preliminary evaluation to decision makers
 Step 16: Secure support from decision makers to implement recommended change internally
 Step 17: Identify next steps
 Step 18: Communicate findings

The second pilot study used a modified version of the Rosswurm and Larrabee Model (Figure 3) to implement EBP. This pilot also utilized a mentorship program and was designed to enable nurses in the hospital to understand and implement an evidence-based approach to practice (Thurston & King, 2004). Ten nursing teams devoted six hours a month for one year to identify a problem and work through the six-step EBP model. Participants were provided in-depth education (question formulation, research process, research design) and hands-on experience during half-day meetings held every six to eight weeks over one year.

Both pilot studies employed quantitative and qualitative surveys; unfortunately, each had a low response rate but yielded several positive results related to clinician and manager satisfaction. The Johns Hopkins Model demonstrated high staff satisfaction with: (1) clarity of the process (91%), (2) usefulness to practice (92%), (3) adequacy of training (90%), (4) feasibility for practicing nurses (87%), and (5) overall satisfaction with the EBP process (95%). Managers in both studies indicated that staff demonstrated enthusiasm for the process, renewed sense of professionalism and accomplishment, confidence with the EBP, improved staff morale, increased interest in nursing, and an increased willingness to question clinical practices. The following barriers to introducing EBP emerged and were successfully addressed: (1) staff "buy-in," (2) low levels of research knowledge and skill, (3) insufficient evidence available in the literature, (4) time constraints, and (5) lack of hospital-university partnerships.

Meaning to Staff: In both studies, staff raised concerns arose regarding the potential discrepancy between the needs of the clinical nurses and the priorities of the EBP process. The development of relevant and meaningful questions was facilitated by the inclusion of nursing staff in the initial formulation of relevant questions which drew heavily on their insight, clinical expertise, and needs. By involving staff in the initial development, the program gained significant "buy-in" and contributed to enthusiasm for the EBP.

Research Knowledge and Skills: Both studies did not require prior research experience in order to participate in the process, thereby attracting nurses with a wide range of research knowledge and skills. However, the lack of experience with research created tensions among staff. For example, in the Johns Hopkins model, nurses reflected feelings of inadequacy when attempting to analyze the research studies that they uncovered in the search process. To address this issue, educational sessions were designed to introduce participants to basic research methods in order to increase the comfort level of many of the nurses. The

FIGURE 3. Models for Implementing Evidence-Based Practice

Rosswurm & Larrabee Model (1999)		Thurston & King (2004) Modification	
Step One	Assess need for change by collecting and comparing data, identifying practice problem	Step One	Publicize program—stimulate discussion/identification of practice problems
Step Two	Link problem to intervention and outcome using standardized classification systems and language	Step Two	Ongoing discussion re: problem and decision to submit question to EBP Program
Step Three	Synthesize best evidence by searching research literature, critiquing, rating, and synthesizing best evidence, assessing feasibility	Step Three	Identify, critiquing and judging the evidence by accessing and critiquing the research, seeking clinical expertise and stake holder input, benchmarking, summarizing—decision re: change/no change
Step Four	Design practice changes by defining protocol change, planning a pilot/demonstration including implementation, education, resources needed	Step Four	Design and implement the change through colleague involvement and education, procedure/policy changes, ensuring stakeholder support, planning evaluation
Step Five	Implement and evaluate the practice change including evaluation of pilot and decision to adapt/adopt/reject change	Step Five	Monitoring and evaluating the change through quality monitoring system and patient data; continued staff education and wider communication
Step Six	Integrate and maintain change by communicating to stakeholders, in-		

mentor component in both programs proved extremely beneficial to reducing initial feelings of inadequacy. The mentors were available and accessible throughout the process, responding to questions or concerns in a timely manner. This consistent feedback and support prevented the nurses from becoming frustrated or discouraged.

Insufficient Evidence: Thurston and King (2004) reported that the lack of published evidence related to their search questions limited the opportunities for participants to fully critique and rate the evidence using the EBP protocols. This limitation was also experienced by participants and one site used this discovery to emphasize that change does not need to occur if research is too limited to support a change.

Time Constraints: As noted in the literature, time constraints on line staff create the most obvious barrier to the implementation of EBP. However, in both of these pilot studies, staff were given paid leave from their day-to-day responsibilities in order to participate. The participants clearly valued the time and felt it indicated strong administrative support. These two factors of time and administrative support were critical to the success of the program.

Hospital-University Partnerships: In both studies, the hospitals worked in partnership with a local university which provided significant technical support in the form of mentors, publications, and scholarly expertise while the hospitals provided clinical expertise and experience.

Findings Related to the Macro Approach

The macro approach is best illustrated by the National Implementing Evidence-Based Project (EBP Project) which is a nation-wide project to assist staff who work with severe mentally ill adults and have limited access to evidence on effective services (Torrey et al., 2005). A group of stakeholders identified six practices that are currently supported by rigorous research; namely collaborative pharmacologic treatment, assertive community treatment, family psycho-education, supported employment counseling, illness management and recovery skills training, and integrated dual disorders treatment for substance abuse and mental illness. The main goal of the EBP project was to create resources to facilitate the implementation of these six practices. The project was divided into three phases: (1) development of implementation packages, (2) pilot test the implementation packages and modify as necessary, and (3) the implementation process. The packages contained teaching material, resource kits, videos, demonstration skills, workbooks, and implementation tips.

Phase one consisted of designing and creating the implementation strategy and package by a team of stakeholders. This strategy used a planned change approach to develop an intensive program that was sensitive to site-specific conditions. For example, different parts of the implementation packages were designed to address motivation for change, enabling change, and reinforcing change. All sites were asked to identify one person who understood the specific culture and situation of the site in order to translate the implementation package into the local circumstances. Once these implementation strategies were developed, the implementation packages were created with input from researchers, clinicians, program managers, consumers, and family members.

Phase two involved the identification of eight states to participate in the pilot test. Each state agreed to develop a selection process to obtain three to five agencies per practice area. Each agency was given the implementation package as well as on-site training programs and year-long consultation by a trainer. While research reports account for the early stages of phase two, there are no published results on the progress of implementation. However, four major observations were reported by trainers and consultants: (1) *research is not a priority in the agency.* The organizational culture of many of the implementing agencies is not naturally oriented towards the use of research evidence. Such evidence is not highly valued in many agency cultures. Therefore, changing practices based on such research is difficult, (2) *EBP needs to address immediate and previously identified needs.* For example, those agencies that already identified employment as a service delivery need were eager to embrace the Supported Employment intervention. However, those packages that addressed un-recognized needs were difficult to promote and proved difficult to implement. For example, Integrated Dual Disorders Treatment package was difficult to promote in sites that did not perceive substance abuse to be an obstacle for their clients, (3) m*ixing unanticipated changes with the complexity of EBP* requires more time than anticipated. The implementation of a new practice involves unanticipated changes and shifts in the philosophy of care, finance, daily operations, or personnel issues. The trainers in the EBP project found that implementing the new practice required time spent educating staff about the EBP philosophy before promoting procedural changes, and (4) *the importance of leadership* provided by the trainers or consultants. Having a confident and competent site trainer/consultant is critical to successful implementation.

Combination Approach

Dickinson et al. (2004) reported on a three-year project that introduced EBP into a mental health organization using a combination of micro and macro approaches. The project goal was to change the culture of the organization in order to effectively facilitate the introduction of EBP and maintain it on an ongoing basis.

The project began with the formation of a steering group comprised of clinicians representing a variety of disciplines working in various settings (including day hospitals, community rehabilitation, residential centers, and continuing care facilities). Nine teams consisting of 180 staff were created. The steering group administered a survey to identify staff needs and found three major areas of need: (1) education (knowledge, skills, and technical advice to conduct research), (2) resources (access to evidence or other resources), and (3) organizational supports (the need to work as "teams").

The steering group first addressed education by conducting formal training sessions, including two workshops led by external facilitators. Additional informal training and support was provided on each stage of the EBP process (e.g., critical analysis of evidence, target setting, implementation of change based on evidence, monitoring, feedback, and developing recommendations). Financial resources were secured to allow the introduction of internet facilities, journal subscriptions, and paid time to participate in the process. Throughout the process, the steering group conducted regular team-building activities to address team dynamics and support.

The limited evaluation of EBP in mental health setting is based primarily on the observations of the steering group members and on a low response to a staff survey (25%). After one year of implementing EBP processes, five of the nine teams had completed the EBP cycle and implemented new changes based on critically assessed evidence in the areas of discharge process and the use of standardized assessment protocols. The remaining four teams (out of nine) encountered delays in the first year and were unable to complete a full EBP cycle. Additional support was given to these four teams during the second and third years but the teams had still failed to complete the EBP cycle. In all four of these teams, problem identification and target setting had taken place but change and implementation had not occurred. It is unclear if the five successful teams continued to implement EBP beyond their initial success.

The delays in the process by the four teams were attributed to: (1) staff transfers, (2) leadership ambivalence, (3) lack of team cohesion, and (4) insufficient time. In comparing the two groups of teams, the group that successfully implemented changes served more stable clients, possibly allowing them more time within the workday to focus on the EBP process. The limited findings from the staff survey included the following impediments to the EBP process: (1) personal factors (poor motivation, lack of confidence, and lack of knowledge) and (2) organizational factors (limited access to resources, poor teamwork, insufficient time, staff transfers, and disruptive staffing schedules).

CONCLUSIONS AND RECOMMENDATIONS

In comparing all three approaches, it would appear the micro approach had the most successful outcomes, while the macro and combination ran into more obstacles. However, it is important be cautious about drawing conclusions based on these three demonstration projects. The micro approaches relied heavily on informal surveys of practitioners to assess their experiences. While the satisfaction of practitioners with the implementation model and improved knowledge and skill are important, there is no evidence yet that EBP has improved practice related to client outcomes or been sustained within the agency. The incomplete findings from the macro approach make it difficult to draw any concrete conclusions. While lessons can be drawn from all three approaches, there is no conclusive evidence that one approach is more effective than another.

Incorporating EBP into the daily practices of an organization is complex. It requires involvement of all staff levels, adequate resources, strong planning, and the development of an evidence-based culture. Drawing on lessons learned from the literature as well as the implementation pilot studies, there are several important elements to consider as a social service agency seeks to implement EBP. In order to assess the organizational readiness of a social service agency for implementing EBP, a specially designed assessment tool is featured in Figure 4. The major components of the tool include a four-point scale to assess organizational capacity, organizational culture, staff capacity, and the implementation plan. These four components are defined through the use of the following questions:

Organizational Capacity: Does the organization have the financial and human resources needed to implement EBP? Does the organization

FIGURE 4. Assessing Organizational Readiness for Implementation of Evidence-Based Practice

		Not even close	Some way to go	Nearly There	We're there
A. Organizational Capacity		1	2	3	4
1.	There is leadership support from top management in the form of a designated change manager or champion				
2.	The mission reflects a commitment to being a learning organization and is linked to EBP				
3.	Human resources are adequate and available to introduce and sustain EBP				
4.	Financial resources are adequate and available to introduce and sustain EBP				
5.	Change at this time is appropriate and feasible in the life of the organization				
		Section Total:			
B. Organizational Culture/Climate					
1.	Staff understand the mission and goals of the organization as it relates to EBP				
2.	There is cohesiveness and trust among all staff				
3.	Staff are given high levels of autonomy in their work and encouraged to question				
4.	There are open lines of communication in place				
5.	Risk-takers are rewarded				
		Section Total:			
C. Staff Capacity					
1.	Professional growth and development is desired by staff				
2.	Staff have confidence needed to acquire new skills				
3.	One or more staff currently show interest or skills in EBP				
4.	Staff are not overstressed with other responsibilities or tasks				
5.	Staff are comfortable with research methods				
		Section Total:			
D. Implementation Plan					
1.	There is a mechanism to involve all staff (at all levels and across all program) in the phases of implementation				
2.	There is a cohesive team of implementers (oriented, trained, and supported)				
3.	There is capacity to implement an EBP training program				
4.	Resources are available to pilot an implementation process				
5.	There is capacity to "stay the course" for 3-5 years in order to evaluate the impact				
		Section Total:			

Directions for mapping the four scores:

Sum the total score for each section. Plot the results on the corresponding line (e.g. if the total for component A is 16, place a dot on the circle marked 16 on the axis labeled "A" and then do the same for the other three components) and then connect the dots. This gives a visual display of the organizational strengths (highest scoring component) and areas for continued development (lowest scoring component) prior to embarking on a process to implement EBP.

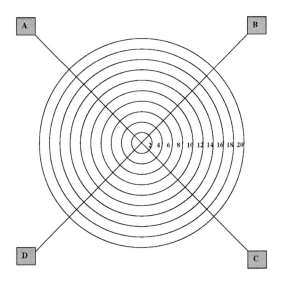

Adapted from (2006) Firm Foundations: A practical guide to organizational support for the use of research. Research in Practice. www.rip.org.uk

have resources to support staff devoting a significant amount of time to acquiring, assessing, and applying the research to practice? Does the organization have the financial means to support the required trainings or other inputs needed?

EBP Culture: Can the culture of the organization support EBP? For example: (1) how clear is the agency's mission and goals among staff, (2) what is the nature of staff cohesiveness and autonomy?, (3) how open are the lines of communication, (4) how open is staff to change, (5) what are the levels of job stress, (6) how are risk-takers rewarded, and (7) how are continuous quality improvement feedback systems utilized?

Staff Capacity: What is the capacity of staff to acquire, assess, apply, and adapt research into practice? Where is capacity already sufficient? Where are staff members currently implementing these steps? Where do staff need additional training? With these strengths and limitations, how are ways identified to strengthen the gaps and build upon the strengths?

The response to the questions in Figure 4 can be plotted to create a visual description of strengths and areas for improvement. The tool is designed for multiple stakeholders to complete in order to foster dialogue about the results.

In summary, the development, implementation, and sustainability of EBP within an organization require participation and engagement of all stakeholders at all levels of the organization. In order to begin the process of implementing EBP, it is important to bring together multiple disciplines and levels of staff, especially line staff in order to draw upon their expertise and perspectives on workload and client issues. Implementation of EBP cannot be accomplished alone; line staff need manager support and managers need line staff. The implementation of EBP is a change that may involve shifts in organizational practices, structures, and resource allocation. These changes may appear radical and unfamiliar to some staff members who may be skeptical and need space to address their questions. Leaders of the EBP implementation process need to be prepared to give tangible meaning to the purpose of the shifts. Time spent on orientation and training can provide staff with a more complete understanding and appreciation of EBP and thereby alleviate fears and feelings of inadequacy. The steps for implementing EBP identified in this analysis suggest that implementation is not a linear process with well-tested action steps. Rather, it is complex and requires considerable discussion, planning, field-testing, and oversight by everyone involved.

REFERENCES

Arad, S., Hanson, M., & Schneider, R. J. (1997). A framework for the study of relationships between organizational characteristics and organizational innovation. *Journal of Creative Behavior, 31*(1), 42-58.

Austin, M. J., & Claassen, J. (2006). *Impact of organizational change on organizational culture: The prospects for introducing evidence-based practice.* Berkeley, CA: Bay Area Social Services Consortium, Center for Social Services Research, School of Social Welfare, University California, Berkeley.

Barratt, M. (2003). Organizational support for evidence-based practice within child and family social work: a collaborative study. *Child & Family Social Work, 8*(2), 143-150.

Barwick, M. A., Blydell, K. M., Stasiulis, E., Ferguson, H. B., Blase, K., & Fixsen, D. (2005). *Knowledge transfer and evidence-based practice in children's mental health.* Toronto, Ontario: Children's Mental Health Ontario.

Cameron, K. S., & Quinn, R. E. (1999). *Diagnosing and changing organizational culture.* Reading: Addison-Wesley.

Canadian Health Services Research Foundation. (2001) *Is research working for you? A self-assessment tool (draft for pilot testing).* Ottawa, Ontario. http://www.chsrf.ca/other_documents/working_e.php

Damanpour, F. (1988). Innovation type, radicalness, and the adoption process. *Communication Research. Special Issue on Innovative Research on Innovations and Organizations, 15*(5), 545-567.

Danielson, C., & Wiggenhorn, W. (2003). The strategic challenge for transfer: Chief learning officers speak out. In E. Holton & T. Baldwin (Eds.), *Improving learning transfer in organizations.* San Francisco, CA: John Wiley & Sons, Inc.

Diamond, M. A. (1996). Innovation and diffusion of technology: A human process. *Consulting Psychology Journal: Practice and Research, 48*(4), 221-229.

Dickinson, D., Duffy, A., & Champion, S. (2004). The process of implementing evidence-based practice: The curate's egg. *Journal of Psychiatric & Mental Health Nursing, 11*(1), 117-119.

Frambach, R. T., & Schillewaert, N. (2002). Organizational innovation adoption: A multi-level framework of determinants and opportunities for future research. *Journal of Business Research: Special Marketing Theory in the Next Millennium, 55*(2), 163-176.

Frey, G. A. (1990). A framework for promoting organizational change. *Families in Society, 71*(3), 142-147.

Gambrill, E. (1999). Evidence-based practice: An alternative to authority-based practice. *Families in Society, 80*(4), 341-350.

Gerrish, K., & Clayton, J. (2004). Promoting evidence-based practice: An organizational approach. *Journal of Nursing Management, 12*, 114-123.

Gibbs, L. E., & Gambrill, E. (2002). Evidence-based practice: Counterarguements to objections. *Research on Social Work Practice, 12*, 452-476.

Gira, E., Kessler, M., & Poertner, J. (2004). Influencing social workers to use research evidence in practice: Lesons from medicine and the allied health professions. *Research on Social Work Practice, 14*(2), 68-79.

Handy, C. (1995). *The age of paradox.* Boston: Harvard Business School Press.

Hodges, S. P., & Hernandez, M. (1999). How organizational culture influences outcome information utilization. *Evaluation & Program Planning, 22*(2), 183-197.

Hodson, R. (2003). Leading the drive for evidence-based practice in services for children and families: Summary report of a study conducted for research in practice.

Huczybski, A. & Lewis, J. (1980). An empirical study into the learning transfer process in management training. *Journal of Management Studies.* 17, 227-240

Jaskyte, K., & Dressler, W. W. (2005). Organizational culture and innovation in nonprofit human service organizations. *Administration in Social Work, 29*(2), 23-41.

Khademian, A. K. (2002). *Working with culture: How the job gets done in public programs.* Washington, D.C: CQ Press.

Lawler, J., & Bilson, A. (2004). Towards a more reflexive research aware practice: The influence and potential of professional and team culture. *Social Work & Social Sciences Review, 11*(1), 52-69.

Lehman, W. E., Greener, J. M., & Simpson, D. D. (2002). Assessing organizational readiness for change. *Journal of Substance Abuse Treatment, 22*(4), 197-209.

Lemon Osterling, K. & Austin, M. J. (2006). *The dissemination and utilization of research for promoting evidence-based practice.* Berkeley, CA: Bay Area Social Services Consortium, Center for Social Services Research, School of Social Welfare, University California, Berkeley.

Mathieu, J., Tannenbaum, S. & Salas (1990). A causal model fo individual and situational influences on training effectiveness measures. In M. Teachout (Chair), *Understanding and evaluating training effectiveness: Multiple perspectives.* Symposium conducted at the Fifth Annual Conference for the Society of Industrial and Organizational Psychology, Miami.

Mullen, E., & Bacon, W. (2000). *A survey of practitioner adoption and implementation of practice guidelines and evidence-based treatments.* Paper presented at the Developing Practice Guidelines for Social Work Intervention: Issues, Methods, and Research Agenda, St. Louis.

Mullen, E., Bellamy, J., & Bledsoe, S. (2004). *Implementing evidence-based practice (EBP) in social work: A pilot study.* Paper presented at the Inter-Center Network for the Evaluation of Social Work Practice, University of Applied Sciences Solothurn, Northwestern, Switzerland.

Mullen, E., Schlonsky, A., Bledsoe, S., & Bellamy, J. (2005). From concept to implementation: Challenges facing evidence-based social work. *Evidence & Policy, 1*(1), 61-84.

Newhouse, R., Dearholt, S., Poe, S., Pugh, L. C., & White, K. M. (2005). Evidence-based practice: A practical approach to implementation. *The Journal of Nursing Administration, 35*(1), 35.

Noe, R & Schmitt, N. (1986). The influence of trainee attitudes on training effectiveness: Test of a model. *Personnel Psychology*, 39, 497-523.

Nutley, S., & Davies, H. T. (2000). Making a reality of evidence-based practice: Some lessons learned from the diffusion of innovations. *Public Money & Management, 20*(4), 35-42.

Nutley, S., Walter, I., Percy-Smith, J., McNeish, D., & Frost, S. (2004). *Improving the use of research in social care practice.* London, UK: Social Care Institute for Excellence.

Oxman, A. D., Thomson, M. A., Davis, D. A., & Haynes, R. B. (1995). No magic bullets: A systematic review of 102 trials of interventions to improve professional practice. *Canadian Medical Association Journal, 153*(10), 1423-1431.

Pawson, R., Boaz, A., Grayson, L., Long, A., & Barnes, C. (2003). *Types and quality of knowledge in social care.* London, UK: Social Care Institute for Excellence.

Pearlmutter, S. (1998). Self-efficacy and organizational change leadership. *Administration in Social Work, 22*(3), 23-38.

Proctor, E. K. (2004). Leverage points for the implementation of evidence-based practice. *Brief Treatment & Crisis Intervention, 4*(3), 227-242.

Proehl, R. A. (2001). *Organizational change in the human services*. Thousand Oaks, CA: Sage Publications, Inc.

Robbins, V., Collins, K., Liaupsin, C., Illback, R. J., & Call, J. (2003). Evaluating school readiness to implement positive behavioral supports. *Journal of Applied School Psychology, 20*(1), 47-66.

Rogers, E. M. (1995). *The diffusion of innovations* (Fourth edition ed.). New York: Free Press.

Rosswurm, M. & Larrabee, J. (1999). A model for change to evidence-based practice. *Image: Journal of Nursing Scholarship*, 31(4), 317-322

Sackett, D. L., Straus, S. E., Richardson, W. S., Rosenberg, W., & Haynes, R. B. (1997). *Evidence-based medicine: How to practice and teach EBM* (Second ed.). Edinburgh: Churchill-Livingstone.

Schein, E. (1985). *Organizational culture and leadership: A dynamic view*. San Francisco, CA: Jossey-Bass.

Sheldon, B., & Chilvers, R. (2000). *Evidence-based social care: A study of prospects and problems*. Lyme Regis: Russell House Publishing.

Sheldon, B., & Chilvers, R. (2002). An empirical study of the obstacles to evidence-based practice. *Social Work & Social Sciences Review, 10*(1), 6-26.

Smith, D. (2004). *Social work and evidence-based practice*. London, UK: Jessica Kingsley.

Thurston, N. E., & King, K. M. (2004). Implementing evidence-based pratice: Walking the talk. *Applied Nursing Research, 17*(4), 239.

Torrey, W. C., Lynde, D. W., & Gorman, P. (2005). Promoting the implementation of practices that are supported by research: The national implemeting evidence-based practice project. *Child & Adolescent Psychiatric Clinics of North America, 14*(2), 297.

Tozer, C., & Bournemouth, S. (1999). 20 questions: The research needs of children and family social workers, *17* (Vol. 1).

Wenger, E., McDermott, R., & Snyder, W. M. (2002). *Cultivating communities of practice*. Boston, MA: Harvard Business School Press.

The Dissemination and Utilization of Research for Promoting Evidence-Based Practice

Kathy Lemon Osterling, PhD
Michael J. Austin, PhD

SUMMARY. Social service practitioners and researchers have long been aware of the gap between research and practice. The evidence-based practice movement has brought increasing attention to the role of empirically based interventions within social service practice, however, effective methods of research dissemination and utilization have received relatively little attention. This article describes factors related to dissemination and utilization of research within human service agency settings, including those factors related to: (1) individual practitioners, (2) the organization, (3) the nature of research, and (4) how research is communicated. The implications of these factors for dissemination and utilization of research are also identified. Ultimately, effective dissemination and utilization of research will involve considerable collaboration between researchers and practitioners. If they are to reach the shared goal of improved interventions and client outcomes, effective collaboration will require both practi-

Kathy Lemon Osterling is Assistant Professor, School of Social Work, San Jose State University, San Jose, CA. Michael J. Austin is Professor, School of Social Welfare, University of California, Berkeley, CA.

The authors would like to acknowledge Jennette Claassen MSW Graduate Student Researcher for her assistance in searching and retrieving literature for this article.

tioners and researchers to make changes to their practice and to their research.

KEYWORDS. Evidence-based practice, research dissemination, research utilization, research-practice collaboration, individual factors, organizational factors

INTRODUCTION

Social service practitioners and researchers have long been aware of the gap between research and practice. Some scholars suggest that researchers and practitioners live in two separate worlds that rarely meet (Eisele & Gamm, 1981). Indeed, studies suggest that practitioners generally do not utilize research in their work with clients (Rosen, 1994). Conversely, researchers have traditionally done little to disseminate research findings or work with practitioners to implement evidence-based interventions (Huberman, 1990). Over the past few years, the evidence-based practice (EBP) movement has brought increasing attention to the role of empirically-based interventions within social service practice. The move toward EBP is shaping much of the current social work discourse, however despite increasing attention to EBP, relatively little attention has been given to effective dissemination and utilization methods. As social problems become more entrenched, it is critical for social service practitioners to become more strategic and systematic in their efforts to serve vulnerable populations. Effective dissemination and utilization of research has the potential to improve social service practice as well as outcomes for clients. In fact, the call for the integration of research into social work practice is featured in the Code of Ethics of the National Association of Social Workers (1999):

> Social workers should critically examine and keep current with emerging knowledge relevant to social work. Social workers should routinely review the professional literature and participate in continuing education relevant to social work practice and social work ethics . . . (4.01b). Social workers should base practice on recognized knowledge, including empirically based knowledge . . . (4.01c).

While there is general agreement that using research to guide decision-making in social service practice is both beneficial and ethical, it is less clear how to disseminate and utilize research. The process of effective dissemination and utilization of research findings is multifaceted and goes far beyond simply publishing or reading journal articles (Gira, Kessler, & Poertner, 2004). Dissemination and utilization is considered to be a complex process involving the influence of numerous factors (Rogers, 2003). The purpose of this analysis is to provide a framework for understanding the factors related to effective dissemination and utilization of research within human service agency settings in order to identify future directions in the form of dissemination and utilization strategies. Ultimately, effective dissemination and utilization of research will involve considerable collaboration between researchers and practitioners (Huberman, 1990). In an effort to bridge the gap between the two worlds of research and practice, such collaboration will require practitioners to make adjustments to their practice and researchers to make adjustments and to their research.

The methodology used to identify literature for this review and analysis is consistent with systematic review procedures. Studies were selected based on pre-determined search terms, databases to be searched and an inclusion and exclusion criteria. Twelve academic databases were searched including those related to psychology, sociology, social work, and social services. Research institute Websites were also searched and a snowball method was also used in which additional materials were identified from primary reference lists of other studies.

FACTORS RELATED TO DISSEMINATION AND UTILIZATION OF RESEARCH

This analysis of the dissemination and utilization of research begins with the definitions of these two processes. Dissemination includes a range of activities designed to transfer knowledge to a target audience; for example, the distribution of written materials, in-service training events, or feedback to practitioners on the use of best practices (Gira et al., 2004; Lavis, Robertson, Woodside, McLeod, & Abelson, 2003). The concept of utilization is generally defined as putting the research to use in practice. Reid and Fortune (1992) define five types of utilization: (1) instrumental utilization occurs when research is used to make decisions or alter practices; (2) conceptual utilization takes place when research is used to enhance insight about an issue, without actually influencing practice or decisions; (3) persuasive utilization involves the use of research to support a particular position; (4) methodological utilization includes the use of specific research or assessment tools; and (5) indirect utilization includes the use of theories, practice models or procedures that are the result of research but do not involve actual familiarity with the research itself. Instrumental utilization related to decision-making appears most frequently in discussions of dissemination and utilization.

While dissemination is a distinctly different activity from utilization, even highly effective dissemination techniques do not ensure that research will be utilized (Rodgers, 1994). For both dissemination and utilization to take place, multiple factors need to be addressed (Backer, 2000; Dal Santo, Goldberg, Choice & Austin, 2002; Rodgers, 1994). One of the most useful frameworks for understanding the multiple factors related to dissemination and utilization was developed by Rogers (2003) and includes the following factors: (1) characteristics of the individual (i.e., the practitioner), (2) characteristics of the organization, (3) characteristics of the innovation itself (i.e., the research), and (4) the nature of the communication (i.e., how the research is communicated). These factors, individually and collectively, can either act as barriers or facilitators to effective dissemination and utilization. They are summarized in Figure 1 and described in more detail in the next several sections.

INDIVIDUAL FACTORS

While there is limited research on practitioner characteristics that facilitate dissemination and utilization within the field of social services, several studies have addressed the role of individual characteristics within the health professions, most notably in nursing where the "Barriers Scale" has been utilized (Funk, Champagne, Wiese, & Tornquist, 1991). Based on Roger's diffusion of innovation theory, this scale includes items related to the individual, the organization, the research and the communication. Studies of nurses have found certain characteristics of practitioners that operate as barriers to research utilization; namely, (1) being unaware of research (Carroll, Greenwood, Lynch, Sullivan, Ready, & Fitzmaurice, 1997), (2) being isolated from knowledgeable colleagues with whom to discuss research (Carroll et al., 1997; Kajermo, Norstrom, Krusebrant & Bjorvell, 1998), and (3) not feeling capable of evaluating the quality of research (Carroll et al., 1997;

FIGURE 1. Factors Related to Dissemination and Utilization

I. Individual Factors

Barriers
- Isolation from knowledgeable colleagues with whom to discuss research (Carroll et al., 1997; Kajermo et al. 1998)
- Not being able to evaluate the quality of research (Carroll et al., 1997; Parahoo, 2000)
- Not being aware of research (Carroll et al. 1997)

Facilitators
- Background in research methods (Kajermo et al. 1998)
- Positive attitude toward research (Grasso et al., 1989; Estabrooks et al. 2003; Estabrooks, 1999)
- Positive attitude toward a particular EBP (McFarlane, 2001)
- Higher educational level (Michel & Sneed, 1995)
- "Belief suspension:" Willingness to use research when it contradicts prior knowledge (Estabrooks, 1999)
- Number of in-service trainings attended (Estabrooks, 1999)
- A critical thinking disposition (Profetto-McGrath, 2003)

II. Organizational Factors

Barriers
- Not enough time on the job to read research or implement new ideas (Carroll et al., 1997; Humphris, et al. 2000, Kajermo et al. 1998; McCleary & Brown, 2003; Parahoo, 2000; Rodgers, 1994)
- Staff and management not supportive of implementation of research (Carroll et al. 1997; McCleary & Brown, 2003; Parahoo, 2000)
- Not enough authority to change practices (Carroll et al., 1997; Kajermo et al. 1998: McCleary & Brown, 2003; Parahoo, 2000)

Facilitators
- In-service trainings on research methods and skills in searching for appropriate literature (Carroll et al., 1997; Humphris et al. 2000; Kajermo et al. 1998; Parahoo, 2000)
- In-service trainings on how to promote EBP or use research in practice settings (Barratt, 2003; Humphris et al. 2000)
- Providing scheduled time for reading research and discussing it with colleagues (Barratt, 2003; Carroll et al., 1997; Humphris et al. 2000; Kajermo et al. 1998; Parahoo, 2000)
- Strong leadership that prioritizes the use of research; improving administrative and organizational support for research utilization (Barratt, 2003; Carroll et al., 1997; Parahoo, 2000)
- Acceptance of the need to change practices (McFarlane, et al., 2001)
- Addressing resource and operational barriers directly (McFarlane et al. 2001; Parahoo, 2000)

III. Research Factors

FIGURE 1 (continued)

Barriers

- Research does not appear generalizable to local practice context (Carrion et al. 2004; Dal Santo, 2002; Hoagwood et al. 2001; Kajermo et al. 1998; Parahoo, 2000)
- Confusion about what constitutes evidence (Barratt, 2003)
- Confusion about conflicting results in the literature (McCleary & Brown, 2003)
- Time lag between research and practice (Beyer & Trice, 1982)

Facilitators
- Relevant research that incorporates the realities of the local practice setting (Carroll et al. 1997; Kajermo et al. 1998)

IV.   Communication Factors

Barriers
- Lack of availability or access to research reports or articles (Bryar et al., 2003; Carrion et al., 2004; Carroll et al., 1997; Kajermo et al. 1998; McCleary & Brown, 2003; Parahoo, 2000; Rodgers, 1994)
- Implications of research for practice are not made clear (Dal Santo et al. 2002; Kajermo et al. 1998; McCleary & Brown, 2003; Parahoo, 2000; Rodgers, 1994)
- Relevant literature is not compiled in one place (Bray et al., 2003; Kajermo et al. 1998; McCleary & Brown, 2003)
- Statistical analyses are not understandable (Bryar et al., 2003; Carrion et al., 2004; Carroll et al., 1997; Kajermo et al. 1998; McCleary & Brown, 2003; Parahoo, 2000)
- Research is not presented in an easily understandable fashion (Barrett, 2003; McCleary & Brown, 2003; Rodgers, 1994)
- Differing priorities and backgrounds of researchers and practitioners (Rosen, 1983; Shrivastava & Mitroff, 1984)
- Power dynamics between researchers and practitioners (Maurrasse, 2001)

Facilitators
- Presenting results in a user-friendly and understandable way (Barratt, 2003; Carroll et al., 1997; Grasso et al., 1989; Kajermo et al. 1998; Parahoo, 2000)
- Access to databases or libraries in order to access research (Barratt, 2003; Carroll et al., 1997)
- Researcher-practitioner collaborations that incorporate shared missions and goals (Carise et al. 2002)
- Researcher-practitioner collaboration that is characterized by strong links between researchers and practitioners, regular discussions of progress reports (Beyer & Trice, 1982; Huberman, 1990)
- Involvement of senior managers in the planning and implementation of research projects (Dal Santo et al. 2002)

Parahoo, 2000). Carrion, Woods and Norman (2004) surveyed forensic mental health nurses in the United Kingdom and found that 57 percent of nurses were unaware of the research, 57 percent felt isolated from knowledgeable colleagues with whom to discuss research, and 57 percent reported not feeling capable of evaluating the research. Similar findings were reported by Bryar, Closs, Baum, Cooke, Griffiths,

Hostick et al. (2003) in their survey of nurses, midwives, and health visitors in the United Kingdom. Depending on the locality, between 45-64 percent of nurses were unaware of the research; between 44-59 percent felt incapable of evaluating the research; and between 37-60 percent reported feeling isolated from knowledgeable colleagues with whom to discuss research.

Certain individual-level characteristics have also been linked to the facilitation of research utilization. Kajermo et al. (1998) found that nurses who had an educational background in research methods perceive fewer barriers to utilization of research than those without this educational background. Michel and Sneed (1995) also found that nurses with a master's degree reported greater research utilization than those with a bachelor's degree. Other research suggests that the attitudes of practitioners can affect dissemination and utilization. McFarlane, McNary, Dixon, Hornby, and Cimett (2001) examined predictors of dissemination of family psychoeducation practices in mental health centers in Maine and Illinois and found that when staff perceived the intervention more positively in the beginning stages of the utilization process, there was a greater likelihood of utilization.

Overall attitudes toward research in general are also predictive of utilization. Grasso, Epstein, and Tirpodi (1989) examined the process of research utilization within a residential treatment center serving adolescents and found that a positive attitude toward research was one factor that predicted research utilization and that pro-research attitudes were also related to research training within the agency as well as the previous education of the practitioner. Estabrooks (2003) conducted a systematic review of individual determinants of research utilization among nurses and found that the most frequently replicated result was related to the attitudes of practitioners toward research. Similarly, Estabrooks (1999) surveyed nurses in Canada and found that attitudes toward research were significantly related to research utilization. Other individual-level factors that predicted research utilization included the number of in-service training events attended in the previous year (e.g., the more events attended, the greater the research utilization), and a willingness to use research even when it contradicts prior knowledge (referred to as "belief suspension"). In addition, Profetto-McGrath, Hesketh, Lang and Estabrooks (2003) evaluated the role of a critical thinking in the utilization of research among nurses in Canada. They defined a disposition toward critical thinking as "attributes or habits of minds integrated into individuals' beliefs or actions that are conducive to critical thinking" (pg. 323) and found that practitioners who are most likely to utilize research were: (1) inquisitive, (2) open-minded, (3) able to seek out the best available information (even when it contradicts their own beliefs), (4) analytical, (5) systematic, and (6) were prudent in their judgments.

ORGANIZATIONAL FACTORS

Organizational factors related to work pressures and a lack of time on the job frequently act as a barrier to research utilization. Using the Barriers Scale, studies have found between 51-80 percent of nurses report that there is not enough time on the job to read research and between 55-85 percent of nurses report that there is not enough time to implement new ideas (Bryar et al., 2003; Carrion et al., 2004; Carroll et al., 1997; Kajermo et al., 1998; McCleary & Brown, 2003; Parahoo, 2000). Additionally, Rodgers (1994) used qualitative methods to identify factors influencing the use of research among nurses and identified a lack of time to read research as a major contributor to a lack of research utilization. In the process of implementing evidence-based practice among occupational therapists, Humphris, Littlejohns, Victor, O'Halloran, and Peacock (2000) found that the three most frequently noted barriers involved workload pressures, time limitations and insufficient staff resources.

In addition to time and workload constraints, other major barriers include organizational structure, a lack of organizational support for research dissemination and utilization, and a lack of authority to change practices. Aarons (2004) found that mental health workers in "low bureaucracy" settings (e.g., programs that are under contract with a county) were more open to using evidence-based practice than those within "high bureaucracy" settings (e.g., programs within the county), suggesting that organizational structure may impact research utilization. Research also suggests that between 50-57 percent of nurses report that other staff who are not supportive of research utilization become barriers and between 57-75 percent of nurses report that they do not have enough authority to change practices (Bryar et al., 2003; Carrion et al., 2004; Carroll et al., 1997; McCleary & Brown, 2003; Parahoo, 2000).

The factors that facilitate research utilization can minimize common organizational barriers, such as providing scheduled time for reading research and discussing it with colleagues. Carroll et al. (1997) found that 64 percent of nurses reported that the utilization of research would increase if there was time to read and implement research findings and 52 percent reported that providing colleagues with support networks and mechanisms to discuss research would increase research utilization.

Likewise, Parahoo (2000) found that nurses requested time to reflect on and think about research findings, as well as time to attend courses or to conduct their own research. Similar findings were noted by Barratt (2003) in her study on organizational support for evidence-based practice within child and family social service settings with respect to staff needing regular time away from their normal work duties in order to read and synthesize research. However, managers also reported that providing scheduled time for staff to read research may not be realistic within the constraints of social service practice.

The use of in-service and pre-service training to facilitate an understanding of research and evidence-based practice can also improve research utilization. Kajermo et al. (1998) and Parahoo (2000) found that training and educating nurses in research methods and skills related to searching literature and implementing and evaluating change could improve their research utilization. Carroll et al. (1997) found that 50 percent of nurses reported that increasing their knowledge about research would facilitate research utilization. In addition, there is evidence to suggest that social workers may require additional training in order to implement evidence-based practices. Barratt (2003) found managers of social service agencies reported that they needed training in order to develop the abilities to promote evidence-based practice in their organizations.

The dissemination and utilization of research can also be facilitated by changing aspects of organizational culture so that the use of research becomes a priority. Barratt (2003) found that 90 percent of social service workers reported that senior level managers should be responsible for ensuring that evidence-based practice be disseminated and utilized throughout agencies. Likewise Parahoo (2000) found that nurses reported that managers who were "knowledgeable" and "research aware" were viewed as the most important facilitators of research dissemination and utilization. Nurses often attributed non-utilization of research to the lack of support from managers and reported that a supportive organizational culture in which organization leaders listened to staff and provided positive feedback helped to facilitate research utilization. Moreover, Carroll et al. (1997) found that 53 percent of nurses reported that improving support and encouragement from top management would increase research utilization.

Organizational leaders who address both resource and operational barriers as well as cultivate a culture that recognizes the need to improve practices are clearly in a position to support research utilization.

Parahoo (2000) found that the improvement of staffing levels (related to adequate patient coverage) was reported by nurses to be a factor that facilitates research utilization. Poor staffing levels were viewed as contributing to low morale among nurses and a general lack of interest in research innovations. Nurses also reported that hiring a staff member to help facilitate access to research and assist staff in integrating research into practice would also facilitate research utilization. In addition, McFarlane et al. (2001) found that the utilization of a new psychoeducation intervention was greatest in mental health centers that directly addressed resource and operational barriers; for example, successful utilization can be seen in staff behaviors that reflected a recognition that new interventions would require a change in existing practices as well as attitudes.

RESEARCH FACTORS

The nature and relevance of available research also impacts research dissemination and utilization. Between 45-67 percent of nurses report that a barrier to research utilization is that research results are often not generalizable to their setting (Bryar et al., 2003; Carrion et al., 2004; Kajermo et al. 1998; Parahoo, 2000). In addition, Dal Santo et al. (2002) found that managers may be somewhat suspicious of research because of its general inability to take into consideration external policies that affect practice, as well as the resource limitations of social service agencies.

Moreover, in their discussion of evidence-based practice in child and adolescent mental health services, Hoagwood, Burns, Kiser, Ringeisen and Schoenwald (2001) suggest that the research community does not generally address the match between a particular evidence-based treatment and the context in which the intervention will be delivered. Efficacy research is typically conducted within tightly controlled laboratory-type settings that seek to factor out the impact of "nuisance variables," such as comorbidity of diagnoses or system-level factors such as payment systems and service availability. However, within real-world practice settings, the influence of so-called "nuisance variables" may be critical to the success of an intervention (Hoagwood et al., 2001). In addition, research on the efficacy of interventions has often been criticized for a general failure to attend to the influence of race/ethnicity on the success of an intervention (United Advocates for Children of California [UACC], 2005). Yet, within social service settings, many of which serve a culturally diverse population, information on the efficacy of an intervention for various racial/ethnic groups can be critical. Researchers have attempted to address this problem by conducting "effectiveness" research on interventions that have proven to be successful in efficacy research. Effectiveness research is intended to test an efficacious intervention within "real-world" settings. Yet, in general, research is still lacking on the effectiveness of interventions with particular populations, and "real-world" settings can often vary greatly between localities, making application of interventions to unique practice settings problematic. Indeed, Kajermo et al. (1998) found that nurses reported their use of research could be facilitated by "more realistic and relevant research [that is] closer to reality" (pg. 804).

The general confusion about what constitutes evidence and the prevalence of conflicting findings in the literature can also leave practitioners unclear about whether a particular intervention is actually useful and should be disseminated and utilized. Barratt (2003) found that social service staff were generally confused about the nature of evidence and whether the term evidence-based practice refers to just published research or also includes unpublished administrative data, theory or expert opinion. Approximately 93 percent of the sample felt that it was crucial for organizations to develop a shared understanding of what constitutes the 'best evidence' in social service settings. Nurse practitioners also report that conflicting results in the research literature can be a barrier to research utilization (McCleary & Brown, 2003).

The timing of research may also affect dissemination and utilization. Beyer and Trice (1982) suggest that there is often a time lag between research and practice and that problems with coordinating relevant research with the needs of decision-makers and practitioners can hinder utilization. Even recently completed research can become irrelevant in the ever-changing practice setting that must respond to new political pressures, funding constraints, policy changes and shifting client populations. Correspondingly, the generally slow pace of research may not be able to keep up with the changing nature of practice due to limited funding, lengthy procedures for protecting human subjects, and the use of time-consuming research methods.

COMMUNICATION

The way in which research is compiled, presented and communicated can directly affect the way that research is utilized by practitioners. The lack of availability or access to research can be a barrier to its use in practice. For example, between 32-78 percent of the nurses in several studies report that research reports and articles are not readily available and therefore not utilized in their practices, while between 48-66 percent report that research literature is not available in one location for easy access (Bryar et al., 2003; Carrion et al., 2004; Carroll et al., 1997; Kajermo et al., 1998; McCleary & Brown, 2003; Parahoo, 2000). In addition, the way in which research reports are written and presented can act as a barrier to their use in practice. For example, between 48-73 percent of nurses report that statistical analyses are not understandable and between 42-64 percent report that the implications of research for practice are not made clear in research reports (Bryar et al., 2003; Carrion et al., 2004; Kajermo et al., 1998; McCleary & Brown, 2003; Parahoo, 2000). Similarly, Dal Santo et al. (2002) found that social service practitioners reported that a barrier to research utilization was that research reports often do not translate general recommendations into specific action steps that agencies can implement, a process usually completed by agency staff.

Not surprisingly, research also suggests that addressing many of the barriers related to accessing research and increasing its understandability can facilitate research dissemination and utilization. Barratt (2003) found that 100 percent of surveyed social service staff felt that research evidence should be presented in a form that is readily understandable to practitioners. Grasso et al. (1989) also found empirical support for the usefulness of user-friendly research; research reports that were easily comprehensible and useful were more effectively utilized in residential children's centers. In addition, practitioners also suggest that having easy access to databases or libraries can facilitate their use of research (Barratt, 2003; Carroll et al., 1997). Research that is concise, understandable and written specifically for implementation within health care agencies can greatly facilitate the use of research by nurses (Carroll et al., 1997; Kajermo et al., 1998; Parahoo, 2000).

Research organizations have not adequately responded to the need to tailor research reports for use in agency settings. In assessing the extent to which research organizations engage in activities to transfer knowledge to their target audiences, Lavis et al. (2003) found that that 60 percent of research organizations tailor dissemination activities to specific audiences, approximately 50 percent spend time with their target audience discussing research or implications of the research for practice, 39 percent dedicate resources to get to know their target audience, and just

20 percent dedicate resources to skill-building among their target audience.

The differing priorities, backgrounds and ideologies of researchers and practitioners may also interfere with effective communication. Rosen (1983) notes that social service practitioners with a humanistic stance toward the alleviation of social problems and an individualized approach to client self-actualization may favor subjective and experiential sources of knowledge. In contrast, researchers are often described as seeking an objective understanding of the world that places importance on measurable phenomena, technical knowledge, theories and rationality (Shrivastava & Mitroff, 1984).

Such differing perspectives may contribute to communication and collaboration problems between researchers and practitioners. Fisher, Fabricant and Simmons (2004) suggest that the expertise and technical knowledge of researchers can conflict with the non-technical and informal nature of knowledge valued by community partners. Some scholars suggest that a power imbalance exists between the status of university researchers and that of community practitioners that can lead to mistrust and stifled communication (Maurasse, 2001). For example, Fisher et al. (2001) note: "When university . . . faculty . . . . cite statistics or refer to sources (in order) to document points or use a language that is foreign to almost anyone outside of their field of study, its impact may be to reduce rather than open dialogue" (p. 29).

Involving practitioners in the research process and strengthening collaboration between researchers and practitioners may help address some of these communication barriers and power imbalances. Dal Santo et al. (2002) found that involvement of agency staff, especially senior staff in the development and implementation of research projects improved both dissemination and utilization of the research findings. In a study of linkages between researchers and practitioners in Switzerland, Huberman (1990) found that the following five types of linkages were related to dissemination and utilization of research: (1) "Hello-Goodbye," (2) "Two Planets," (3) "Standoff," (4) "Mutual Engagement," and (5) "Synergy." Each of these types in defined in Figure 2.

Clearly, the "mutual engagement" and "synergy" collaborations were the most effective in producing research that was ultimately welcomed by practitioners and disseminated within practice settings. Practitioners described the following factors as particularly important to increasing their understanding of the research or ensuring that the findings were put to practical use: (1) interim reports on study findings, (2)

FIGURE 2. Different Types of Relationships Between Researchers and Practitioners

1) *"Hello-Goodbye"*: No collaboration or communication between researchers and practitioners before, during, or after the study where findings were disseminated to a "passive target audience" whose priorities had not been addressed in the research and there was no communication between the researchers and the practitioners eighteen months after the study was completed.

2) *"Two Planets"*: Weak collaboration between practitioners and researchers throughout and after the study reflected episodic contacts that focused on providing training or technical assistance in order to carry out the study where "largely decorative" advisory groups were involved in the research (e.g. met infrequently, lacked a concrete purpose, did not understand research findings, and engaged in few, if any, dissemination activities). Eighteen months after the study was completed both practitioners and researchers were waiting for the other to disseminate findings.

3) *"Standoff"*: Moderate collaboration that remained stable throughout the study period and afterwards, but that ultimately did not directly affect utilization (e.g. the researchers did not consult with the practitioners in the development of the study's focus or while the study progressed leading practitioners to feel that the researchers were "out of touch" with their practice setting and to perceive the findings with suspicion). The dissemination strategy was simply to send the final report to the practitioners who did little to disseminate the findings; there was no contact between researchers and practitioners eighteen months after the study completion.

4) *"Mutual Engagement"*: Weak initial collaboration that grew in strength throughout the course of the study based on frequent informal contacts and a series of interim reports that were concise, easily understandable and discussed in meetings between

researchers and practitioners which helped to neutralize power imbalances and created enthusiasm on the part of both practitioners and researchers to disseminate findings.

5) *"Synergy"*: Well-established collaboration prior to the implementation of the study and these linkages were "activated" during and after the study (e.g. regular discussions of interim reports, frequent informal contacts, meetings to discuss study findings and plan for dissemination, and efforts to use data within practitioner staff meetings and training events).

personal contacts with researchers, (3) co-worker involvement in the study, (4) extensive conversations with researchers before dissemination, (5) attitude changes regarding the value and use of research, and (6) continuous contacts between workers' supervisors and researchers. Huberman (1990) concluded that collaborations that lead to greater dissemination and utilization are characterized by frequent contacts during the study and concerted effort to prepare locally-relevant and user-friendly reports that are of use to practitioners.

IMPLICATIONS FOR DISSEMINATION AND UTILIZATION OF RESEARCH

It is clear that the dissemination and utilization of research findings is a complex process that is influenced by the characteristics of individuals, organizations, research and communication. Most of the research on dissemination and utilization focuses on individual-level interventions that feature passive dissemination approaches (e.g., distributing written materials or attending lecture-style conferences) that generally do not result in actual utilization of research findings by practitioners (Bero, Grilli, Grimshaw, Harvey, Oxman, & Thomson, 1998; Gira et al., 2004; Grimshaw, Shirran, Thomas, Mowatt, Fraser Bero et al., 2001; Oxman, Thomson, Davis, & Haynes, 1995). Other dissemination strategies identified by Oxman et al. (1995) are somewhat more effective and they include outreach visits by experts (i.e., a trained person to provide information on research) and the use of local opinion leaders (i.e., trusted persons in the professional community who have the ability to influence people). There is also some evidence to suggest that audit and feedback approaches can be useful; for example, an expert reviews the ways in which practitioners work with their clients in order to provide feedback on the connection between the actions of practitioners and research on best practices (Gira et al., 2004). Although some discrete individual-level approaches to the dissemination of research may be moderately effective in leading to research utilization, most studies suggest that effective dissemination and utilization of research usually involves a combination of different and complimentary strategies (Bero et al., 1998; Gira et al., 2004; Grimshaw et al., 2001; Oxman et al., 1995).

Although research has addressed dissemination and utilization on the individual-level, attention to other factors, including the organization, the nature of the research and the nature of the communication are also critical elements in how information is disseminated and whether or not it is utilized. Some scholars suggest that "sustained interactivity" between researchers and practitioners has the potential to address multiple barriers to dissemination and utilization on the individual and organizational level, as well as barriers related to the nature of the research and communication. Huberman (1994) defines sustained interactivity as a collaborative process between researchers and practitioners in which strong interpersonal links are formed throughout the course of a research study. Such a strategy has the potential to improve communication between researchers and practitioners as well as to improve dissemination and utilization in other areas as well. Indeed, some scholars suggest that strong linkages between researchers and practitioners are the most effective means through which to achieve dissemination and utilization of research (Beyer & Trice, 1982; Huberman, 1994). Figure 3 provides an overview of the potential benefits of practitioner-research collaborations.

As noted earlier, the use of research in practice is hindered by the practitioner's lack of awareness of research, lack of ability to evaluate research, and feelings of isolation from knowledgeable colleagues (Bryar et al., 2003; Carrion et al., 2004; Carroll et al., 1997; Kajermo et al., 1998; Parahoo, 2000). Conversely, research utilization on the individual level appears to be facilitated by the positive attitude of practitioners toward research and the use of critical thinking skills (Estabrooks, 1999; Grasso et al., 1989; Profetto-McGrath et al., 2003). Strong practitioner-researcher collaboration may have the potential to address these barriers and facilitators.

On the individual level, practitioner-researcher collaborations can provide practitioners with research findings on particular topics of in-

FIGURE 3. Benefits of Practitioner-Researcher Collaborations

Level	Benefits
Individual	• Researchers can provide practitioners with overviews of research findings. Such syntheses may increase practitioner awareness of research, access to research and encourage practitioners to evaluate the quality and applicability of research • Researchers can participate in training events related to the use of critical thinking skills and the role of research in practice
Organizational	• The compilation of research findings by researchers can enhance staff's time to read and reflect on research • Ongoing practitioner-researcher collaborations require commitment from agency leaders; such commitment had the potential to increase organizational and leadership support for the use of research in practice.
Research	• Collaborations can ground research within the realities of local contexts
Communication	• Collaborations can help researchers to tailor research reports to the practice community • Increased accessibility to research reports • Reduction in power imbalances

terest in their practice setting based on collecting and synthesizing multiple studies (Schiller & Malouf, 2000). Such syntheses can increase the practitioner's awareness of research, access to research, and participation in evaluating the quality and applicability of research. In addition, practitioner-researcher collaborations also provide an opportunity for researchers to participate in training events related to discussing the role of research in practice and helping practitioners expand their use of critical thinking skills. The skill set that is common to both researchers and practitioners involves critical thinking skills. Figure 4 includes an array of critical thinking skills needed for the effective dissemination and utilization of research.

On the organizational level, barriers to dissemination and utilization include workload pressures, lack of time to read research or implement new ideas, and lack of organizational or leadership support (Bryar et al., 2003; Carrion et al., 2004; Carroll et al., 1997; Kajermo et al., 1998; McCleary & Brown, 2003; Parahoo, 2000). It is clear that research dissemination and utilization can be facilitated by providing on-the-job time for reading and discussing research, training and education programs, and strong organizational and leadership support for structured and sustained collaborations between researchers and practitioners (Barratt, 2003; Carroll et al., 1997; Kajermo et al., 1998; Parahoo, 2000). The compilation and discussion of research findings can greatly enhance the staff's time to read and reflect on research.

FIGURE 4. Major Skill Sets in the Critical Thinking Process*

I.   Clarifying – What is being stated?
- Clarify problems
- Clarify issues, conclusion, or beliefs
- Identify unstated assumptions
- Clarify and analyze the meanings of words and phrases
- Clarify values and standards

II.   Analyzing – What does it mean?
- Identify significant similarities and differences
- Recognize contradictions and inconsistencies
- Analyze/evaluate arguments, interpretations, beliefs, or theories
- Distinguish relevant from irrelevant questions, data, claims, or reasons
- Detect bias
- Evaluate the accuracy of different sources of information ("evidence")
- Use sound criteria for evaluation
- Compare perspectives, interpretations, or theories
- Evaluate perspectives, interpretations, or theories

III,   Applying – How can it be applied?
- Compare with analogous situations; transfer insights to new contexts
- Make well-reasoned inferences and predictions
- Refine generalizations and avoid oversimplifications
- Compare and contrast ideas with actual practice
- Raise and pursue root or significant questions
- Make interdisciplinary connections
- Analyze or evaluate policies or actions

IV.   Owning – How do the results of critical thinking apply to my situation?
- Evaluate one's own reasoning process
- Explore thoughts underlying feelings and feelings underlying thoughts
- Design and carry out critical tests of concepts, theories, and hypotheses
- Discover and accurately evaluate the implications and consequences of a proposed action

----

*Abstracted from "Examples of Critical Thinking Skills" (p 129), Gibbs, L & Gambrill, E. (1999) *Critical thinking for social workers*. Thousand Oaks, CA: Pine Forge Press. Based on Ennis, R.H. (1987). A taxonomy of critical thinking dispositions and abilities. In J.B. Baron & R.J. Steinber (Eds) *Teaching thinking skills: Theory and practice*. NY: Freeman. Paul, R.(1993). *Critical thinking: What every person needs to survive in a rapidly changing world*. Santa Rosa, CA: Foundation for Critical Thinking

On the research level, studies suggest that research is not perceived to be generalizable to local settings, fails to consider external policies and resource limitations that affect practice, and arrives too late to be utilized due to the time lag between research and practice (Beyer & Trice, 1982; Bryar et al., 2003; Carrion et al., 2004; Dal Santo et al., 2002; Kajermo et al., 1998; Parahoo, 2000). Jensen, Hoagwood & Trickett

(1999) note that community collaborations help to bridge the gap between research conducted in tightly controlled settings and the realities of real-world practice settings. They suggest six principles for successful collaboration between university researchers and community partners, including: (1) a broad focus on the applicability of the research to the population under consideration; (2) integrating the perspectives of community collaborators within the research; (3) a thorough assessment of outcomes relevant to the local context; (4) flexibility to address local needs and conditions; (5) modification of research methods; and (6) the use of long-term commitments beyond the current project.

There is some evidence to suggest that research grounded in the reality of local contexts is more likely to be disseminated and utilized. Simons, Kushner, Jones and James (2003) evaluated the impact of a program in the United Kingdom that was expressly aimed at encouraging teachers to use research, as well as conduct their own research. Collaborations between teachers and researchers from university departments of education found that teachers more likely to adopt the new practice when they saw a connection between a new practice and the context in which the evidence for the new practice arose. These findings suggest that the closer the link between research and the local contexts in which practitioners work, the more likely the research is to be utilized.

As noted earlier, the communication factors that act as a barrier to research dissemination and utilization include the inaccessibility of research, incomprehensible statistical analyses, unclear research implications, and inadequate communications due to differing perspectives between practitioners and researchers (Bryar et al., 2003; Carrion et al., 2004; Carroll et al., 1997; Dal Santo et al., 2002; Fisher et al., 2004; Kajermo et al., 1998; McCleary & Brown, 2003; Parahoo, 2000; Rosen, 1983). Factors that facilitate communications include user-friendly and understandable research reports, easy access to research information, and effective and sustained contact between researchers and practitioners (Barratt, 2003; Carroll et al., 1997; Grasso et al., 1989; Huberman, 1990; Kajermo et al., 1998; Parahoo, 2000).

CORE ELEMENTS OF EFFECTIVE PRACTITIONER-RESEARCHER COLLABORATIONS

The establishment of strong collaborations between practitioners and researchers has the potential to improve research dissemination and utilization. A synthesis of the literature on effective collaboration, especially among researchers and practitioners is summarized in Figure 5 and includes four core elements: (1) incentive to collaborate, (2) shared values, trust, open communication, and respect, (3) ability to collaborate, and (4) capacity to build and sustain collaboration.

Incentive to Collaborate: Robertson (1998) notes that a necessary precondition to effective collaboration is an incentive to collaborate among all parties. Most notably, collaboration is often motivated by a need to gain access to resources or to use resources more efficiently. In the case of practitioner-researcher collaborations, a clear incentive for practitioners is to gain access to research and experts who can provide evidence relevant to practice. Researchers have incentives to collaborate with practitioners in order to improve the quality of the research and suggest areas of inquiry that may be new to researchers. Indeed, effective practitioner-researcher collaborations involve a high degree of reciprocity (Huberman, 1994). Such collaborations balance the flow of incentives as research informs practice and practice informs research.

Shared Values, Trust, Open Communication and Respect: The differing backgrounds and experiences of researchers and practitioners need to be addressed so that both parties can create an environment that reflects shared values, trust, open communication and respect. Both researchers and practitioners need to overcome biases and come to an understanding that although researchers and practitioners use different methods, both parties are interested in the same outcomes, namely improving services and client outcomes (Carise, Cornely & Gurel, 2002) Similarly, Robertson (1998) suggests that shared values create a willingness to collaborate and help to establish trust among collaborators. Trust is created by open communication among all parties and can lead to feelings of reciprocity in the collaboration. Correspondingly, open communication and mutual respect are often fostered by frequent contacts and communication between parties (Lane, Turner, & Flores, 2004; Robertson, 1998). For example, Lane et al. (2004) found that respect for the unique perspectives and pressures facing both practitioners and researchers led to open communication. Successful communications were characterized by both practitioners and researchers asking questions and listening to one another, informal sharing of meals and shared rides to meetings that provided opportunities to address disagreements and to develop compromises.

Ability to Collaborate: While the ability to collaborate (i.e., knowledge and skills) is a necessary prerequisite to effective collaboration, additional work on top of the regular work duties of researchers and

FIGURE 5. Core Elements of Effective Practitioner-Researcher Collaborations

Element	Description
Incentive to Collaborate	• Practitioners can gain access to research and experts who provide evidence relevant to practice • Researchers can use practitioner feedback to improve the quality of research and suggest areas of inquiry that researchers may not be aware of
Shared Values, Trust, Open Communication and Respect	• Both researchers and practitioners need to overcome biases and come to an understanding that both parties are interested in improving services and client outcomes • Shared values create a willingness to collaborate and help to establish trust among collaborators • Trust results from feelings of reciprocity and is created by open communication and respect
Ability to Collaborate	• Skills and knowledge are required in order to collaborate • Collaborations typically involve additional work on top of regular work duties
Capacity to Build and Sustain Collaboration	• Successful collaboration involves the use of systems and mechanisms to help coordinate activities and duties • Mechanisms to build and sustain collaborations include: 1) the use of supraorganizational forums (e.g. parties from several collaborations come together to discuss successful collaboration and make decisions regarding their own collaborations), 2) a broker or strategy maker to coordinate activities, 3) the use of multiple communication channels, and 4) the establishment of guidelines to govern duties, activities and decision-making

practitioners is also required (Robertson, 1998). In addition, Carise et al. (2002) found that both practitioners and researchers required preparation before engaging in a collaborative research project, especially when evaluating the implementation of a new system that requires researchers to understand the practice setting and the experiences of practitioners. Such preparation is needed in order to prepare staff for future changes in their practices and prepare researchers to work effectively with practitioners.

Capacity to Build and Sustain Collaboration: Successful collaboration also involves the use of the following systems and mechanisms, identified by Robertson (1998) to help coordinate activities and duties: (1) forums to bring together the parties from several collaboratives to discuss experiences and learn from each other, (2) brokers to coordinate activities, (3) multiple communication channels, including the use of a board of directors, and (4) guidelines to govern duties, activities and decision-making related to the use of agency resources needed to conduct a study and the ownership of data collected in the study (Anderson, 2001). In their discussion of a successful researcher-practitioner collaboration, Lane et al. (2004) found that effective collaboration was facilitated by "conscious and continuous effort" on the part of researchers and practitioners to ensure that the collaboration was successful, especially in light of a variety of competing demands on the time and attention of both parties.

CONCLUSION

The gap between research and practice can be detrimental to both the quality of social service practice, as well as the quality of social service research. Research can inform practice, just as practice can inform research. While the EBP movement has brought increasing attention to the importance of using the best evidence to serve vulnerable populations, less attention has been given to the development of effective dissemination and utilization methods. Numerous interacting factors related to individuals, organizations, the nature of research and the nature of communication are involved in the dissemination and utilization process.

This analysis suggests that effective collaborations require both practitioners and researchers to change the ways they engage one another. In essence, practitioners need to shift from such statements as "Tell us what you found AND what we should do differently" to "Involve us in the research process so that we can share in the data interpretation and develop our own conclusions about what we should be doing differently." In a similar fashion, researchers need to shift from such statements as "Tell us what you want to know and we'll tell you what we found" to "How can we both use research to improve outcomes for clients and strengthen current practice?" Based on the shared goals of improving interventions and client outcomes, practitioner-researcher partnerships will need to focus more attention on improving the dissemination and utilization of research if they are to reach these goals.

REFERENCES

Aarons, G. A. (2004). Mental health provider attitudes toward adoption of evidence-based practice: The Evidence-Based Practice Attitude Scale (EBPAS). *Mental Health Services Research, 6*(2), 61-74.

Anderson, S. G. (2001). The collaborative research process in complex human services agencies: Identifying and responding to organizational constraints. *Administration in Social Work, 25*(4), 1-19.

Backer, T. E. (2000). The failure of success: Challenges of disseminating effective substance abuse prevention programs. *Journal of Community Psychology, 28*(3), 363-373.

Barratt, M. (2003). Organizational support for evidence-based practice within child and family social work: A collaborative study. *Child and Family Social Work, 8,* 143-150.

Bero, L. A. Grilli, R., Grimshaw, J. M., Harvey, E., Oxman, A. D., & Thomson, M. A. (1998). Closing the gap between research and practice: An overview of systematic reviews of interventions to promote the implementation of research findings. *British Medical Journal, 317,* 465-468.

Beyer, J. M. & Trice, H. M. (1982). The utilization process: A conceptual framework and synthesis of empirical findings. *Administrative Science Quarterly, 27,* 591-622.

Bryar, R. M., Closs, S. J., Baum, G., Cooke, J., Griffiths, J., Hostick, T., Kelly, S., Knight, S., Marhsall, K., Thompson, D. R. (2003). The Yorkshire BARRIERS project: Diagnostic analysis of barriers to research utilization. *International Journal of Nursing Studies 40,* 73-84.

Carise, D., Cornely, W., & Gurel, O. (2002). A successful researcher-practitioner collaboration in substance abuse treatment. *Journal of Substance Abuse Treatment, 23,* 157-162.

Carrion, M., Woods, P., & Norman, I. (2004). Barriers to research utilization among forensic mental health nurses. *International Journal of Nursing Studies, 41,* 613-619.

Carroll, D. L., Greenwood, R., Lynch, K., Sullivan, J. K., Ready, C., & Fitzmaurice, J. B. (1997). Barriers and facilitators to the utilization of nursing research *Clinical Nurse Specialist, 11*(5), 207-212.

Dal Santo, T., Goldberg, S., Choice, P, & Austin, M. J. (2002). Exploratory research in public social service agencies: As assessment of dissemination and utilization. *Journal of Sociology and Social Welfare, 29*(4), 59-81.

Eisele, F. R., & Gamm, L. (1981). Research utilization: Reaching decision makers. *Children and Youth Services Review, 3,* 291-303.

Ennis, R.H. (1987). A taxonomy of critical thinking dispositions and abilities. In J.B. Baron & R.J. Steinber (Eds). *Teaching thinking skills: Theory and practice.* NY: Freeman.

Estabrooks, C. A. (2003). Individual determinants of research utilization: A systematic review. *Journal of Advanced Nursing, 43*(5), 506-520.

Estabrooks, C. A. (1999). Modeling the individual determinants of research utilization. *Western Journal of Nursing Research, 21*(6), 758-772.

Fisher, R., Fabricant, M. & Simmons, L. (2004). Understanding contemporary university-community connections: Context, practice, and challenges. *Journal of Community Practice, 12*(3/4), 13-34.

Funk, S. G., Champagne, M. T., Wiese, R. A., & Tornquist, E. M. (1991). Barriers: The Barriers to research utilization scale. *Applied Nursing Research, 4,* 39-45.

Gibbs, L & Gambrill, E. (1999) *Critical thinking for social workers.* Thousand Oaks, CA: Pine Forge Press.

Gira, E. C., Kessler, M. L. & Poertner, J. (2004). Influencing social workers to use research evidence in practice: Lessons from medicine and the allied health professions. *Research on Social Work Practice, 14*(2), 68-79.

Grasso, A. J., Epstein, I., & Tripodi, T. (1989). Agency-based research utilization in a residential child care setting. *Administration in Social Work, 12*(4), 61-80.

Grimshaw, J. M., Shirran, L., Thomas, R., Mowatt, G., Fraser, C., Bero, L., Grilli, R., Harvey, E., Oxman, A., & O'Brien, M. A. (2001). Changing provider behavior: An overview of systematic reviews of interventions. *Medical Care, 39*(8) II-2-II-45.

Hoagwood, K., Burns, B. J., Kiser, L., Ringeisen, H., & Schoenwald, S. K. (2001). Evidence-based practice in child and adolescent mental health services. *Psychiatric Services, 52*(9), 1179-1189.

Huberman, M. (1994). Research utilization: The state of the art. *Knowledge and Policy: The International Journal of Knowledge Transfer and Utilization, 7*(4), 13-33.

Huberman, M. (1990). Linkage between researchers and practitioners: A qualitative study. *American Educational Research Journal, 27*(2), 363-391.

Humphris, D., Littlejohns, P., Victor, C., O'Halloran, P., & Peacock, J. (2000). Implementing evidence-based practice: Factors that influence the use of research evidence by occupational therapists. *British Journal of Occupational Therapy, 63*(11), 516-522.

Jensen, P. S., Hoagwood, K., & Trickett, E. J. (1999). Ivory towers or earthen trenches? Community collaborations to foster real-world research. *Applied Developmental Science, 3*(4), 206-212.

Kajermo, K. N., Nordstrom, G., Krusebrant, A., & Bjorvell, H. (1998). Barriers to and facilitators of research utilization, as perceived by a group of registered nurses in Sweden. *Journal of Advanced Nursing, 27,* 798-807.

Lane, J., Turner, S., & Flores, C. (2004). Researcher-practitioner collaboration in community corrections: Overcoming hurdles for successful partnerships. *Criminal Justice Review, 29*(1), 97-114.

Lavis, J. N., Robertson, D., Woodside, J. M., McLeod, C. B., & Abelson, J. (2003). How can research organizations more effectively transfer research knowledge to decision makers? *The Millbank Quarterly, 81*(2), 221-248.

Maurrasse, D. J. (2001). *Beyond the campus: How colleges and universities form partnerships with their communities.* New York: Routledge.

McCleary, L. & Brown, G. T. (2003). Barriers to paediatric nurses' research utilization. *Journal of Advanced Nursing, 42*(4), 364-372.

McFarlane, W. R., McNary, S., Dixon, L., Hornby, H., & Cimett, E. (2001). Predictors of dissemination of family psychoeducation in community mental health centers in Main and Illinois. *Psychiatric Services, 52*(7), 935-942.

Michel, Y. & Sneed, N. V. (1995). Dissemination and use of research findings in nursing practice. *Journal of Professional Nursing, 11*(5), 306-311.

National Association of Social Works (1999). *Code of Ethics.* Washington DC: Author.

Oxman, A. D., Thomson, M. A., Davis, D. A., & Haynes, R. B. (1995). No magic bullets: A systematic review of 102 trials of interventions to improve professional practice. *Canadian Medical Association Journal, 153*(10), 1423-1431.

Parahoo, K. (2000). Barriers to, and facilitators of, research utilization among nurses in Northern Ireland. *Journal of Advanced Nursing, 31*(1), 89-98.

Paul, R. (1993). *Critical thinking: What every person needs to survive in a rapidly changing world.* Santa Rosa, CA: Foundation for Critical Thinking

Profetto-McGrath, J. Hesketh, K. L. Lang, S., & Estabrooks, C. A. (2003). A study of critical thinking and research utilization among nurses. *Western Journal of Nursing Research, 25*(3), 322-337.

Reid, W. J., & Fortune, A. E. (1992). Research utilization in direct social work practice. In A. J. Grasso, & I. Epstein (Eds.). *Research utilization in the social services* (pp. 97-116). New York: Hawthorne.

Robertson, P. J. (1998). Interorganizational relationships: Key issues for integrated services. In J. McCrosky, & S. D. Einbinder (Eds.). *Universities and communities: Remaking professional and interprofessional education for the next century* (pp.67-87). Wesport CT: Praeger.

Rodgers, S. (1994). An exploratory study of research utilization by nurses in general medical and surgical wards. *Journal of Advanced Nursing, 20*, 904-911.

Rogers, E. (2003). *Diffusion of innovations.* 5th Ed. New York: Free Press.

Rosen, A. (1994). Knowledge use in direct practice. *Social Service Review,* 561-577.

Rosen, A. (1983). Barriers to utilization of research by social work practitioners. *Journal of Social Service Research, 6*(3/4), 1-15.

Schiller, E. P. & Malouf, D. B. (2000). Research syntheses: Implications for research and practice. In R. M. Gersten, E. P. Schiller, & S. Vaughn, (Eds.). *Contemporary special education research: Syntheses of the knowledge vase on critical instructional issues. The LEA series on special education and disability* (pp. 251-262). Mahwah, NJ: Lawrence Erlbaum Associates.

Shrivastava, P., & Mitroff, I. I. (1984). Enhancing organizational research utilization: The role of decision makers' assumptions. *Academy of Management Review, 9*(1), 18-26.

Simons, H., Kushner, S., Jones, K., & James, D. (2003). From evidence-based practice to practice-based evidence: The idea of situated generalisation. *Research Papers in Education 18*(4), 347-364.

United Advocates for Children of California (2005). Children's mental health and evidence based practices: Preliminary thoughts and issues. Sacramento CA: Author. Dissemination and Utilization of Research

Impact of Organizational Change on Organizational Culture: Implications for Introducing Evidence-Based Practice

Michael J. Austin, PhD
Jennette Claassen, MSW

SUMMARY. Evidence-based practice (EBP) seeks to integrate the expertise of individual practitioners with the best available evidence within the context of the values and expectations of clients. Prior to implementing EBP, it is important to understand the significance that organizational change and organizational culture play. This article seeks to explore the literature associated with both organizational change and organizational culture. The analysis of organizational culture and change draw upon findings from both the private, for-profit sector, and the public, non-profit field. It is divided into four sections: organizational change and innovation, organizational culture, managing organizational culture and change, and finally, applying the findings to the implementation of EBP. While the audience for this analysis is managers in public and nonprofit human service organizations who are considering implementing EBP into their work environment, it is not intended to provide a "how to" guide, but rather a framework for critical thinking.

Michael J. Austin is Professor and Jennette Claassen is Research Assistant, School of Social Welfare University of California, Berkeley.

KEYWORDS. Evidence-based practice, organizational change, organizational culture, private, for-profit, public, non-profit

INTRODUCTION

Evidence-based practice (EBP) seeks to integrate the expertise of individual practitioners with the best available evidence within the context of the values and expectations of clients (Sackett, Straus, Richardson, Rosenberg, & Haynes, 1997; Gambrill, 1999). While scholars have identified multiple requirements for research evidence to impact practice and policy related to the nature of evidence as well as its dissemination and utilization, this analysis focuses on the action steps needed at the organizational level to introduce a change that can impact the culture of the organization (Davies & Nutley, 2002; Kitson, Harvey, & McCormack, 1998).

Based on the U.K. experiences, EBP appears to be an innovation that requires several changes at the organizational level, including (a) ideological and cultural changes, (b) technical changes, such as changing the content or mode of service delivery in response to evidence about the effectiveness of interventions, and (c) changes in organization and management to support EBP (Hampshire Social Services, 1999; Hodson, 2003). To achieve these changes, a combination of approaches at the micro, macro, and organizational levels appears to be the most effective (Hodson, 2003). "Micro" approaches alter the attitudes, ways of working and behaviors of individual practitioners, while "macro" approaches redesign key systems, such as systems for the dissemination of evidence or systems for developing policy. "Organizational approaches" integrate micro and macro strategies while removing impediments to new ways of working through the redesign of routines and practices. Organizational approaches also supply the supportive structures that are necessary to sustain EBP processes at every level of the organization (Center for Evidence-based Social Services, 2004).

Evidence-based practice appears to operate best within an organizational context that supports practitioners at each stage of the EBP process. The process itself involves the following steps: (a) becoming motivated to apply evidence-based practice, (b) converting information needs into a well-formulated answerable question, (c) achieving maximum efficiency by tracking down the best evidence with which to answer the question (which may come from the clinical examination, the diagnostic laboratory, the published literature or other sources), (d) critically appraising the evidence for its validity and applicability to clinical practice, (e) applying the results of this evidence appraisal to policy/practice, (f), evaluating performance, and (g) teaching others to do the same (Sackett et al., 1997).

The modification of agency cultures may also be necessary to support and sustain evidence-based practice. The modification of an agency's culture needs to include strategies that address the reality that practitioners generally do not have time to consult the research literature to guide practice decision-making due to an overwhelming volume of information, lack knowledge about searching techniques, lack of time, and lack access to information and libraries. In essence, what does management need to do to build and sustain the supports for evidence-based practice? What do supervisors need to do to assist line staff in the process of adopting evidence-based practice? And what adjustments do line staff members need to make to incorporate evidence-based practice into their daily routines? (Johnson & Austin, forthcoming).

In order to understanding the significance that organizational change and organizational culture play in successfully implementing EBP, it is important to review the research associated with these two concepts. This analysis of organizational culture and organizational change draws upon findings from both the private, for-profit sector, and the public, non-profit field. It is divided into the following four sections: organizational change and innovation, organizational culture, managing organizational culture and change, and finally, applying the findings to the implementation of EBP. While the audience for this analysis are managers in public agencies who are considering implementing EBP into their work environment, it is not intended to provide a "how to" guide, but rather, a framework for critical thinking.

Consistent with the EBP principles of a systematic review, this structured review of the literature located references using pre-determined search terms, database searches, and inclusion and exclusion criteria noted in the Appendix. The inclusion and exclusion criteria were based on three broad areas: (1) organizational change processes that facilitate positive organizational change, (2) organizational culture and (3) the management of organizational culture and change within the human service field. Due to the limited amount of citations related to the human services, additional sources are included related to the public and private sector, medicine and nursing, and public administration. Additional articles were included using a snowball method in which supplementary materials were identified from primary reference lists of other studies. A total of 107 articles were identified in the initial search. Sixty-one full articles were retrieved based on abstracts that seemed promising and a total of 43 were found to be relevant to the topic.

CHANGE AND INNOVATION

Human service agencies are becoming increasingly aware of the need to make changes in the way they are structured and managed. Human service agencies need to contend with declining funding, increased demand for more accountability, and an ever-shifting public agenda. Creative and flexible organizational cultures are needed to respond to these significant changes in public programs. Research findings from the literature on organizational change and organizational culture can be helpful in identifying concepts and findings to use in assessing the challenges faced by human service organizations. While much of the organizational change literature draws from the for-profit sector, Robertson and Seneviratne (1995) found that the strategies and processes transcend the organizational type and have similar implications for the non-profit and public sectors. The major components of the research literature on organizational change and innovation are summarized in Figure 1 related to definitions, types of change, degree of change, facilitators and inhibitors of change, staff receptivity, and staff readiness.

DEFINITION OF CHANGE AND INNOVATION

With the understanding that innovation involves a process of moving an organization from its current state to that of a new and different state, this analysis considers innovation and change to be interchangeable concepts and therefore the term "change" is used throughout. Change is defined as the adoption of an idea or behavior-whether a system, process, policy, program, or service-that is new to the adopting organization (Aiken & Hage, 1971; Daft, 1982, Damanpour & Evan, 1984). Damanpour (1988) defined organizational change as either responding to changes in its environment or as "a preemptive action" (p. 546). A change within an organization does not need to be an original or novel but simply a new idea within that particular working environment that may or may not prove to be successful (King, 1992).

FIGURE 1. Major Dimensions of Organizational Change

I.   Definition: a process by which an organization identifies, examines, and implements a new idea.

II.   Types of change: two main types of change are *administrative* (process) and *technical* (product), where administrative changes refer to the organizational structure and administrative processes (mainly occurring at the management level and less at the basic work activities of the organization) and technical changes are the changes in products, services, production, or process technology and affect the work activities of the organization.

III.   Degree of change: two major degrees, *fundamental* departure from existing practices (radical reorientation, non-routine, ultimate, core, transformative, and high risk) and *minor* adjustments to existing practices (routine, instrumental, peripheral, incremental, and low risk)–See Figure 2

IV.   Facilitators and inhibitors of change: since size alone may not inhibit or facilitate change, successful adoption of change in an organization includes the following characteristics: 1) simplicity of the change, 2) degree that it is similar to previous practices, 3) advantage of change is clearly articulated and understood (e.g., improved outcomes, increased financial gains), 4) rolled out in stages or small steps, and 5) readily observable to those being asked to implement the change.

V.   Staff receptivity and resistance: organizational change can be experienced by staff as: 1) personal loss and feelings of inadequacy, 2) lack of competence and self-confidence, and 3) frustration related to a lack of understanding and knowledge.

VI.   Staff readiness: The three factors related to staff readiness are: 1) what is important for change to occur?, 2) what is necessary but not always sufficient for change to occur?, and 3) what change is appropriate in the current situation?.

In developing a way to explain change, researchers have divided change into two distinct categories; namely, product and process (Poole, Ferguson, & Schwab, 2005; King, 1992). Product changes are the outputs and services that are distinctly different from the previous outputs. Process changes are changes in the technology, such as new tools or ways of working which increase the quality of a service or the working environment (Poole, Ferguson, & Schwab, 2005, p. 102). For the purposes of this analysis, change is viewed as a process by which an organization identifies, examines, and potentially implements a new idea.

The process of change includes individual and organizational factors that affect the generation and adoption of a new idea in an organization. Organizational factors have received the most attention with respect to the structural facilitators and barriers that promote and sustain organizational change (Jaskyte & Dressler, 2005; Frank, Zhao, & Borman, 2004; Arad, Hanson, & Schneider, 1997). Individual factors have received less attention, resulting in major gaps in our understanding of the human process involved in change (Diamond, 1995; Jaskyte & Dressler, 2005).

The major organizational factors that influence change can be divided into three major categories: (1) types of change (2) degree of change and 3) structural facilitators of and barriers to change. The type and degree of organizational change are important to understand because they have differing rates of disruption and adoption in an organization (Damanpour, 1988; Frey, 1990; Pearlmutter, 1998). Damanpour (1988) notes that all types of change do not have identical attributes, their adoption is not the same, and they do not relate equally to the same predictor variables. As a result of these differences, it is necessary to differentiate between the various types of organizational change.

The two main types of change are administrative (process) and technical (product). They represent a general distinction between the social structures operating within an organization and the technology used by the organization (Damanpour, 1988). While the terms, administrative and technical, are more commonly used within the for-profit sector, the concepts are transferable to the nonprofit and public human service sector (Pearlmutter, 1998; Jaskyte & Dressler, 2005). Administrative changes refer to the organizational structure and administrative processes, mainly occurring at the management level and less at the basic work activities of the organization. Examples of administrative changes in human service organizations include the creation of a new employee/volunteer incentive/reward system, a new recruitment system, or a new performance evaluation system (Jaskyte & Dressler, 2005). Technical changes are the changes in products, services, production, or process technology and affect the work activities of the organization. Examples of technical change in human service organizations involve the introduction of new service programs or delivery systems (Jaskyte & Dressler, 2005).

Degree of Change

In addition to the type of change, it is important to note the degree of change created within an organization. Researchers have described an array of organizational change from minor to radical. For example, Burke & Litwan (1992) used the terms "incremental" and "transformative" where incremental aims at fixing a problem, modifying a procedure, or making an adjustment while transformative changes aim to alter the fundamental structure, systems, or strategies of the organization. Normann (1971) used the terms "variation" and "reorientation"; the former describing refinements or modifications and the latter referring to fundamental changes in existing products or services. Knight (1967) and Nord and Tucker (1987) both used the terms "routine" and "non-routine" to describe the degree of change. Routine suggests only minor changes while non-routine are changes in the internal or external environment of the agency. Grossman (1970) distinguished between "instrumental" and "ultimate" change with instrumental involving those factors that facilitate change and ultimate referring to the change itself. Singh, House, and Tucker (1986) used "peripheral" and "core" to describe the different degrees. Peripheral changes in an organization are flexible and involve less institutional change. Core changes are those that change the least flexible aspects of an organization (i.e., goals, authority, and resources acquisition). Finally, Frey (1990) distinguished between "low risk" and "high risk" degrees of change. Low risk refers to those changes that have relatively little cost. High risk includes those changes that cannot easily be terminated or reversed, must be implemented in entirety, or conflict with the dominant values of the organization.

The varying degrees of change are described in Figure 2. Despite the differing terminology, these terms all resemble one another. Reorientation, non-routine, ultimate, core, transformative, and high risk are all considered radical innovations because they produce fundamental changes in the activities of the organization and represent a departure from existing practices. The concepts of variation, routine, services instrumental, peripheral, incremental, and low risk reflect minor degrees of change from the original state. For human service agencies, minor change involves the development of new changes to meet client needs, hiring staff to implement those changes, and the extension of hours of operation to provide the services (Pearlmutter, 1998). The minor changes seek to improve what is already in place and are viewed as less threatening to staff and easiest to manage (Proehl, 2001). Damanpour (1988) found that minor changes in organizations tend to be initiated by staff occupying the lower levels in the hierarchy of the organization. In

FIGURE 2. Degree of Change

Is the change Incremental or Transformative?

Incremental aims at fixing a problem, modifying a procedure, or making an adjustment

Transformative changes aim to alter the fundamental structure, systems, or orientation and strategies of the organization

Variation refers to refinements and modifications, especially to a product or service

Reorientation refers to a fundamental change in existing product or service

Is the change Routine or Non-Routine?

Routine suggest only minor changes in products, services, or production process

Non-Routine introduces change in the internal or external environment of the adopting organization

Is the change Instrumental or Ultimate?

Instrumental facilitate the adoption of the ultimate innovations at a later point

Ultimate are the ends in themselves

Is the change Peripheral or Core?

Peripheral are flexible and involve less institutional change (location, staff turnover)

Core are the changes that are least flexible of all organizational features (goals, authority, resource acquisition)

Is the change Low Risk or High Risk?

Low Risk includes those that have relatively little loss of relative costs if the innovation is introduced or implemented

High Risk includes the changes that cannot be terminated or reversed, must be implemented in entirety, and conflict with dominant values of the organization.

essence, line workers tend to initiate small changes that enhance work activity but do not introduce large changes in organizational structure.

A change in mission, a new service delivery system, or provision of service to an unserved population would constitute radical change (Pearlmutter, 1998). Damanpour (1988) also stresses that workers higher in the organizational hierarchy initiate radical changes because radical change causes deeper changes in roles, status, and behavior of members of an organization. These substantial changes can create shifts in structure, roles, and power as well as produce feelings of anxiety and fear among lower level workers. Radical change is the most threatening, difficult to control, and introduces the most unknown outcomes (Proehl, 2001). As a result, the introduction of a radical change needs to anticipate and address the conflict in roles, power, and status that accompany the change process.

Radical and minor changes are not necessarily mutually exclusive because some changes fall in the middle of the continuum. Prior to the introduction of a change, a manager needs to assess the degree of change required by locating it on the continuum. This will shape the strategy for introducing and implementing the change. Drawing on the frameworks developed by Frey (1990) and King (1992), a manager can assess the location of a future change on the continuum from the perspective of risk and novelty. Risk is the relative costs that might be incurred if a proposed change fails to meet its objectives or the potential negative consequences of adopting the change. Risk can be assessed at all levels within the organization in order to determine its potential impact. The first aspect of risk is the amount of conflict the change may introduce within the organization. A change that conflicts with the dominant values of the organization or its members is considered a high-risk innovation. The more the change promotes the perceived values of the majority of the organization, the closer it resembles the minor change domain of the continuum. Secondly, changes need to be assessed in terms of their implementation requirements. Changes implemented in small stages or in one department may involve lower risk and, therefore, represent a minor change. However, comprehensive changes involving substantial shifts are considered high-risk. Thirdly, changes that cannot be terminated without incurring substantial costs are considered high-risk, radical changes.

Facilitators and Inhibitors

With the understanding of the types and degree of change, the next step is to determine the factors that facilitate or inhibit the adoption of a change; namely factors associated with the change itself and factors associated with organizational characteristics (Arad, Hanson, and Schneider, 1997; Frambach & Schillewaert, 2002). While the organizational change literature identifies the important role that organizational factors have in facilitating or inhibiting the change process, there is considerable debate about the most influential factors. Arad, Hanson, and Schneider (1997) note only a subset of the relevant factors are found in most studies which makes it difficult to draw solid conclusions regarding which factors are more influential in the change process.

While the importance of organizational characteristics continues to be debated in the literature, the size of the organization is frequently cited as a positive factor associated with successful change (Kaluzny, Veney, & Gentry, 1974; Kimberly and Evanisco, 1981; Mohr, 1969). While some claim that larger organizations experience a greater need to change and have the resources to enter into different change processes, others perceive smaller organizations as more flexible and able to support new changes. These differing perceptions "may be largely attributable to the correlation of organization size with other variables, such as structure, strategy, and culture" (Frambach & Schillewaert, 2002, p. 165). Size alone may not inhibit or facilitate change and the negative relationship sometimes found between size and innovation might be explained by other organizational variables (Arad, Hanson, & Schneider, 1997).

In addition, leadership is identified as a characteristic that can inhibit or facilitate change depending on the qualities and attributes of each leader. Some have argued that leadership is the most important factor affecting change (King, 1992; Osborne, 1998; Shin & McClomb, 1998). Many of the qualities of leaders who encourage change are viewed as transformational where charisma is used to stimulate an environment of learning and risk as well as a supportive environment for staff. While leadership is continually cited as a major facilitator of change, Jaskyte and Dressler (2005) found that transformational leadership was not necessarily correlated with the organization's ability to implement change.

In addition to leadership, there are important characteristics associated withof successful and sustainable change are also associated with the change itself. Roger's seminal work (1995) on diffusion of innovation is linked to the sustainability of change and Rogers (1995) identified the following five major characteristics in the context of sustaining and diffusing innovations:

Relative advantage. The perceived advantage that the change has over the current practice. Various stakeholders affected by the change may view the relative advantage of a particular change differently.

Compatibility. The similarity between the change and the previous practice. The more consistent the change is with prior work, the higher likelihood the change will be sustained.

Complexity. The simplicity of implementing the change determines its sustainability. Simple changes are more likely to be adopted than complex ones.

Trialability. The ability of the change to be implemented in stages rather than in its entirety.

Observability. Changes that are seen as having an immediate effect on workers will be implemented faster and potentially sustained longer Based on theses characteristics of change, the successful adoption of change in an organization would include the following characteristics: (1) simple, (2) similar to previous practices, (3) clearly articulated and understood advantage (e.g., improved outcomes, increased financial gains), (4) tried out in stages or small steps, and (5) readily observable to those being asked to implement the change.

Even with an understanding of the type and degree of change and the barriers as well as facilitators that promote change, there is little evidence of a clear, simple process. While minor changes tend to follow a linear and relatively simple process, radical changes tend to be multifaceted and move in non-linear patterns (Pelz, 1983, as cited in King, 1992).

Staff Receptivity and Resistance

Before addressing the emotional dynamics that accompany an organizational change process, it is important to identify some of the organizational factors associated with the resistance to change. While human nature may naturally push people towards resistance in order to maintain the status quo, workers tend to resist change when the change is seen as a threat to their professional practices, status, or identity (Lawler & Bilson, 2004). For example, if the change is perceived as a modification of practice, the previous form of practice may be perceived as of little value (Horwath & Morrison, 2000). If the change is presented as a *continuation of previous practice*, the resistance can be decreased. To reduce resistance, the change needs to retain some of the prior elements of the working environment in order to reassure workers that their previous work style was valid. As Pearlmutter (1998) notes, "For people to be able to deal with enormous and complex change-seeming chaos-they need to have something to hold on to that is stable. Although paradoxical, it is this principle that reminds us that change and innovation are managed by individual people, whose life experiences have taught them that, in order to change, they must have some stability, some place of comfort that remains" (p. 28).

Despite the substantial amount of research on organizational change, much of it ignores the human side of change (Diamond, 1996; Jaskyte & Dressler, 2005). Staff within organizations can experience change in one or more of the following three ways: (1) personal loss and feelings of inadequacy (Diamond, 1996), (2) lack of competence and self-confidence (Pearlmutter, 1998; Kayser, Walker, & Demaio, 2000), and (3) frustration related to a lack of understanding and knowledge (Tozer & Ray, 1999; Zell, 2003). While people in organizations are able to change, adapt, learn, and unlearn as they find new ways to operate within their workspace, it is important to understand how staff experience change and the methods used for increasing staff acceptance and support of change.

The connection between the resistance to change and the psychological aspects of work environments, various responsibilities require cognitive shifts in the naming and framing of the emotions (related to competence and self-confidence) that can affect their self-esteem at work (Diamond, 1996). In their study of organizational change and self-confidence, Kayser, Walker, & Demaio (2000) found that self-confidence and self-competence are derived from years of practice experience, lack of distracting outside responsibilities, and age. Those practitioners with more years of practice and more experiences with organizational change felt less anxious and more positive about dealing with change. Learning new skills in addition to navigating organizational change may be more difficult for novice practitioners.

In addition to self-confidence and self-competence, workers can also exhibit high degrees of self-efficacy, "the belief in one's capability to perform a specific task" (Gist, 1997, p. 472 as cited in Pearlmutter, 1998, p. 25). Self-efficacy, as defined by Bandura (1982) includes "judgments of how well one can execute the courses of action required to deal with prospective situations." Bandura described experiences and motivation as the cognitive processes that create personal efficacy. In other words, if people believe they can succeed at a task, they will engage in the task with more confidence and assurance that they can complete the task. If, on the other hand, they take on the task with the belief that they cannot succeed, they will avoid or resist the activity.

All three factors (self-confidence, self-competence, and self-efficacy) play a key role in a worker's response and openness to change. The successful adoption of organizational change depends on an individual's openness to learning and change, which in turn, requires minimal defensiveness and adequate levels of self-esteem. The higher the levels of self-confidence, self-competence, and self-efficacy, the lower the levels of unconscious defensiveness (Diamond, 1996). It is the defensive and adaptive tendencies that sustain the status quo and usually block learning and change.

For staff, the psychological aspect of change can also involve emotional and cognitive loss similar to the experiences of death and dying (Zell, 2003; Diamond, 1996). Organizational change often brings with it strong feelings of shock, frustration, anger, and helplessness where staff can experience periods of denial, anger, bargaining, depression, and finally acceptance of a proposed change (Zell, 2003; Diamond, 1996). Kübler-Ross (1969) identified the following five stages associated with the dying process: (1) denial and isolation (e.g., feelings of shock, disbelief, and numbness, (2) anger (e.g., venting rage and resentment about the situation often at those close to the individuals), (3) bargaining (attempt to delay, postpone, or stop the process), (4) depression (managing feelings of reactive or anticipatory loss), and (5) acceptance (opportunity to approach the inevitable with dignity). These concepts can be applied to the process of organizational change. For example, the introduction of change can lead workers to re-examine where they are, where they have been, and where they are going, both personally and organizationally (Diamond, 1996). The initial introduction of change can bring about feelings of loss relate to familiar work methods and the comfort of routine (Diamond, 1996; Zell, 2003). As Diamond (1996) has noted, the introduction of new technology in a public service agency requires staff to proceed through a grieving process in order to accept an innovation or change; in essence, "workers attach themselves emotionally to the predictability of organizational structures and procedures, and that attachment is severed with the introduction of change" (p. 227).

In recognition of the loss that workers feel, organizations need to provide transitional space for workers to confront their fears and anxieties related to the organizational change. This space can be used to support workers through the acknowledgment of loss but also to guide them into recognition of the potentially positive outcomes associated with the change. Workers need "opportunities to express anger and frustration and also to envision the success of the change process" (Nicholls &

McDermott, 2002 p.140). With this understanding of workplace grief related to a change process, managers need to develop strategies to assist workers, individually and collectively, through such loss and grief in a timely manner.

Readiness for Change

While the introduction of a new idea or change into an organization has the potential to be embraced and implemented, it also has the potential to fade out or not take root (Jaskyte & Dressler, 2005; Arad, Hanson, & Schneider, 1997; Frambach & Schillewaert, 2002). There is growing consensus that, "readiness is likely to be a major factor in determining whether an innovation will be effectively implemented and sustained" (Robbins, Collins, Liaupsin, Illback, & Call, 2003, p. 53).

With the ability to measure whether a change has the potential for implementation, organizations are better able to evaluate the readiness of their organizations and staff for the introduction of a change (Robbins et al., 2003). While there is readily available advice for managers regarding an organization's readiness to introduce change, very few models or tools exist that provide a systematic way to assess their organizations (Dixon, 2005; Hodges & Hernandez, 1999; Atherton, 2002; Robbins et al., 2003; Horwath & Morrison, 2000; Lehman, Greener, & Simpson, 2002). Whether managers choose to use formal assessment tools or informal practices, "it is important that those managing change have a clear understanding of where their organization stands" (Dixon, 2005, p. 2) prior to the introduction of change.

In order to ensure the successful introduction and maintenance of change, it is important to examine the readiness for change within the organization from the individual as well as the organizational perspective (Frambach & Schillewaert, 2002). Several models for assessing organizational readiness were found in the literature (Davis & Salasin, 1975; Horwath & Morrison, 2000; Lehman, Greener, & Simpson, 2002). Each model views the introduction of change from the perspective of the actors involved and the various stages of the process. The Horwath and Morrison (2000) audit model, developed in the context of child welfare services, stresses the importance of discussions with staff, other agencies or departments, and all others directly or indirectly affected by the potential change. Horwath and Morrison (2000) note that, "direct consultation often refines the picture gained from paper-based analysis and provides essential insight not only to the degree of congruence between policy and practice, but also about underlying professional attitudes and responses to change. In addition, consultation engages staff at an early stage in the process. Skipping this element carries with it the danger that subsequent prescriptions about change may be based on a partial or inaccurate view of how the current state of practice might increase staff resistance to change" (p. 249). Horwath and Morrison developed a three-part framework that reflects the overall outcome to safeguard children and promote general welfare that includes: (1) practitioner needs, (2) agency capacity, and (3) collaborative arrange- ments.

In contrast to the more informal audit model, Lehman, Greener, and Simpson (2002) developed a comprehensive assessment of organizational readiness in the form of the Organizational Readiness for Change (ORC) instrument. Originally designed for use in drug abuse treatment organizations, it was redesigned in 2003 for social service agencies but its reliability and validity in these organizations have not yet been reported. The instrument focuses on motivation and personality attributes of program leaders and staff, institutional resources, staff attributes, and organizational climate. The three factors identified by the instrument are: (1) what is important for change to occur, (2) what is necessary but not always sufficient for change to occur, and (3) what change is appropriate in the current situation. The major elements of the assessment are highlighted in Figure 3.

In contrast to the first two models, Davis and Salasin (1975) developed a different conceptual model as a way to assess organization readiness for change in mental health settings. The AVICTORY model is an acronym for eight elements thought to be predictive of organizational readiness for implementing change: Ability, Values, Information, Circumstances, Timing, Obligation, Resistance, and Yield (Figure 4). The AVICTORY model assesses both the organizational readiness and the individual readiness to implement a particular change. The model was used by Robbins et al. (2003) to identify schools that were ready to introduce significant organizational change.

Comparing the models, several areas of overlap are highlighted in Figure 5. Using the elements from the Lehman, Greener, and Simpson's (2002) model, each model was analyzed and categorized according to their assessment elements. Several elements were seen in all three models (staffing and training needs related to the new innovation, adaptability and resistance of staff reflected in previous change processes, and current stress levels of staff). In comparing the AVICTORY and ORC models and their similarities, additional overlaping elements include the need for change, pressure for change, adequate office space, com-

FIGURE 3. Organizational Readiness for Change (Social Agency): Assessment Elements*

Elements of Organizational Readiness

I. Motivation
- Program needs (need guidance with mission, goals, staff roles, etc.)
- Training needs (need more training in various skill sets)
- Pressure for change (coming from clients, staff, funding sources, etc.)

II. Resources
- Offices (space, equipment, etc.)
- Staffing (qualifications, turnover, sufficient skills, etc.)
- Training (priorities, conference travel support, etc.)
- Computer access (equipment, data systems, etc.)
- E-Communications (internet access, utilization, policy limitations, etc.)

III. Staff Attributes
- Growth (professional development, literature for updating, etc.)
- Efficacy (effectiveness, confidence, competence, etc)
- Influence (knowledge sharing, advice seeking, etc.)
- Adaptability (ease of learning, experimental, etc.)
- Satisfaction (valuing work, feeling appreciated, etc.)

IV. Organizational Climate
- Mission (staff confusion, planning, link with job duties, etc.)
- Cohesion (teamwork, friction, etc.)
- Autonomy (rules and limitations, freedom to innovate, etc.)
- Communication (formal and informal, valuing of inquiry, etc.)
- Stress (job pressures, balance of workloads, etc.)
- Change (encouragement to experiment, ease of change, etc.)
- Leadership (effectiveness of top management and board, participation in organizational planning, recognition of staff concerns, etc.)

*TCU Survey of Organizational Functioning (2003), Institute of Behavioral Researcl Fort Worth, TX

puter needs/access, consistency with mission, current communication levels, and a review of the reaction to previous change. Two key elements were addressed by both AVICTORY and the Audit but not by ORC; namely, adequate and accurate information about the change and the predicted response of the external environment. AVICTORY also addressed the area of adequate financial resources, which the other two

FIGURE 4. AVICTORY* Elements

Element	Description
Ability	Assess the organization's ability to commit resources, including human, informational, and financial, necessary for implementation of the innovation.
Values	Assess the congruence of the values of the organizational constituencies (e.g., school staff, families, students, and community agency staff) within the main ideas that underlie the innovation.
Information	Assess the quality and credibility of the innovation and the availability of information sufficient to support it.
Circumstances	Assess the environmental and organizational attributes that influence change (e.g., well-defined roles, satisfactory, interpersonal relationships)
Timing	Assess the dynamic environment and organizational factors which may influence implementation or use of the innovation
Obligation	Assess the degree to which key persons in the organization have a felt need or obligation to alter or enhance current practices.
Resistance	Assess the presence of various forms of resistance to the innovation
Yield	Assess the presence of incentives for engaging the new approach.

*Davis, H., & Salasin, S. (1975). The utilization of evaluation. In E. Streunig, & M. Guttentag (Eds.), *Handbook of evaluation research*. Beverly Hills, CA: Sage

models did not address. All three models addressed many of the barriers and facilitators identified by organizational change researchers.

In reviewing the various models for assessing readiness for change, it is clear that assessments need to include both individual and organizational perspectives as well as external and internal stakeholders. Individual stakeholders include all levels of staff (i.e., management, middle-management, and line staff) whose perceptions of organizational readiness should include most, if not all, of the following topics:

- Motivation for change (staff, program, and pressures)
- Adequate resources (human, financial, training, equipment, skills)
- Staff attributes related to capacity, resistance, influence
- Organizational climate
- External and internal stakeholders' perceptions of changels invovled lements of both the individual an

For managers leading their organizations through a change process, the following aspects of organizational change need to be taken into account: (1) the type of change, (2) the degree of change, (3) the facilitators and inhibitors of change, (4) staff perceptions related to the emotional process associated with change (e.g., perceived understanding of the change, nature of potential resistance and the ease of adopting the change), and (5) organizational and individual readiness for change.

FIGURE 5. Comparison of Three Models Related to Readiness for Change

Domain	Organizational Readiness for Change[1]	AVICTORY[2]	Audit of Readiness[3]
Motivation for change			
Program need	*	*	
Immediate training needs	*		*
Pressures for change	*	*	
Incentives		*	
Resources			
Office space	*	*	
Staffing	*	*	*
Training	*	*	*
Computer access	*	*	
E-communication	*		
Financial		*	
Informational		*	*
Staff attributes			
Professional growth	*		
Efficacy	*		*
Influence	*		
Adaptability/Resistance	*	*	*
Organizational Climate			
Mission	*		
Cohesion	*	*	
Autonomy	*		
Communication	*	*	
Stress	*	*	*
Change	*	*	
External			
Constituencies		*	*

[1] Lehman, W. E. K., Greener, J. M., & Simpson, D. D. (2002)

[2] Davis, H., & Salasin, S. (1975)
[3] Horwath, J., & Morrison, T. (2000)

Organizational change takes place within the context of an organization's culture. However, research on organizational cultures has received far less attention than organizational change in the research literature. Research on organizational culture is complex and requires lengthy timeframes for data collection and analysis. As a result, the literature for understanding the organizational culture of social service agencies is even more limited. The next section provides an overview of organizational culture and its implications for guiding organizational change.

ORGANIZATIONAL CULTURE

Scholars and practitioners in the public and private sector have long recognized the role and importance of culture on organizational performance (Khademian, 2002). However, only in the past few decades has the organizational change literature begun to explore the relationship between organizational culture and organizational change. While the empirical research is limited, the research agenda includes organizational values, expectations and assumptions that exist within an organization (Jaskyte & Dressler, 2005; Hodges & Hernandez, 1999). The older models of change and innovation, which focus heavily on structural and environmental explanations for innovation or change, provide an incomplete picture of the forces and energy driving the organization. Public programs are also beginning to recognize the importance of acknowledging and understanding culture as a key element in the effective management of change. Khademian (2002) reports that understanding organizational culture "is an essential ingredient for understanding why government programs perform the way they do" (p. 5). There is a growing need to focus on culture as an important ingredient in the management of change.

While progress has been made in defining organizational culture, managers need practical tools for understanding how to enhance or modify organizational cultures. For example, Smircich (1983) notes that organizational cultures can be viewed as a set of factors brought into an organization (by senior and middle management) or as factors that the organization produces in the form of an "adaptive or regulatory mechanism" that brings staff together into a social structure. In the case of an adaptive mechanism, organizational culture can be unconsciously generated, interactional, and implicit whereby the culture is a negotiated process rather than the result of authoritative dictates from above (Hodges, 1997). Whether organizational culture is viewed from the top or the bottom of the organization, changes in the organization can lead to a change in the organizational culture that can make it more or less supportive of organizational outcomes.

It is clear that understanding the culture of the organization is a key element in any organizational change process. Foster-Fishman (1995) noted that the complexity of culture and its interaction with change requires multiple perspectives that simultaneously considers the consistent, differentiated, fragmented, and ambiguous parts of culture. Martin (1992) described these perspectives in the following way: (1) the integrated perspective views cultures are consistent and monolithic, (2) the differentiated perspective occurs where aspects of culture are inconsistent and multiple subcultures are present, and (3) the fragmented perspective includes how the ambiguous aspects of culture and subcultures respond differently to change.

While public social service agencies reflect all three features of organizational culture, the fragmented perspective allows for a more in-depth look at the interaction between organizational change and organizational culture. For example, Foster-Fishman (1995) noted that it is important to examine the ambiguous meanings associated with change and how the current culture supports and maintains that ambiguity because accepting ambiguity as an essential feature of organizational cultures can facilitate our understanding of how culture interactions with organizational change. She applied this perspective to three dimensions of change: (1) the desirability of the proposed change, (2) the capacity of the organization to accomplish a change, and (3) and the perceptions of the members of the organization regarding both the desirability of change and the organization's capacity for managing change. Because members of an organization perceive their organizational lives through their own cognitive interpretive lens (Bartunek, 1984), their perceptions of organizational change are influenced by these lenses or frameworks.

Foster-Fishman (1995) identified three key factors that can impact the organizational culture; namely, (1) the views of staff that are either compatible or incompatible, (2) the different views of organizational life and the proposed change held by subgroups or sub-cultures within the organization, and (3) the existence of consistent and inconsistent organizational practices. In essence, managers need to understand the interaction between cognitions of staff related to their readiness for change, the different way that groups of staff may react, and the nature of current organizational practices, especially when introducing evidence-based practice and how this change contradicts or builds upon current practice.

DEFINING ORGANIZATIONAL CULTURE

The organization culture literature includes extensive debates about "what culture is, how to identity it, how it influences organizational behavior, and how to examine culture in order to better understand it" (Khademian, 2002). The most common definition of organization culture is that it is a set of the beliefs, values, and meanings that are shared by members of an organization (Hodges & Hernandez, 1999; McLean, 2005; Jaskyte & Dressler, 2005). While this definition is simple, the concept of organizational culture is more complex.

Schein's (1992) pioneering work on organizational culture has helped to identify the elements within an organization that create the organizational culture. He uses the iceberg metaphor to describe elements of culture; namely, those elements that appear under the waterline or those that remain invisible. Figure 6 outlines his framework for understanding organizational culture. The three levels of culture include: (1) *basic assumptions*, namely the fundamental dynamics of how the organization and its members relate to the environment, time, space, reality, and each other which often fall below the level of consciousness and tend to dictate and motivate the behavior, (2) *values and beliefs* which reflect what members believe "ought to be" the work of the organization in the form of easily articulated ideologies, attitudes, and philosophies, and (3) *cultural artifacts* are the most visible layer of culture within the organization and include the languages used, stories told, ceremonies performed, rewards given, symbols displayed, heroes remembered, and history recalled. As organizations attempt to change or modify their culture, it is important to understand and analyze the three layers (basic assumptions, values and beliefs, and cultural artifacts). Sustainable changes in organizational cultures involve understanding and changing the basic assumptions (deepest layer), then addressing the values and beliefs, and, finally, dealing with the third layer of cultural artifacts.

In the following section on analyzing organizational culture, several major domains are addressed; namely, facilitators and inhibitors of change, types of organizational cultures, and the management of organizational cultures.

ORGANIZATIONAL CULTURE FACILITATORS AND INHIBITORS OF CHANGE

A comprehensive review of the literature on organizational culture and innovation by Jaskyte and Dressler's (2005) revealed that research-

FIGURE 6. Three Levels of Culture

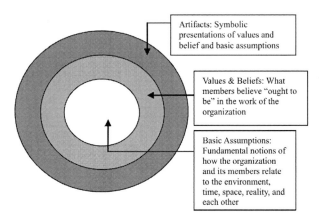

Artifacts: Symbolic presentations of values and belief and basic assumptions

Values & Beliefs: What members believe "ought to be" in the work of the organization

Basic Assumptions: Fundamental notions of how the organization and its members relate to the environment, time, space, reality, and each other

ers have focused primarily on the positive attributes of organizational culture by identifying organizational values, norms, beliefs, and assumptions. Less attention had been given to the emerging debate about the role of organizational culture in facilitating or inhibiting change. While there is agreement that organizational culture has an impact, it is not clear what role it plays in facilitating change. On one side of the debate is the argument that strong, homogenous organizational cultures are essential for organizations to introduce, implement, and sustain changes because a strong culture can exert a greater degree of control over employee behaviors and beliefs, and therefore change within the organization is easier (Denison, 1990; Pervaiz, 1998; Peters & Waterman, 1982). On the other side of the debate is the conviction that strong cultures are problematic for the introduction and maintenance of change because a strong culture creates uniformity, loyalty, and commitment and potentially "cult-like" behaviors that can inhibit an organization's ability to respond to change (Nemeth, 1997). In a study of thirty-two nonprofit service agencies Jaskyte and Dressler's (2005) found that homogenous cultures might not be appropriate for fostering change. "The higher the cultural consensus on such values as stability, security, low level of conflict, predictability, rule orientation, team orientation, and working in collaboration with others, the less innovative the organization may be" (p. 35). The organizations with weaker cultural consensus placed higher value on willingness to experiment, pursuing opportunities, and taking risks. According to Martin (1992) the discrepancy in the two theories can be explained by the role that strong organizational cultures can play in alleviating anxiety, helping control the uncontrollable, bringing predictability, and clarifying ambiguity. These characteristics, at the same time, can control any kind of behavior that might disrupt organization harmony and predictability and thereby block the introduction and maintenance of change.

TYPE OF ORGANIZATIONAL CULTURES

In assessing an organization's readiness for change, it is important to understand the types of organizational cultures that range from very informal to formal, rigid structures. Managers need to determine if the organization is open and capable of change, or if the culture needs modifications before implementing a change. While theorists have divided types of organizational culture differently, several similarities exist among the models. Both Handy (1993) and Cameron and Quinn (1999) identified the "clan" or "club" culture that places a high value on the *informal*, family-type atmosphere where relationship, cohesion, and teamwork are emphasized. Many of these organizational cultures were created by charismatic and visionary individuals who made quick decisions and changes based on minimal discussion or planning. Historically, community-based organizations tend to foster this type of organizational culture. The second type of organizational culture is the formal, role-oriented culture. Labeled "role culture" (Handy, 1993) or "hierarchy culture" (Cameron and Quinn, 1999), this type of organizational culture is very *formal* with a structured work environment that stresses stability, efficiency, and order. Organizational members are given clear procedures for completing their work and enjoy a sense of security and stability. The order and stability of this organizational culture prevent chaos or uncertainty from entering the work environment, thereby resisting the instability that change can create. Many public human service organizations cultivate this formal organizational culture. Additional organizational cultures include those that are results-oriented, driven, and strive to remain *competitive* within the market. This organizational culture type creates an intense working condition where the leaders are demanding and the pressure is extreme. Very few human service organizations reflect this type of organizational culture (Proehl, 2001). Public human service organizations lean towards the formal culture and employ staff members who arc vcry comfortable with the security that the organizational culture offers. However, the formal culture may not promote critical thinking and can be resistant to change. As organizations anticipate periods of change, it is important for managers to find ways to modify the organizational culture to one that promotes more comfort with the instability associated with the change process.

MANAGING ORGANIZATIONAL CULTURES

Public human service organizations were built to reduce error, increase efficiency, and improve the reliability of services (Cahn, 2004). They were praised for being impervious to change, assuring that each member of the agency dispersed equal and accountable services to the public. By maintaining routines and reducing exposure to risk, public organizations were seen as implementing the will of the people and public employees were expected to competently carry out the wishes of the people as expressed by elected officials by limiting their own discretion (Cahn, 2004). This approach to organizational processes, while successful in many regards, has frequently created a culture that is either unwilling or unable to support the autonomy and risk-taking needed to create cultures that are accepting of change. By warding off any kind of potential chaos or uncertainty that is often associated with change, human service workers are rarely encouraged to challenge the status quo, exercise discretion, or to take risks. Organizational cultures with little room for dissent can inhibit the introduction or implementation of change and thereby generate considerable resistance.

Most of the literature on managing organization culture features the for-profit sector and very little of the literature features the nonprofit sector. Since managing an organization's culture is seen as crucial to the improvement of overall performance (Khademian, 2002), private sector managers have come to see the management of organizational culture as a top priority. Public sector managers, on the other hand, have been constrained in their efforts to manage the organization's culture. The constraints include rules for contracting, hiring and firing, budgeting, goal setting, and benchmarking for accountability. While several human service organizations have built upon their organizational culture to promote the use of effective management techniques, a debate has emerged around the capacity of managers to actually modify organizational cultures (Hodges & Hernandez, 2002; Lawler & Bilson, 2004; Khademian, 2002; Jasktye, 2005; Arad, Hanson, & Schneider). The debate revolves around the feasibility of managing, shaping, or changing an organization's culture (Hodges & Hernandez, 1999; Khademian, 2002).

On one side of the debate are those who see the elements of organizational culture as a set of processes to be managed. "Managers, increasingly interested in the effective and efficient ways to manage their organizations, have begun referring to organizational culture as a management-directed phenomenon and a tool for organizational adaptation and change (Hodges & Hernandez, 1999, p. 185). They view organizational culture as a set of factors linked to organizational performance, and the process of creating of an organizational culture is seen as a top-down, management-directed function. Based on these views, supporters of the idea that organization culture can be managed take the following positions: 1) "a unifying culture can be used to weave together the work of an organization and enhance performance and, second, the top priority of a leader is to mold and maintain a unifying culture" (Khademian, 2002, p. 18) and 2) "the only thing of real importance that managers do is to create and manage culture" (Schein, 1985 as cited in Hodges & Hernandez, 2002, p. 185).

In contrast to the view that culture can be managed are those who see organizational culture as "implicit, interactional and unconsciously generated at all levels of an organization" (Smircich, 1983 as cited in Hodges & Hernandez, 2002, p. 185) with little possibility of being managed in the public sector (Khademian, 2002). While social scientists acknowledge the significant impact culture has on organizational change, they also agree that culture is highly resistant to change. For example, "Anthropological perspective on organizational culture, with its focus on interpretive processes, suggests that managers face difficulty in explicit attempts to change organizational culture because they cannot completely control the complex interactions that produce culture throughout an organization" (Hodges & Hernandez, 1999, p. 185). The complex interactions between the internal aspects of organizational life and the external environment of changing public policies are the largest influences on an organization's culture and this interaction cannot be easily managed (Khademian, 2002). In fact, these environment factors are often seen as creating the culture of the organization.

Strategies for managing organizational cultures: Even though there is little empirical evidence on either side of the debate, Khademian (2002) developed a way of addressing both sides of the issue with a framework for public sector managers that builds upon two basic premises: (1) culture evolves from the efforts to "conduct a public task with specific resources and skills in a complex environment" (p. 43) where the three roots of organizational culture are tasks, resources, and environment, and (2) public managers influence and help shape culture by managing the process of integrating the three roots in order to create a "common understanding (or commitment) held by people working together in an organization or program" (p. 3). The work of the organization depends on a mix of tasks (services) and resources (financial and human) that exist in a complex and changing environment. Within the expectations, constraints, and legacies of a complex internal and external environment, Khademian (2002) identified six strategies for understanding and managing the culture of public organizations (see Figure 7).

Strategy 1 and 2 involves a manager stepping back from daily activities in order to "soak and poke" around the organization in order to identify the connections between existing commitments and the roots (tasks, resources, and environment). To guide the process of identifying program commitments (Khademian, 2002), several questions are posed for managers to ask themselves:

- What language is used to explain organizational improvements and failures?
- What stories are told and what kinds of examples given?
- How do people behave in an emergency or problem situation and who has authority or exercises influence in such circumstances?
- What language is used to describe the real power and responsibilities within the agency beyond the formal organizational authority and responsibility?

Strategy 3 encourages managers to be clear about their future directions and to use practice and experimentation to reach their goal. Managers seeking change begin by gaining an understanding of the connection between the commitments of the organization and its roots. Managers seeking to promote change need to understand the existing commitments and how those commitments need to change. Articulating the changes can help participants see the task and understand the direction. Strategy 4 focused on the internal process related to a mix of resources and tasks with the external dynamics whereby participants from outside the organization need to be included in the process. Strategy 5 focuses on the efforts of managers to coordinate the integration of tasks, resources, and the environment. Strategy 6 highlights the importance of recognizing change, even if incremental in nature, and finding ways to preserve the change and foster more of the same (e.g., sustainability).

FIGURE 7. Strategies for Understanding and Managing Culture

Strategy 1:	Identify the commitments that form the existing culture
Strategy 2	Identify the connections between the roots of culture and commitments
Strategy 3	Think about what needs to change and articulate the change.
Strategy 4	Understand the management of cultural roots as an inward, outward, and shared responsibility.
Strategy 5	Relentlessly practice and demonstrate the desired changes in culture
Strategy 6	Capitalize on incremental change and institutionalize it

Role of leaders in managing organizational cultures: The vast majority of organizational culture and change literature refer to the role of leaders in understanding and managing change, especially the role of transformative leadership (Pearlmutter, 1998; King, 1992; Osborne, 1998; Shin & McClomb, 1998). Leaders who display characteristics of individualized consideration, inspiration, oriented to the future, coalition building, risk-taking, and effective communications are better able to introduce and sustain change within their organizations (Pearlmutter, 1998; Jaskyte & Dressler, 2005). According to Khademian (2002), leaders who are skeptical about the feasibility of managing organizational culture will be less successful in changing their cultures because they see environment as the overwhelming factor in trying to manage the culture of the organization. Those leaders who are less skeptical about the manageability of culture perceive the primary role of a leader as managing the culture by shaping the values and organizational philosophies, thereby helping the organization to define priorities, acceptable behavior, and valued outcomes.

In Khademian's (2002) review of programs that successfully managed organizational change, she noticed a consistent set of leadership characteristics that took into account the roots of the culture (tasks, environment, and resources) and managed their interrelationship with organizational commitments. The seven characteristics for facilitating change include:

- Listen and learn from the information gathered.
- Look for ways to broaden the base of participation.
- Identify and provide resources to enable all participants to excel.
- Practice continuous evaluation.
- Target authority structures within and without the program.
- Be relentless.

In addition to managerial leadership, there is considerable research on the role of opinion leaders. Rogers (1995) was the first to explore the role of individuals, termed opinion leaders, on the dissemination and diffusion of new concepts. He focused on the concept of adopting new ideas and the ways in which practitioners are influenced by the judgments of colleagues, and, therefore, more likely to accept the change. While several research studies suggest social pressure is effective in reducing resistance to change (Davis, Thomson, Oxman, & Yaynes, 1995), others are more cautious in supporting these conclusions. O'Brien et al., 1999 have noted that using local opinion leaders results in mixed effects on professional practice and suggested that further research on the process of identifying opinion leaders and under what conditions are they able to influence the practice of their peers. This call for research is complicated by the lack of a common, unified definition of opinion leaders (Locock, Dopson, Chambers, Gabby, 2001).

In an extensive literature review and research study exploring the role of opinion leaders within a health care setting, Locock et al. (2001) discovered several key findings related to opinion leaders. First, in most cases, the opinion leaders emerged throughout the process rather than being identified prior to the change efforts. Opinion leaders were described as those individuals who command respect, know what they are talking about, and/or understand the realities of practice (Locock et al., 2001). There are at least two types of opinion leaders; namely, *expert opinion* leaders who are a credible authority able to articulate the change in a confident, knowledgeable manner and the *peer opinion* leader who can relate to the everyday problems facing the practitioners and draw upon a high level of trust among them. Locock et al. (2001) also raised concerns about ambivalent or resistant opinion leaders. While opinion leaders are helpful in persuading colleagues to accept a change, they can also work against the change. Opinion leaders can also lack the enthusiasm for a change and, therefore, drain the enthusiasm from the entire staff.

It is clear that the debate about the manageability of organizational cultures will continue. However, it is widely agreed that culture involves basic assumptions, values and belief, and the artifacts operating within the organization. Understanding the types of cultures that exist and the ways each culture promotes or resists change can help administrators to more effectively manage their organizations. Khademian presented a framework to assist managers by connecting the organizational commitments (culture) to the roots (environment, resources, tasks). Given this analysis of the research on organizational culture, the following questions can assist managers in applying the concepts of organizational culture to a human service organization:

- What type of culture exists within your agency?
- What are some examples of the key values and beliefs held by staff within the agency?
- What commitments does the agency maintain? How are these commitments reflected in the mission statement?
- In what ways does your agency's culture promote change? Hinder change?
- Who are the opinion leaders in your agency? In the past, how have them been used to facilitate change?

In addition to understanding the ways in which staff members and others may think about change within the culture of the organization, managers also need to assess their own schemata. If they see themselves as fostering an "innovation-supportive organizational environment" (Chandler, G, Keller, C. & Lyon, D. 2000), then they need to consider the following values identified by Subramiam and Ashkanasy (2001): (1) being innovative and willing to experiment with new ideas, (2) being opportunistic and not constrained by many rules, and (3) willing to take risks.

CONCLUSION

It is important for managers of human service organizations to understand the significance of both organizational culture and organizational change for the process of implementing evidence-based practice. This analysis and synthesis of the research on organizational change and culture is summarized in Figure 8.

The top tier of the flow chart identifies the importance of understanding the basic aspects of organizational culture and organizational change. Organizational change is divided into two large types: administrative and technical. Administrative refers to the organizational structure and administrative process (e.g., the creation of a new employee reward system or new performance evaluation system). Technical changes are those changes in services or process technology that affect the daily work activities (e.g., a new service delivery system or new intervention). In addition to the type of change, the degree of change is critical and can range from minor change (e.g., improve what is already in place) to radical change (e.g., changes to the core of the agency related to mission, allocation of resources, or shifts in authority). Radical change can be the most difficult for staff to handle and may create feelings of anxiety and fear. Changes in organizations often fail to take root due to resistance from staff that can be attributed to such factors as: (1) levels of self-esteem and self-efficacy levels, (2) experiences of loss, and (3) threats to professional capacity. Staff members with low levels of self-efficacy and self-esteem do not handle change well. Asking people to change their duties, work environments, and responsibilities can be challenging for those with little confidence in themselves and their ability to adapt to the changes. Another significant aspect of resistance is the staff's sense of loss that accompanies significant levels of change. Staff members need time to grieve the loss of the old idea and welcome the new idea. Change that is unfamiliar to staff can create a sense of fear and a threat to their professional practices, status, and identity. Change that builds upon previous work can reassure staff that they are capable of completing the tasks and can provide less resistance.

The organizational culture is best described using the following three levels of culture Schein's (1992): (1) *basic assumptions* about how the organization and its members relate to the environment, time, space, reality, and each other, (2) *values and beliefs* which reflect what members believe "ought to be" the work of the organization and are captured in easily articulated ideologies, attitudes, and philosophies, and (3) *cultural artifacts* include the languages used, stories told, ceremonies performed, rewards given, symbols displayed, heroes remembered, and history recalled. In addition to understanding the elements of culture, it is important to analyze the type of culture operating within the agency; namely, informal family-type structures where relationships are highly valued, formal structures that stress stability and predictability, and entrepreneurial structures that are less frequently found in the human services. Identifying the type of organizational culture can assist managers in developing strategies for implementing change.

FIGURE 8. Organizational Change and Culture

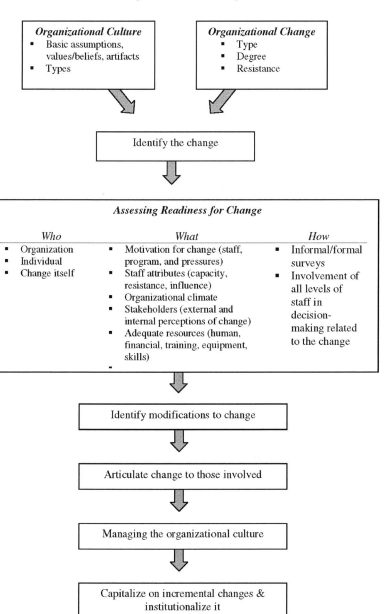

Once there is a baseline understanding of organizational culture and organizational change, managers need to understand the ramifications of the proposed change (e.g., evidence-based practice) in order to begin an organizational assessment and involvement strategy.

Assessment is an important phase of change and one that is often skipped or only partially implemented. Assessment includes an evaluation of the readiness for organizational change, the individuals (staff), and the change itself. All three levels are crucial to gather a complete picture of the readiness to implement change, especially the sources of organizational support and resistance. Without assessing the readiness for organizational change (e.g., motivation for change, adequate resources, staff attributes, organizational climate, and stakeholders), it is difficult to distinguish how the type and degree of change will affect the organization.

The motivation relates to staff perceptions of a need to change. Unless the financial, human, equipment and training needs are adequately addressed before embarking on a change, resistance will increase. Important staff attributes include the staff's capacity to implement the change, different areas of staff resistance, and the views of opinion leaders. Lastly, an assessment of the internal and external stakeholders includes external partners who may be affected by the change and internal departments working within the same organization. More effective change implementation strategies can emerge by including all voices in the assessment of organizational readiness for change.

Once the assessment is completed and appropriate modifications are made to the change process, managers can begin to clearly articulate the change to those involved so that participants can see the task ahead and understand the direction. As the implementation of change begins, Khademian (2001) reminds managers of the importance of understanding the process in the context of the organization's culture, the external environment, and all the individuals involved in the change. Even small changes need to be recognized, celebrated, preserved and fostered throughout the organization.

REFERENCES

Aiken, M., & Hage, J. (1971). The organic organization and innovation. *Sociology, 5*(1), 63-82.

Arad, S., Hanson, M., & Schneider, R. J. (1997). A framework for the study of relationships between organizational characteristics and organizational innovation. *Journal of Creative Behavior,* 31(1), 42-58.

Atherton, C. (2002). Changing culture not structure: Five years of research in practice in child care. *MCC: Building Knowledge for Integrated Care,* 10(1), 17-21.

Bandura, A. (1982). Self-efficacy mechanism in human agency. *American Psychologist,* 37(2), 122-147.

Bartunek, J.M. (1984). Changing interpretive schemes and organizational restructuring: The example of a religious order. *Administrative Science Quarterly,* 29, 355-372.

Burke, W. W., & Litwin, G. H. (1992). A causal model of organizational performance and change. *Journal of Management,* 18(3), 523-545.

Cahn, K. D. C. (2004). Getting there from here: Variables associated with the adoption of innovation in public child welfare. *Dissertation Abstracts International, A: The Humanities and Social Sciences,* 65 (3), 1114-A-1115-A. (Available from UMI, Ann Arbor, MI. Order No. DA3127385.)

Cameron, K. S., & Quinn, R. E. (1999). *Diagnosing and changing organizational culture.* Reading: Addison-Wesley.

Center for Evidence-based Social Services. (2004). Becoming an evidence-based organization: Applying, adapting, and acting on evidence–module 4. *The Evidence Guide: Using Research and Evaluation in Social Care and Allied Professions.* Exeter, UK: University of Exeter. www.ex.ac.uk/cebss

Chandler, G. Keller, C. & Lyons, D. (2000). Unraveling the determinants and consequences of an innovation-supportive organizational culture. *Entrepreneurship Theory and Practice,* 25(1), 59-76.

Daft, R. L. (1982). Bureaucratic versus nonbureaucratic structure and the process of innovation and change. *Research in the Sociology of Organizations, 1,* 129-166

Damanpour, F. (1988). Innovation type, radicalness, and the adoption process. *Communication Research. Special Issue on Innovative Research on Innovations and Organizations, 15*(5), 545-567.

Damanpour, F., & Evan, W. M. (1984). Organizational innovation and performance: The problem of "organizational lag." *Administrative Science Quarterly, 29*(3), 392-402.

Davies, H. & Nutley, S. (2002). Evidence-based policy and practice: Moving from rhetoric to reality, *Discussion Paper 2. Scotland: St Andrews University, Research Unit for Research Utilization.* www.st-andrews.ac.uk/~ruru/RURU%20 publications%20list.htm

Davis, H., & Salasin, S. (1975). The utilization of evaluation. In E. Streunig, & M. Guttentag (Eds.), *Handbook of evaluation research.* Beverly Hills, CA: Sage.

Davis, D. A., Thomson, M. A., Oxman, A. D., & Haynes, R. B. (1995). Changing physician performance: A systematic review of the effect of continuing medical education strategies. *Journal of the American Medical Association,* 274(9), 700-705.

Denison, D. R. (1990). *Corporate culture and organizational effectiveness.* New York: John Wiley and Sons.

Diamond, M. A. (1995). Organizational change as human process, not technique. *National Institute of Drug Abuse Research Monograph,* 155, 119-131.

Diamond, M. A. (1996). Innovation and diffusion of technology: A human process. *Consulting Psychology Journal: Practice & Research, 48*(4), 221-229.

Dixon, G. (n.d.) *Evidence-based practices (A three-part series): Moving science into service–steps to implementing evidence-based practice.* Retrieved June 2005 from http://www.scattc.org/pdf_upload/Beacon003.pdf

Foster-Fishman, P. G. (1995). The influence of organizational culture on the adoption and implementation of an empowerment philosophy. (Doctoral dissertation, www.il.proquest.com/umi/]). *Dissertation Abstracts International Section A: Humanities & Social Sciences, 56* (1-A), 0266.

Frambach, R. T., & Schillewaert, N. (2002). Organizational innovation adoption: A multi-level framework of determinants and opportunities for future research. *Journal of Business Research. 55*(2), 163-176.

Frank, K. A., Zhao, Y., & Borman, K. (2004). Social capital and the diffusion of innovations within organizations: The case of computer technology in schools. *Sociology of Education, 77*(2), 148-171.

Frey, G. A. (1990). A framework for promoting organizational change. *Families in Society, 71*(3), 142-147.

Gambrill, E. (1999). Evidence-based practice: An alternative to authority-based practice. *Families in Society: The Journal of Contemporary Human Services, 80*(4), 341.

Grossman, J. B. (1970). The supreme court and social change. *American Behavioral Science, 13*(4), 535-551.

Hampshire Social Services (1999). *Evidence-based practice in Hampshire Social Services: Notes on our strategy.* Hampshire, UK: Hampshire Social Services.

Handy, C. (1993). *Understanding Organizations.4th Ed.* London: Penguin Books Ltd.

Hodges, S. (1997). *Information pathways: How organizational culture influences the utilization of outcome measures in the Texas Children's Mental Health Plan.* Doctoral Dissertation, Tampa, Fl: University of South Florida, Department of Anthropology

Hodges, S. P., & Hernandez, M. (1999). How organizational culture influences outcome information utilization. *Evaluation & Program Planning, 22*(2), 183-197.

Hodson, R. (2003). *Leading the drive for evidence based practice in services for children and families: Summary report of a study conducted for research in practice.* UK: Research in Practice. Available at *http://www.rip.org.uk/devmats/leadership.html*

Horwath, J., & Morrison, T. (2000). Identifying and implementing pathways for organizational change-using the framework for the assessment of children in need and their families as a case example. *Child & Family Social Work, 5*(3), 245-254.

Jaskyte, K., & Dressler, W. W. (2005). Organizational culture and innovation in nonprofit human service organizations. *Administration in Social Work, 29*(2), 23-41.

Johnson, M. A., & Austin, M. J. (forthcoming). Evidence-based practice in the social services: Implications for organizational change. *Administration in Social Work.*

Kaluzny, A. D., Veney, J. E., & Gentry, J. T. (1974). Innovation of health services: A comparative study of hospitals and health departments. *Milbank Memorial Fund Quarterly, 52*(1), 51-82.

Kayser, K., Walker, D., & Demaio, J. (2000). Understanding social workers' sense of competence within the context of organizational change. *Administration in Social Work, 24*(4), 1-20.

Khademian, A. K. (2002). *Working with culture: How the job gets done in public programs.* Washington, DC: CQ Press.

Kimberly, J. R., & Evanisko, M. J. (1981). Organizational innovation: The influence of individual, organizational, and contextual factors on hospital adoption of technological and administrative innovations. *Academy of Management Journal, 24*(4), 689-713.

King, N. (1992). Modelling the innovation process: An empirical comparison of approaches. *Journal of Occupational & Organizational Psychology, 65*(2), 89-100.

Kitson, A., Harvey, G., & McCormack, B. (1998). Enabling the implementation of evidence-based practice: A conceptual framework. *Quality in Health Care, 7*, 149-158.

Knight, K. E. (1967). A descriptive model of the intra-firm innovation process. *Journal of Business, 40*, 478-496.

Kübler-Ross, E. (1969). *On death and dying.* New York, NY: Collier Books/ Macmillan Publishing Co.

Lawler, J., & Bilson, A. (2004). Towards a more reflexive research aware practice: The influence and potential of professional and team culture. *Social Work & Social Sciences Review, 11*(1), 52-69.

Lehman, W. E. K., Greener, J. M., & Simpson, D. D. (2002). Assessing organizational readiness for change. *Journal of Substance Abuse Treatment, 22*(4), 197-209.

Locock, L., Dopson, S., Chambers, D., & Gabbay, J. (2001). Understanding the role of opinion leaders in improving clinical effectiveness. *Social Science and Medicine, 53*(6), 745-757.

Martin, J. (1992). *Culture in organizations: Three perspectives.* New York, NY: Oxford University Press.

McLean, L. D. (2005). Organizational culture's influence on creativity and innovation: A review of the literature and implications for human resource development. *Advances in Developing Human Resources, 7*(2), 226-246.

Mohr, L. B. (1969). Determinants of innovation in organizations. *American Political Science Review, 63*(1), 111-126.

Nemeth, C. J. (1997). Managing innovation: When less is more. *California Management Review, 40*(1), 59.

Nicholls, D., & McDermott, B. (2002). Collaboration to innovation: Facilitating the introduction of intensive child and adolescent psychiatry treatment teams. *Australasian Psychiatry, 10*(2), 139-143.

Nord, W. R., & Tucker, S. (1987). *Implemeting routine and radical innovations.* Lexington, MA: Lexington Books.

Normann, R. (1971). Organizational innovativeness: Product variation and reorientation. *Administrative Science Quarterly, 16*(2), 203-215.

O'Brien, M. A., Oxman, A. D., Haynes, R. B., Davis, D. A., Freemantle, N. & Harvey, E. L. (1999). *Local opinion leaders: Effects on professional practice and healthcare outcomes.* Retrieved June 2005 from: http://www.mrw.interscience. wiley.com/cochrane/clsysrev/articles/CD000125/framc.html

Osborne, S. P. (1998). Naming the beast: Defining and classifying service innovations in social policy. *Human Relations, 51*(9), 1133-1154.

Pearlmutter, S. (1998). Self-efficacy and organizational change leadership. *Administration in Social Work, 22*(3), 23-38.

Pervaiz, K. A. (1998). Culture and climate for innovation. *European Journal of Innovation Management, 11*, 30-47.

Peters, T. J., & Waterman, J. R. H. (1982). *In search of excellence: Lessons from america's best-run companies.* New York, NY: Warner Books.

Poole, D. L., Ferguson, M., & Schwab, A. J. (2005). Managing process innovations in welfare reform technology. *Administration in Social Work, 29*(1), 101-106.

Proehl, R.A. (2001). *Organizational Change in the Human Services.* Thousand Oaks, CA: Sage Publications

Robbins, V., Collins, K., Liaupsin, C., Illback, R. J., & Call, J. (2003). Evaluating school readiness to implement positive behavioral supports. *Journal of Applied School Psychology, 20*(1), 47-66.

Robertson, P. J., & Seneviratne, S. J. (1995). Outcomes of planned organizational change in the public sector: A meta-analytic comparison to the private sector. *Public Administration Review, 55*(6), 547.

Rogers, E. (1995). Diffusion of Innovations. 4th Ed. New York: Free Press.

Sackett, D. L., Straus, S. E., Richardson, W. S., Rosenberg, W., & Haynes, R. B. (1997). *Evidence-based medicine: How to practice and teach EBM (2nd ed.).* Edinburgh: Churchill-Livingstone.

Schein, E. H. (1992). *Organizational culture and leadership: A dynamic view.* 2nd Ed. San Francisco, CA: Jossey-Bass.

Shin, J., & McClomb, G. E. (1998). Top executive leadership and organizational innovation: An empirical investigation of nonprofit human service organizations (HSOs). *Administration in Social Work, 22*(3), 1-21.

Singh, J. V., House, R. J., & Tucker, D. J. (1986). Organizational change and organizational mortality. *Administrative Science Quarterly*, 31(4), 587-611.

Smircich, L. (1983). Concepts of culture and organizational analysis. *Administrative Science Quarterly*, 28, 339-358.

Subramaniam, N. & Ashkanasy, N. (2001). The effects of organizational culture perceptions on the relationship between budgetary participation and managerial job-related outcomes. *Australian Journal of Management*, 26(1), 35-54.

Tozer, C. & Bournemouth, S. (1999). *20 questions: The research needs of children and family social workers*, 17(1) from http://www.elsc.org.uk/socialcareresource/rpp/articles/1711999art3.htm

Zell, D. (2003). Organizational change as a process of death, dying, and rebirth. *Journal of Applied Behavioral Science, 39*(1), 73-96.

APPENDIX. BASSC Search Protocol

Structured review on best practices for instituting a model of evidence-based practice into agency environments: three broad areas: 1) organizational change, change processes that facilitate positive organizational change, 2) organizational culture and 3) the management of organizational culture and change.

Search Terms

organi?ational change OR organi?ational culture OR organi?ational behavi*r OR organi?ational development OR organi?ational climate AND evidence base OR evidence-base

organi?ational change OR organi?ational culture OR organi?ational behavi*r OR organi?ational development OR organi?ational climate AND child welfare

organi?ational change OR organi?ational culture OR organi?ational behavi*r OR organi?ational development OR organi?ational climate AND social service

organi?ational change OR organi?ational culture OR organi?ational behavi*r OR organi?ational development OR organi?ational climate AND human service

organi?ational change OR organi?ational culture OR organi?ational behavi*r OR organi?ational development OR organi?ational climate AND innovation

organi?ational innovation

innovation process

organi?ational creativity

dissemination OR diffusion AND evidence based

organi?ational change process

APPENDIX (continued)

Databases

Academic databases for books and articles
Pathfinder or Melvyl
ArticleFirst
Current Contents Database
ERIC
Expanded Academic ASAP
Family and Society Studies Worldwide
PAIS International
PsychInfo
Social Science Citation Index
Social Services Abstracts
Social Work Abstracts
Sociological Abstracts

Systematic Reviews

Cochrane Collaboration
Campbell Collaboration

Reference lists from primary & review articles

Research Institutes
Mathmatica
Urban Institute
RAND
GAO
National Academy of Sciences
Chapin Hall
CASRC (San Diego)
Brookings Institute
Manpower Demonstration Research Corporation
Annie E. Casey Foundation

Conference proceedings

PapersFirst (UCB Database)
Proceedings (UCB Database)

Dissertation Abstracts

DigitalDissertations (UCB database)
Professional Evaluation Listserves
EVALTALK
GOVTEVAL
ChildMaltreatmentListserve

Internet

Google
Dogpile

Experts / personal contacts

Knowledge Management: Implications for Human Service Organizations

Michael J. Austin, PhD
Jennette Claassen, MSW
Catherine M. Vu, MPA
Paola Mizrahi, BA

SUMMARY. Knowledge management has recently taken a more prominent role in the management of organizations as worker knowledge and intellectual capital are recognized as critical to organizational success. This analysis explores the literature of knowledge management including the individual level of tacit and explicit knowledge, the networks and social interactions utilized by workers to create and share new knowledge, and the multiple organizational and managerial factors associated with effective knowledge management systems. Based on the role of organizational culture, structure, leadership, and reward systems, six strategies are identified to assist human service organizations with implementing new knowledge management systems.

Michael J. Austin is Professor, Jennette Claassen is Research Assistant, Catherine M. Vu is Research Assistant, and Paola Mizrahi is Research Assistant, all at School of Social Welfare, University of California at Berkeley, Berkeley, CA 94720.

KEYWORDS. Knowledge management, human services, organizational factors, managerial factors, tacit knowledge, explicit knowledge

INTRODUCTION

The focus of evidence-based practice is on the practitioner's use of evidence to meet the service needs of clients. The focus of client information and practitioner knowledge is on the organization and how well it manages information and knowledge. Organizations have come to realize that their greatest asset is the knowledge of their workers. Knowledge and intellectual capital represent the wealth of an organization, especially human service organizations. The term "knowledge management" first appeared in the literature of the for-profit sector in the early 1980s in an effort to capture the resources buried in their workforce and research community. This development prompted researchers to examine the knowledge that exists within businesses and understand how that knowledge is used (Hansen, Nohria, and Tierney, 1999). Consulting companies whose main business is collecting, organizing, managing, and disseminating knowledge were pioneers in knowledge management as they sought to identify systems and structures, mainly databases and repositories, to codify and store knowledge for easy access.

In defining knowledge management, Davenport and Prusak (2000) distinguish between the terms "knowledge," "information," and "data." Often times used interchangeable, their definition helps to promote a clear understanding of knowledge management. Data is defined as "unorganized facts," discrete findings that carry no judgement or interpretation. In contrast, information is "data plus context" where data have been organized, patterned, grouped, or categorized. And finally, knowledge is "information plus judgment," a richer and more meaningful perspective derived from experience and the analysis of the data and information. As research on knowledge management progressed, it became clear that knowledge management involved more than information management or information technology. It included linking individuals to each other through systems and structures that helped organizations to recognize, create, transform, and distribute knowledge among all workers (Gold, Malhotra, Segars, 2001). The focus shifted from information technology (managing data and information) to increasing one's understanding of the interactional process of creating and sharing knowledge within organizations (Nonaka, 1994).

In an extensive review of the definitions of knowledge management, Awad and Ghaziri (2004) found the following six common components used to define knowledge management that build upon a foundation of information management: (1) using accessible knowledge from outside (and inside) sources, (2) embedding and storing knowledge, (3) representing knowledge in databases and documents, (4) promoting knowledge growth in the organizational culture, (5) transferring and sharing knowledge throughout the organization, and (6) assessing the value of knowledge assets and impact. Within this working definition of knowledge management, this analysis focuses on all components of knowledge management except information storing and documenting.

While the majority of experience with knowledge management resides in the for-profit sector, recent interest in the public and nonprofit sectors has emerged in relationship to improving service effectiveness and efficiency as well as reducing costs (Haynes, 2005; Edge, 2005; Syed-Ikhsan & Rowland, 2004; McAdam and Reid, 2000; Office of Security Defense, 2002). While focused mainly on information technology, the federal government has several knowledge management projects, including the Federal Knowledge Management Working Group, which seeks to understand knowledge management at the federal level of government. In addition to the benefits of knowledge management in the public sector, there are multiple challenges including: (1) the little support and flexibility in financial reward systems (Office of Security Defense, 2002), (2) isolated nature of public sector work (Murray, 2001), (3) the culture of resistance and hoarding of knowledge (Svieby and Simons, 2002; Murray, 2001, Liebowitz and Chen, 2003), (4) the difficulty in developing and maintaining collaborative cultures (Edge, 2004), and (5) the reduction of centrally allocated resources for managing knowledge (McAdam and Reid, 2000). The limited amount of research on knowledge management in the public sector suggests that implementation strategies need more attention in order to move beyond anecdotal reporting (Edge, 2004). Despite what little we know about knowledge management in the public sector, even less is known about knowledge management in the human services sector.

The process of knowledge management can be viewed from three perspectives: individual, group, and organizational. The individual level includes an understanding of tacit and explicit knowledge and constitutes the first part of this analysis. As individuals create information and acquire knowledge, it needs to be shared through social interactions and exchanges within the organization in order to create new knowledge. Knowledge sharing is addressed in the second section of this analysis. The process of creating and sharing knowledge depends not only on the individual and team level sharing but also on an understanding of the many organizational factors noted in the next sections that underlie the successful implementation of a knowledge management system. And finally, this analysis concludes with a discussion of the implications for implementing knowledge management systems in human services organizations.

THE ROLE OF TACIT AND EXPLICIT KNOWLEDGE IN ORGANIZATIONAL LIFE

It is no longer sufficient to simply employ people who can do the job; we need to understand how they do it as well as the processes that underlie their work (Horvath, 2001; Stenmark, 2000; Tagger, 2005). Intellectual capital is the sum of the knowledge possessed by the employees of an organization. Managing knowledge is the key to maximizing productivity and promoting organizational sustainability (Grossman, 2006).

Horvath (2001) defines knowledge as the recognition that people add value to information by combining it with other information to form new and unique combinations; they refine information for specific uses or generalize it for broader application. Also, people evaluate information for its usefulness and occasionally reframe information to yield new insights. In essence, organizational members provide context, meaning, and purpose to information and move it along a continuum toward what we commonly call knowledge. Therefore, knowledge is defined by Horvath (2001) as *information with significant human value added.* In addition, knowledge is dynamic, created in social interactions amongst individuals and organizations, and depends on particular time and space (Nonaka, 1994). As a result, information becomes knowledge when it is interpreted by individuals, given a context and anchored in the beliefs and commitments of individuals.

According to Augier and Vendelo (1999), knowledge can be viewed in terms of a continuum with tacit knowledge on one end and explicit, or codified, knowledge on the other. The concept of "tacit knowledge" was first defined by Polanyi, although the idea that certain thoughts and knowledge are contained in areas that are inaccessible to a conscious process goes back to at least as far as Helmholtz's work in the 19th century (Nonaka, 1994; Tagger, 2005).

Tacit knowledge is knowledge that exists in the minds of workforce members, manifests itself through their actions, and is not easily articulated. Tacit knowledge can be displayed by experts who make judgments and take actions, usually without making direct reference to a framework that explains what they are doing. Therefore, tacit knowledge is a meaningful and important source of information that influences the decisions and actions of practitioners, often called "know how" (Brown & Duguid, 2001 and Zeira & Rosen, 2000). In contrast, explicit knowledge refers to knowledge that has been captured and codified into manuals, procedures and rules that can be disseminated. It may refer to knowledge that has been learned through explicit instruction or to a skill acquired through practice. While knowledge may be needed to acquire skills, it may no longer be needed once a person becomes adept in exercising them (Brown & Duguid, 2001).

When explicit knowledge is embodied in a language that can be communicated, processed, transmitted and stored, it takes the form of data-based information and evidence-based principles in organizational manuals. In contrast, tacit knowledge is personal and difficult to formalize because it is embedded in action, procedures, commitment, values and emotions and acquired by sharing experiences and observations that are not easily communicated (Nonaka, 1994).

As a result, tacit and explicit knowledge are interdependent, essential to knowledge creation and of equal importance (Nonaka, 1994). Explicit knowledge without tacit insights quickly loses its meaning; where *"know that"* requires *"know how."* Therefore, knowledge is at least two dimensional and created through interactions between tacit and explicit knowledge. Agency-based practice represents the integration and dissemination of both tacit and explicit knowledge (Brown & Duguid, 2001; Madhavan & Grover, 1998).

Extracting Tacit Knowledge

An interesting aspect of tacit knowledge is the inherent tension between its value and its elusiveness. Its high value stems from knowing things we are unable to express; for example, *"We can know more than we can tell"* (Polanyi, 1998, as cited in Nonaka 1994, p.16) and *"We can often know more than we realized"* (Leonard and Sensiper, 1998, p. 114). This realization becomes significant when knowledgeable and skillful people leave an organization. They take with them not only a substantial amount of organization-specific knowledge and information but also tacit knowledge that they acquired on the job and may not have transferred to others (Tagger, 2005). Therefore, one of the goals of identifying tacit knowledge is to capture it contributions to organizational effectiveness, especially before experienced personnel leave the organization.

Horvath (2001) identifies the following reasons to capture and manage tacit knowledge: (a) the need to promote the transfer of best or most promising practices, especially related to how work actually gets done; (b) the need to define core competencies, especially the unique value-added skills that individuals derived from particular situations, experiences and organizational history; and (c) the need to document innovative processes by which organizational problems are defined and solutions developed. The essence of an organization's learning capabilities is often found in the tacit knowledge of its employees because much of the crucial *know how* resides in the minds of the organization's members (Madhavan & Grover, 1998 and Nonaka, 1994).

While some tacit knowledge can never be articulated, it is important to note the two different kinds of tacit knowledge identified by Nonaka (1994): *technical tacit knowledge* that is embodied in skills and can therefore be copied ("know how"), and *cognitive tacit knowledge* that is ingrained in mental models that are taken for granted and can not be easily demonstrated and transferred. Based on the distinction between technical and cognitive, two major definitions of tacit knowledge have emerged: (1) "tacit knowledge is non-codified, disembodied know-how that is acquired via the informal take-up of learned behavior and procedures" (Howells 1996, p. 92); and (2) "tacit knowledge is manifest only in its application and is not amenable to transfer" (Grant 1997, as cited in Seidler-de Alwis & Hartmann, 2004 p. 375). With this distinction in mind, there is likely to be a knowledge hierarchy where a large proportion of our present day explicit knowledge has originally arisen from embedded tacit knowledge that has slowly became codified or articulated over time (Bush and Richards, 2001). In some professions, this development is referred to as "practice wisdom."

The growing interest in tacit knowledge over the last decade has also informed the process of organizational learning (Swarts & Pye, 2002); especially the different ways in which tacit knowledge affects the sharing of knowledge. While much of the literature and research surrounding knowledge management has emphasized the definition and justification for knowledge management, little has been written about knowledge sharing, especially the transfer of tacit knowledge from one individual to another. Because tacit knowledge is gained through experience and revealed through application, it is important for organizations to create opportunities for the sharing of tacit knowledge (Grant, 1996). Thus, the goal of knowledge management is to capture tacit knowledge and encourage workers to share and communicate their knowledge with others at various levels within the organization by using formal and informal networks and creating a culture in which knowledge sharing is supported and encouraged (Awad and Ghaziri, 2004). The urgency of this sharing process can be seen in an organization's leadership succession planning where senior staff members may leave the organization with knowledge management mechanisms in place for transferring their tacit knowledge to their successors.

KNOWLEDGE SHARING IN ORGANIZATIONS

Within an organization, knowledge sharing can occur at three distinct levels: organizational, group, and individual (De Long and Fahey, 2000). While individuals are the primary conduits through which knowledge is created and shared in an organization, organizations cannot create knowledge without the individuals who possess the knowledge and this knowledge creation needs to be harvested by organizations in order to enhance effectiveness and efficiency (Grant,1996; Ipe, 2003; Nonaka and Takeuchi, 1995). Thus, individuals play a critical role in the process of organizational knowledge creation because they provide the knowledge that can be included, augmented, and implemented as a part of the organization's knowledge base.

Knowledge sharing relies heavily on the interactions between individuals within an organization. Ipe (2003) states, "An organization's ability to effectively leverage its knowledge is highly dependent on its people, who actually create, share, and use the knowledge" (p. 341). The sharing of knowledge is a process by which individuals are able to convert their own knowledge into a form that can be understood, absorbed, and used by others. Knowledge sharing allows individuals to learn from one another as well as contribute to the organization's knowledge base (Hendricks, 1999; Cohen and Levinthal, 1990). Knowledge sharing also promotes creativity and innovation as individuals collaborate together, circulate new ideas and contribute to innovation and creativity in organizations. This is the essence of a learning organization.

The goal of a learning organization, then, is to integrate the specialized knowledge of individuals through the following organizational mechanisms: (1) rules and directives; (2) sequencing; (3) routines; and (4) group problem solving and decision making (Grant, 1996). The rules and directives include standards that guide procedures and processes as well as "provide a means by which tacit knowledge can be converted into readily comprehensible explicit knowledge" (Grant, 1996, p. 115). Sequencing refers to the organizational activities needed to gather the input of specialists over time in order to convey knowledge while minimizing the need for communication and coordination. Routines are sets of behavior that "support complex patterns of interactions between individuals in the absence of rules, directives, or even significant verbal communication" (Grant, 1996, p. 115). Routines are used in an organization to provide consistent and task specific performance outcomes. These three mechanisms (rules, sequencing, and routines) need to be balanced with the fourth related to face-to-face meetings or group collaboration. Because group problem solving and decision making require considerable time and resources when trying to communicate tacit knowledge, they are usually reserved for more complex situations (Galbraith, 1973; Perrow, 1967).

Organizational knowledge needs to be viewed as a communal resource whereby communities of practice inside and outside of organizations have a mutual interest in knowledge sharing that involves the following factors: opportunity structures, care, and authenticity (von Krogh, 2002). Opportunity structures are the occasion and benefits of knowledge sharing in the community; for example, narrow opportunity structures involve communicating very specific knowledge through very specific channels with a limited number of people and broad opportunity structures include many relationships in the community with a wide spectrum of interests and knowledge where sharing occurs on a consistent basis through both virtual and physical means (e.g., "knowledge fairs").

The second factor relates to caring as a social norm that includes: (1) trust, (2) tolerance, (3) active empathy, (4) concrete assistance, and (5) authenticity. The more members are able to trust each other and tolerate the differences inherent in each other's knowledge, experience, and behavior, the more likely they will be to share knowledge and cultivate varied interests that can contribute to positive learning in the community. Active empathy is a proactive approach to understanding the knowledge of others and encourages members to share their knowledge. Tangible help reflected in concrete assistance promotes sharing as members offer knowledge based on their own experiences and thereby promote shared learning. And finally, authenticity refers to sharing knowledge "directly from the source in a way that ensures its genuineness, accuracy, validity, and reliability" (von Krogh, 2002, p. 383). The use of knowledge also contributes its authenticity, thereby advancing the knowledge sharing process and furthering its dissemination. In addition, knowledge sharing is enhanced by other social norms in the organization related to incentives to share and the type of knowledge to be shared (Ipe, 2003).

The nature of knowledge includes its value to the individual as well as to the organization (von Hippel, 1994; Weiss, 1999). Knowledge, when viewed as a commodity, creates a sense of ownership among those who possess it. This sense of ownership stems from the associations between knowledge, status, and career advancement opportunities (Andrews & Delahaye, 2000). When the possession of knowledge leads to competition, incentives must be created to encourage members of an organization to participate in knowledge-sharing activities. Incentives to share knowledge can be separated into *internal* factors (e.g., value of knowledge and benefits received from sharing it) and *external* factors (e.g., the relationship with the recipient and the rewards for sharing). Individuals possessing knowledge are highly valued and viewed as powerful and can use knowledge to achieve their desired outcomes that can decrease the incentive to share knowledge among other staff. The mutual benefits of knowledge sharing between individuals, or reciprocity, is also a motivational factor. Reciprocity as a motivation to share knowledge indicates an open relationship between individuals who expect that their contribution to the exchange of knowledge will be mutually beneficial (Ipe, 2003). Reciprocity can also be viewed as a serious threat to knowledge sharing when it arouses a fear of exploitation, a situation where individuals perceive themselves as offering too much knowledge and receiving little benefit in return.

The relationship between sender of knowledge and the recipient of knowledge is an external factor that can impact motivations to share knowledge (Andrews and Delahaye, 2000). For example, the power differential between senders and recipients can influence whether and how knowledge is shared. Huber (1991) found that individuals with lower status are more inclined to share information with those who hold more power within the organization, while those with more power tend to share knowledge amongst colleagues who have similar power statuses.

Rewards are another external factor related to incentive structures. The more benefits (perceived or realized) that individuals receive from sharing knowledge, the more likely they will share and vice versa. When individuals perceive knowledge sharing as being detrimental to their value or status, they are less likely to share. Bartol and Srivastava (2002) identified four mechanisms of knowledge sharing: (1) individual contribution, (2) formal interactions within and between groups, (3) sharing across groups, and (4) sharing through informal means. The first three mechanisms could involve extrinsic promotional opportunities as incentives to foster knowledge sharing, while the reward for the fourth mechanism would be the intrinsic value of increasing one's expertise and the development of new skills.

Opportunities for knowledge sharing can occur both formally and informally. Formal opportunities include occasions that are specifically intended to obtain, exchange, and disseminate information (e.g., symposiums, conferences, and training events that provide a structured means to share primarily explicit knowledge in an efficient manner to a large number of individuals). Informal opportunities are personal interactions with individuals within and between social networks. Knowledge is most likely exchanged through these channels because of interpersonal relationships that encourage trust and build rapport (Ipe, 2003).

ORGANIZATIONAL FACILITATORS
OF KNOWLEDGE MANAGEMENT

As managers understand the difference between tacit and explicit knowledge and the structures needed to promote knowledge sharing, they position themselves to identify ways to incorporate knowledge management into the fabric of their organization. Therefore, it is important to identify the organizational factors (structure, leadership, education and awareness) that facilitate knowledge sharing (Riege, 2005; Syed-Ikhsan, 2004, Van Beveren, 2003; Taylor & Wright, 2004). Organization culture is often viewed as the most important influence in determining the success or failure of knowledge management (McDermott & O'Dell, 2001, Mason & Pauleen, 2003, Riege, 2005). While many factors may contribute to the successful implementation of knowledge management, the most important first step is the establishment of a clear connection between the knowledge management strategy and the overall goals of the organization (Riege, 2005).

Organizational Culture

While organizational culture can contribute to promoting successful knowledge management strategies (Dyer, Nobeoka, 2000) it can also be a barrier (Chua & Lam, 2005). In a study of middle managers perceptions of knowledge management, 45% identified organizational culture as the greatest barrier to knowledge management, pointing to lack of trust, communication, and individual sharing as detrimental to successful knowledge management implementation (Mason & Pauleen, 2003). In another survey of large and small companies, an organization's main implementation challenge stemmed from the absence of a "sharing" culture (Chief Information Officer Council, n/d). The creation of an open, innovative, and supportive climate, where ideas are welcome and people are engaged in improving the work environment is essential for successful knowledge sharing and management. Effective knowledge sharing involves learning from mistakes as well as creating space to share, reflect, and generate new knowledge (Taylor & Wright, 2004; Riege, 2005).

The unique demands placed on human service organizations can erode the willingness of staff to reflect on and learn from mistakes (Taylor & Wright, 2004). Trust within an organization is crucial to encouraging knowledge sharing. Staff need to feel free to share insights, experiences, and know-how in order to promote the sharing of knowledge. Trust is an essential part of the knowledge management process by "giving clear impressions that reciprocity, free exchange, and proposing innovations will be recognized and fairly compensated. In contrast, lack of trust encourages employees at all levels to hoard knowledge and build suspicion in people and organizational processes" (Awad & Ghaziri, p. 25)

Drawing upon Schein's (1985) concepts of organizational culture, there are several aspects of culture that can inhibit or facilitate knowledge sharing. A "visible" culture includes all the espoused values, philosophy, and mission that are reflected in the structure, stories, and written statements about the organization while the "invisible" culture is the deeper level of unspoken values and beliefs that guide staff. Organizations that are able to connect the visible and invisible dimensions of their organizational culture to the knowledge sharing process are more likely to succeed. McDermott and O'Dell (2001) suggest that organizations do not need to change their organizational culture prior to introducing knowledge management; rather managers need to understand the invisible and visible dimensions of the organizational culture and build a framework for knowledge management within their existing culture. The process for making this connection between the dimensions of culture and knowledge sharing includes: (1) linking knowledge sharing to practical problem-solving, (2) introducing knowledge management in a way that matches the organization's style, and (3) developing a reward system that support knowledge sharing. The invisible dimensions involve a process of linking the notion of knowledge sharing to a existing core values as well as existing organizational networks.

Ipe (2003) describes another example of how organizational culture influences knowledge sharing and knowledge management by illustrating this overlapping aspect of the nature of knowledge, opportunities structures, and motivations noted in Figure 1. The organizational culture allows for the three elements to interact in a non-linear fashion and allows for the sharing of knowledge within an organization. Ipe argues that an organizational culture that is not supportive of any of the three essential elements will prohibit effective knowledge sharing.

Organizational Structure

There is much discussion in the literature on knowledge management about the benefits and limitations of different organizational structures for knowledge management (van Beveren, 2003; Riege, 2005; Nonaka and Takeuchi, 1995). Some studies suggest that an open and flexible organizational structure promotes information sharing better than the hierarchical, bureaucratic structures (Probst, Raub, & Rombhardt, 2000). Most bureaucratic organizations are often characterized by an upward flow of information (with processing and filtering occurring at each level) and a reluctance to share information downwards or outwards because of a belief that employees do not need the information for improved performance (van Beveren, 2003). In addition, hierarchical organizations tend to have detailed rules and procedures that support the punishment of mistakes and failures and thereby constrain knowledge sharing practices. In contrast, communication flow in relatively flat organizations is not restricted to one-direction, but rather is centered around small functional areas or project teams (Ives, Torrey, & Gordon, 2000).

Most public sector human service organizations reflect strong divisional structures based on groups of practitioners who focus on individual decision-making with clients. There is minimal group decision making or problem-solving when staff are concerned primarily with

FIGURE 1. Knowledge Sharing Between Individuals in Organizations

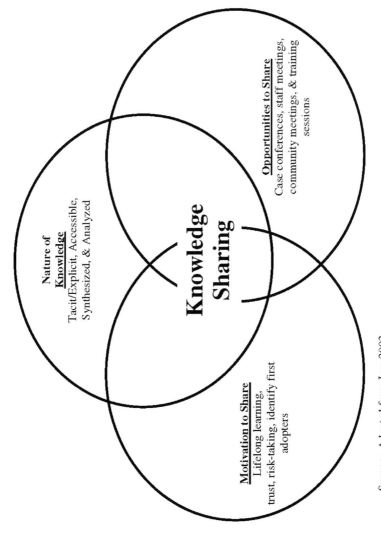

Nature of Knowledge
Tacit/Explicit, Accessible, Synthesized, & Analyzed

Opportunities to Share
Case conferences, staff meetings, community meetings, & training sessions

Knowledge Sharing

Motivation to Share
Lifelong learning, trust, risk-taking, identify first adopters

Source: Adapted from Ipe, 2003

their own caseload. These departmental structures provide for very little internal networking and even fewer informal or formal opportunities to share knowledge across departments (van Beveren, 2003).

Leadership

Top and middle management leadership is crucial to the success of knowledge management. As Mason and Pauleen (2003) noted, knowledge management will only happen when top management is understanding and committed to the process. The lack of senior management support, "buy-in," and encouragement can prevent knowledge management from being infused throughout the organization. Gaining the support of those with access to additional resources, policy, and overall direction can create an environment in which it is expected that staff members will share their knowledge and insight (Riege, 2005). For example, managers need to lead by example in sharing their own failures, lessons learned, and insights.

Education and Reward Systems

Currently, managers and front line staff have a low awareness of the value and benefit of sharing knowledge with one another (Mason and Pauleen, 2003). There is a perception in many organizations that sharing one's knowledge may reduce or jeopardize one's job security (Riege, 2005; Murray, 2001). In some cases, this can result in the hoarding of knowledge (Edge, 2005). Organizations spend the majority of their training time and resources on sharing explicit knowledge, rather than identifying, valuing, and learning to disseminate the tacit knowledge that exists within the organization's workforce.

Effective knowledge management can be found in organizations where knowledge sharing is valued, evaluated, and rewarded (Reige, 2005, McDermott & O'Dell, 2001). For example, to what extent do current reward and evaluation systems encourage shared knowledge? Are knowledge sharing actions praised or do they go unnoticed? The informal reward systems and the formal employee evaluation procedures need to be assessed as part of implementing knowledge management systems. Master and Pauleen (2003) noted that several large companies with established knowledge management strategies focus on formal performance reviews using criteria related to capturing valuable knowledge, archiving it, sharing it, and making use of the knowledge of others. The formality of including the ability to effectively share knowledge in an annual performance review process provides a clear reminder to staff of the organization's commitment to knowledge management.

STRATEGIES FOR IMPLEMENTING KNOWLEDGE MANAGEMENT

The successful implementation of knowledge management involves a cultural transformation within an organization and requires the deliberate actions of management as well as employees (Grossman, 2006). An effective knowledge management initiative represents long-term change and "does not have a beginning and an end. Rather, it is ongoing, organic, and ever-evolving" (Office of Security Defense, 2002). Managers embarking on the implementation of a knowledge management system need to assess a variety of aspects of organizational culture and develop strategies that fit the uniqueness of the organization. McDermott and O'Dell (2001) have identified five lessons for im- plementing knowledge management:

- make a visible connection between knowledge sharing and organizational goals, problems, or expected results
- match the overall style of the organization to the knowledge management program, making knowledge sharing a natural step and building on the strengths of the organization rather than simply replicating practices developed by other organizations
- link knowledge sharing with values held by the organization and employees including expectations, language, and mission
- enhance and build upon natural networks already in existence in the organization
- utilize influential peers to increase knowledge sharing and find ways to build knowledge sharing into routine performance reviews.

While the literature on approaches to implementing knowledge management has grown, the common components continue to include: (1) the creation of knowledge, (2) the capturing knowledge, (3) the organization and refinement of knowledge, and (4) the transferring or dissemination of knowledge throughout the organization (Awad & Ghaziri, 2004; McAdam and Reid, 2000; Edge, 2005; Nonaka and Takeuchi, 1995) For example, knowledge creation includes accessing the knowledge that currently exists within the organization as well as the creation of new knowledge through social interaction. Capturing knowledge involves the organizational value of making knowledge an explicit aspect of organizational life. The organizing and refinement of knowledge deals with the more technical aspects of codifying, filtering, or cataloging knowledge so that others can understand and access it. And finally, dissemination involves orientation and training strategies. Each of these components has multiple strategies for implementation but are beyond the scope of this analysis. Rather, the overall approach and strategies for implementing a knowledge management system are identified.

Organizations have approached a knowledge management system from a multitude of approaches. However, to make forward progress it is generally "advisable to do a number of things along multiple fronts– technical, organizational, cultural–rather than focus on one topic" (Davenport & Prusak, 2000 p.165). Drawing on five lessons identified by McDermott and O'Dell (2001) as well as lessons identified by Davenport and Prusak (2000), the following strategies (in no particular priority) should be considered when implementing a knowledge management system:

Strategy #1: Build a visible connection between knowledge sharing and organizational goals and outcomes

An organization deciding to implement an agency-wide knowledge management system should first assess the visible ways that the organization currently engages in knowledge sharing. Do organizational goals and strategies provide for the use of knowledge sharing? Does the agency explicitly articulate the importance of and use of data-based decision-making? If the organizational mission and service goals do not explicitly state the use of knowledge and knowledge sharing, it will be more difficult to convey to staff the importance of knowledge management. Many successful organizations seeking to implement a knowledge management system have recreated the identity of the organization to include the importance of knowledge sharing. The creation of a brand or tag line in agency publications also conveys a message to staff that knowledge is valued and utilized whenever possible. While some organizations may choose to develop a high profile knowledge management initiative in order to redefine themselves as a knowledge seeking and utilizing organization, others may choose a low-key strategy that infuses knowledge management throughout the organization by connecting knowledge sharing to their departmental goals. For example, if the organizational goal is, "create an integrated, coordinated system of care," a knowledge-inclusive goal could read, "create an integrated, coordinated system of care utilizing the knowledge of all participants."

Successful knowledge management organizations have also started implementation efforts by connecting the importance of knowledge sharing with a problem currently facing the organization. For example, the loss of key personnel and the perceived need to "reinvent the wheel" are problems that can inhibit reaching organizational goals. These concerns can be connected to the concept of improved knowledge management by collecting and disseminating practice wisdom (tacit knowledge) from those exiting the organization (Austin & Gilmore, 1993). Knowledge management can be framed as a strategy to reduce wasted time that prohibits staff from meeting organizational goals.

Strategy # 2: Link knowledge sharing with values held by the organization including expectations, language, recognition, and mission

Similar to the first strategy, the less-visible values that permeate the organization should be identified and assessed in order to develop a strategy for introducing knowledge sharing and knowledge management. If connected to a value already embraced by the staff, the introduction of knowledge sharing can be seen by staff as a way to further their belief in the original value, not necessarily their belief in knowledge sharing. For example, if collaboration is a value already understood and encouraged by the organization, knowledge sharing can be a method for promoting collaboration, thereby also increasing the likelihood that knowledge sharing will be embedded in the organization. As a result, knowledge sharing can strengthen an already existing value. In the same manner, if service efficiency is an organizational value, knowledge sharing can be seen as a strategy to reduce duplication and increase productivity.

The reward and recognition components of staff performance evaluation systems should also be assessed in order to determine their relationship to knowledge sharing values. For example, staff members who know they are being evaluated on their ability to use and share knowledge with their peers will be more likely to embrace the process. Promoting or praising staff based on what they know rather than how they share what they know can encourage a knowledge-hoarding rather than a knowledge sharing environment. A more formal staff recognition system can also be used to increase knowledge sharing. Regular recognition of employees who utilize best practices, share lessons learned, utilize promising practices, or demonstrate knowledge in action can serve as role models for knowledge sharing.

Strategy #3: Tailor the knowledge management system to the style of the organization so that knowledge sharing builds upon the strengths of the organization

One approach to introducing knowledge management into an existing organizational culture is to reflect on past organizational change efforts because organization introduce and respond to change in different ways. For example, in a more formal organizational culture, the change process might include a memo from top management that explains the need for knowledge management mechanisms for sharing, the utilization of staff training and pilot projects to introduce knowledge management, and provides a description of expected outcomes.

Another approach to introducing knowledge management involves the assessment of the learning needs of staff. Using a modified version of a Learning Needs Analysis Tool developed by Clark, Holifield, and Chisholm (2005), managers are able to assess aspects of the organization's culture that can facilitate or inhibit knowledge sharing. For example, the inventory includes the following four aspects of an organization's culture related to knowledge sharing and highlighted in Figure 2: (1) team work, (2) reflection, (3) use of tacit knowledge, and (4) functioning as a learning organization. The *teamwork* component involves the staff's ability and interest in working together by assessing team skills related to levels of trust, strength of communication, and group interaction. The *reflection* component assesses the extent to which personal and professional reflection is viewed as part of everyday work. High levels of reflection involve questioning and extracting one's own knowledge and that of colleagues through open discussion of mistakes, lessons learned, and problem-solving practices. The *use of tacit knowledge* relates to an organization's understanding of tacit knowledge and the degree to which it is valued. High levels of understanding and appreciation can greatly facilitate knowledge sharing. The fourth section related to operating as a *learning organization* includes the staff's perceptions of the organization's commitment to learning, especially the importance of intellectual capital and the promotion of staff development.

FIGURE 2. Staff Inventory for Assessing a Knowledge Sharing Culture

Team Skills

Levels of Trust
- Staff have trust in their colleagues to reflect on personal and professional issues
- There is an atmosphere of trust in the organization
- I have participated in learning dialogues with colleagues I trust

Communication
- Staff are expected to communicate with each other
- Organization supports the development of different communication techniques
- Effective communication is a priority for the organization

Group work
- Staff value the use of working in groups
- Working in groups helps me to advance my skills

Reflection

Open discussion of mistakes
- The organization encourages learning from mistakes
- There is space to share successes and failures
- The organization is one where there is comfort in questioning underlying assumptions

Comfort with colleagues
- Staff are comfortable with open discussion among their colleagues
- Staff have trust and comfort in publicly reflecting on their practice

Dialogue of lessons learned
- Organization encourages sharing and sees learning as part of everyone's job
- There is progressive discussion on what they learn from delivery of services
- Team meetings allow space to reflect on working practices

Problem-solving practices
- Critical reflection is best achieved in a team of colleagues
- The organization is based on reflection, not action
- Staff are encouraged to constantly think about their problem-solving practices

Use of Tacit Knowledge

Level of Understanding
- Organization has made staff aware of what tacit knowledge is
- Tacit knowledge is explained through work activities

Value of Tacit Knowledge
- Tacit knowledge is discussed in the organization as being important for the future
- Updating tacit knowledge important to the sustainability of the organization

Learning Organization

Importance of intellectual capital
- Organization regards individuals as having a key role in developing the organization
- Knowledge based skills are actively pursued by the organization

Promotion of staff development.
- Organization is driven by providing learning opportunities for the individual
- Management acts as a mentor for my learning

***Strategy #4: By identifying the breadth and depth of knowledge that
already exists in the organization, staff can build upon existing sharing
networks to disseminate this knowledge***

Organizations contain large amounts of tacit and explicit knowledge. Yet, staff members often do not know what knowledge exists, where it is located, how it is accessed, and how to effectively disseminate it. The majority of organizations currently have strategies and mechanisms for collecting and storing explicit information, but few have strategies for accessing tacit worker knowledge. A knowledge mapping exercise can serve as a first step in develop an inventory of what tacit knowledge exits among the staff members, where it is located, and how to access it.

Organizations, especially public sector organizations, collect and store data regarding client profiles and services provided. Line staff members collect the data and the information technology departments store and manage the information. Many organizations go a step further and disseminate the information in the form of monthly, quarterly, or annual reports. While many organizations have the explicit data available, they often fall short of translating this data into knowledge that can be utilized by staff. An essential ingredient of a knowledge management system is the capacity to translate existing organizational information into accessible knowledge for all levels of staff. Managers need to model for staff the process of translating information into knowledge for data-based decision-making.

While public sector organizations have repositories for storing internal information that can be translated into explicit knowledge, very few have repositories for the collection of tacit knowledge. The tacit knowledge, most commonly codified in the form of lessons learned, is not collected in many organizations. Often verbally disseminated through informal networks, tacit knowledge needs to be captured and stored in the same fashion as explicit information. Lessons learned from staff can be easily extracted, documented, and disseminated as well as continuously reassessed, altered, and shared. This tacit knowledge can be incorporated into staff orientation and training programs.

In addition to capturing tacit knowledge, it is also important to understand the natural and informal networks that staff members use to find out who knows what, where to get advice, and how to learn more about enhancing their professional practice. Effective informal networks often reflect established trust, open communication, and a mutual obligation to share knowledge. Staff meetings and case conferences are locations where staff share knowledge on a regular basis. Managers may not have access to the informal networks where staff are comfortable questioning, doubting, or sharing lessons learned. In order to identify the most effective networks for introducing knowledge sharing, managers need to know where staff members naturally turn to get knowledge for problem-solving and their preferences for using technology or face-to-face interactions.

Strategy #5: Identify the key knowledge workers within the organization as well as the roles and responsibilities of all staff to increase knowledge sharing

Knowledge management in an organization begins with the staff members who create, hold, and share knowledge. In addition, each organization needs to identify individuals who already function as knowledge workers; namely, someone skilled at transforming experience into knowledge by capturing, assessing, applying, sharing, and disseminating it in order to solve problems and/or achieve outcomes. A knowledge worker is a critical thinker, a continuous learner, an innovative thinker, team player, a creative risk-taker, and someone committed to the value of knowledge (Awad & Ghaziri, 2004). These personal traits are often complemented by systems-oriented skills related to an ability to identify strategies needed to capture and disseminate knowledge, an understanding of barriers and facilitators of knowledge sharing, and an understanding of the technological issues involved in sharing and dissemination. Individuals who possess these skills can be found throughout the agency at all levels. Once identified, these individuals should be recruited to assist in the implementation of knowledge management strategies and empowered to influence others. Knowledge management leaders should assess all levels of the agency to identify (1) who are the natural knowledge workers, (2) who are the potential knowledge workers, and (3) the role and responsibilities of each worker to share knowledge.

While certain individuals are naturally oriented to knowledge sharing, each worker at every level of the organization can play a role in the implementation of a knowledge management strategy. These roles and responsibilities can be incorporated into in-service training, hiring practices, worker expectations, and reward systems. In assessing an organization prior to implementing knowledge management strategies, leaders need to evaluate how well different levels of staff carry out the following roles and responsibilities:

Senior level staff: Since the implementation of knowledge management strategies requires top-level support and leadership, the following roles and responsibilities can help infuse knowledge management throughout the organization:

- *Set an example of being a knowledge user and sharer.* Senior level staff need to provide public examples of how they question, gather, analyze, and utilize data for their decision-making. A transparent decision-making process will begin to increase the value of questioning, brainstorming, exchanging ideas, and making informed decisions.
- *Make visible connections between knowledge sharing and organizational goals.* Senior managers need to find ways to state repeatedly, internally and externally, that knowledge management and organizational learning is critical to achieving the goals of the organization.
- *Link knowledge management to the organization's culture related to mission, values, and expectations.* Infusing knowledge management language throughout the organization will help to transform the culture of the organization in order to feature knowledge sharing as part of everyday problem solving.
- *Allocate resources to knowledge management strategies and infrastructure development.* Allowing staff time to participate in knowledge sharing networks or a knowledge management task force, investing in technology to increase peer sharing, or hiring staff responsible for capturing and disseminating knowledge.

Middle managers: Middle managers play an important role in instilling knowledge management values throughout the agency. They translate the overarching organizational knowledge management strategies into practical activities that support line staff. Middle managers are the enablers, supporters, and champions of knowledge management and need to be able to model the following roles and responsibilities:

- *Ability to extract and document information from staff.* Middle managers are in direct contact with line staff who possess considerable amounts of tacit knowledge. Middle managers should be skilled at extracting important information from their staff. Once extracted, middle managers should be responsible for organizing and disseminating this information as needed.
- *Encourage risk-taking, innovation, and regular review of lessons learned.* Middle managers are responsible for creating open environ-

ments that allow discussion of mistakes, reasons for successes, and continuous dialogue regarding lessons learned.

- *Develop reward structures that encourage sharing.* Middle managers need to develop mechanisms that foster internal and external rewards for sharing, rather than hoarding knowledge.
- *Promote transparency.* Middle managers that are transparent with their own processes related to questioning and doubting, information gathering, and decision-making will increase the value of learning for others.
- *Provide leadership.* Middle managers need to coach and mentor line staff who are exploring, questioning, and seeking opportunities to learn and share.

Line staff: Line staff are responsible for being knowledge learners in their daily interactions with clients, coworkers, and managers. Line staff that display the following are demonstrating a commitment to knowledge management:

- Search out, create, share, and use knowledge in their everyday interactions
- Continuously questioning self and others
- Critically thinking about their approach to work and reviewing past cases for lessons learned (positive and negative)

Strategy #6: Utilize a knowledge management task force or committee to facilitate the implementation of knowledge management strategies

While knowledge management is most successful when it is part of everyone's job, it usually requires the efforts of dedicated staff to embed knowledge management strategies into an organization, especially during the beginning phases of change. Many for-profit organizations have appointed chief knowledge officers (CKOs) whose sole responsibility is to create knowledge management systems. While this approach may be appropriate for the for-profit sector, it may be more appropriate in the non-profit and public sectors to create a knowledge management task force that includes individuals from all levels of the organization. This task force carries similar responsibilities and should be comprised of individuals with similar skills embodied by a CKO. The task force members need to have a vision of how they want knowledge management to function in their agency. They "should spur and catalyze the imagination, encouraging workers to think about the future in improvisational and innovation ways" (Office of Security Defense, 2002, p. 4).

In addition, the task force should be viewed as a change agent with the following mandate: (1) bring a hybrid of management and service delivery expertise to the agency, (2) challenge conventional or traditional approaches to system delivery, (3) understand IT principles, (4) be managers with broad organizational experience, (5) bridge the gap between technology and service delivery, and (6) be avid learners who seek advice, ask questions, and seek new ideas (Office of Security Defense, 2002).

Ideally, a task force within the public sector would include all levels of staff whereby senior managers, middle managers, and line staff would work together to build a knowledge culture and create a knowledge management structure. Such a group could assume the following roles and responsibilities:

- *Advocate for knowledge and learning.* By including knowledge sharing language into everyday language, actions, and work of the organization, it should be possible to see the impact on the mission, values, and goals of the organization. Is there a clear commitment to becoming a learning organization? Do performance evaluation procedures promote knowledge hoarding or knowledge sharing?
- *Design, implement, and oversee the organizations knowledge infrastructure.* Identify where knowledge is currently created, transferred, documented, and stored. Build protocols and mechanisms to document lessons learned.
- *Provide input into the process of knowledge creation and use in the organization.* Support managers in their efforts to include knowledge creation and sharing in their programs (i.e., during staff meetings, case conferences, supervision).
- *Develop strategies to increase the knowledge sharing skills of senior, middle, and direct service staff.*

CONCLUSION

Knowledge management starts as a *process* of understanding the value an agency places on knowledge and gathering a clear picture of where knowledge exists within the agency. Beginning with an agency assessment, managers are able to gauge the organization's commitment to learning, understand the current organizational culture, and gather insight into the current internal inhibitors and facilitators of knowledge

FIGURE 3. Strategies for Implementing a Knowledge Management System in a Human Service Organization

Multiple Strategies

Strategy #1: Build a visible connection between knowledge sharing and organizational goals and outcomes

Strategy # 2: Link knowledge sharing with values held by the organization including expectations, language, recognition, and mission.

Strategy #3: Tailor the knowledge management system to the style of the organization so that knowledge sharing builds upon the strengths of the organization

Strategy #4: By identifying the breadth and depth of knowledge that already exists in the organization, staff can build upon existing sharing networks to disseminate this knowledge.

Strategy #5: Identify the key knowledge workers within the organization as well as the roles and responsibilities of all staff to increase knowledge sharing.

Strategy #6: Utilize a knowledge management task force or committee to facilitate the implementation of knowledge management strategies

Roles and Responsibilities

Senior level staff:
- Set an example of being a knowledge user and sharer
- Make visible connections between knowledge sharing and organizational goals.
- Link knowledge management to the mission, values, and expectations.
- Allocate resources to knowledge management strategies and infrastructure development.

Middle Managers:
- Demonstrate ability to extract and document information from staff
- Encourage risk-taking, innovation, and regular review of lessons learned
- Develop reward structures that encourage sharing
- Promote transparency by modeling their own knowledge sharing processes
- Provide leadership, coaching, and mentoring

Line staff:
- Search out, create, share, and use knowledge in their everyday interactions
- Continuously questioning self and others
- Critically think about their approach to work and review past cases for lessons learned

Knowledge Manager and Representative Task Force Staff:
- Advocate for knowledge and learning.
- Design, implement, and oversee the organizations knowledge infrastructure.
- Provide input into the process of knowledge creation and use in the organization.
- Develop strategies to increase senior, middle, and line staff knowledge and skills in knowledge sharing.

sharing. From this assessment, managers can effectively design a knowledge management initiative that fits the organization.

Since its inception, knowledge management has encountered serious issues, including excessive hype and flawed approaches that have hindered acceptance and limited the potential benefits (CIO Council, n/d).

While numerous knowledge management approaches exist, the consistent recommendation from research is to connect the knowledge management approach to the currently operating *structure of the organization*. Knowledge management can be an elusive, visionary concept that gets lost in the translation of key principles into practice. Connecting the knowledge management initiative to a current organizational priority can increase the likelihood of successful implementation. Equipped with the information from the organizational assessment, managers need to explore different ways of making knowledge management relevant to staff by building something that staff understand and need to change.

Implementing a knowledge management system is a slow process that cannot be forced. There is not a precise beginning and definite ending to a knowledge management initiative. Rather, the process is characterized as one of exploration and experimentation. Agencies that are open to fresh, new ideas and continuously searching for better ways to serve clients should prove to be the most effective and successful in implementing knowledge management processes (see Figure 3, p. 385).

REFERENCES

Andrews, K.M. & Delahaye, B.L. (2000). Influences on knowledge processes in organizational learning: The psychological filter. *Journal of Management Studies, 37(6)*, 797-810.

Augier, M. & Vendelo, T. (1999). Networks, cognition and management of tacit knowledge. *Journal of Knowledge Management, 3(4)*, 252-261.

Austin, M.J. & Gilmore, T. (1993). Executive exit: Multiple perspectives on managing the leadership transition. *Administration in Social Work*, 17(1), 47-60.

Awad, E. & Ghaziri, H. (2004). *Knowledge Management*. New Jersey: Prentice Hall.

Bartol, K. & Srivastava (2002). Encouraging knowledge sharing: The role of organizational reward systems. *Journal of Leadership and Organizational Studies*. 9(1), 64-76.

Brown, J. & Duguid, P. (2001). Knowledge and organization: A social-practice perspective. *Organization Science, 12(2)*, 198-213.

Busch, P., & Richards, D. (2001). Graphically defining articulable tacit knowledge. In P. Eades, & J. Jesse (Eds.), *Selected Papers from Pan-Sydney Area Workshop on Visual Information Processing*: Vol. 2 (pp. 51-60). Sydney: ACS. Retrieved April 10, 2006, from http://crpit.com/confpapers/CRPITV2Busch.pdf.

Chua, A., & Lam, W. (2005). Why KM projects fail: A multi-case analysis. *Journal of Knowledge Management,* 9(3), 6-17.

Clark, T, Holifield, D., & Chisholm. (2005). A continual professional development toolkit for knowledge management in the workplace. *Paper presented at UICEE Conference in Al-*

giers May 2005. Retrieved on June 20, 2006 at http://www.elite.aau.dk/cee_as_wbl/Project_results/Docs/conference%20africa%2005-3.pdf

Cohen, W. & Levinthal, D. (1990). Absorptive capacity: A new perspective on learning and innovation. *Administrative Science Quarterly, 35,* 128-152.

Davenport, T., & Prusak, L. (2000). *Working knowledge: How organizations manage what they know.* Harvard Business School Press.

De Long, D. & Fahey, L. (2000). Diagnosing cultural barriers to knowledge management. *The Academy of Management Executive, 14*(4), 113-127.

Dyer, J. & Nobeoka, K. (2000). Creating and managing a high-performance knowledge-sharing network: The Toyota case. *Strategic Management Journal, 21,* 345-367.

Edge, K. (2005). Powerful public sector knowledge management: A school district example. *Journal of Knowledge Management, 9*(6), 42-52.

Galbraith, J. (1973). *Designing Complex Organizations.* Addison-Wesley: Reading, MA.

Gold, A., Malhortra, A., & Segars, A. (2001). Knowledge Managment: An organizational capabilities perspective. *Journal of Management Information Systems,* 18(1), 185-214.

Grant, R. (1996). Toward a knowledge-based theory of the firm. *Strategic Management Journal, 17,* 109-122.

Grossman, M. (2006). An overview of knowledge management assessment approaches. *The Journal of American Academy of Business, 8(2),* 242-247.

Hansen, M., Nohria, N., & Tierney, T. (1999). *What's your strategy for managing knowledge?* Harvard Business Review (HBR).

Haynes, P. (2005). *New development: the demystification of knowledge management for public services.* Public Money & Management, *4,* 131-135

Hendriks, P. (1999). Why share knowledge? The influence of ICT on the motivation for knowledge sharing. *Knowledge and Process Management, 6*(2), 91-100.

Horvath, J. (2001). Working with tacit knowledge. In J. Cortada, & J., Woods (Eds.), *Knowledge Management Yearbook* (35-50). Butterworth-Heinemann. Retrieved April 5, 2006, from http://www.providersedge.com/docs/km_articles/Working_With_Tacit_K.pdf

Howells, J. (1996). Tacit knowledge, innovation and technology transfer. *Technology Analysis and Strategic Management, 8(2),* 91-106.

Huber, G. (1991). Organizational learning: The contributing processes and the literatures. *Organization Science, 2*(1), 88-115.

Ipe, M. (2003). Knowledge sharing in organizations: a conceptual framework. *Human Resource Development Review, 2*(4), 337-359.

Ives, W., Torrey, B., & Gordon, C. (2000). Knowledge *sharing is a human behavior.* In D. e. a. Morey (Ed.), Knowledge Management. Cambridge, MA: MIT Press.

Leonard, D. & Sensiper, S. (1998). The role of tacit knowledge in group innovation. *California Management Review, 40(3),* 112-132.

Liebowitz, J., & Chen, Y. (2003). *Knowledge sharing proficiencies: The key to knowledge management in Holsapple.* In Handbook on Knowledge Management 1: Knowledge Matters. Springer-Verlag, Berlin.

Madhavan, R., & Grover, R. (1998). From embedded knowledge to embodied knowledge: New product development as knowledge management. *Journal of Marketing, 62(4)*, 1-12.

Mason, D., & Pauleen, D. (2003). *Perceptions of knowledge management: A qualitative analysis.* Journal of Knowledge Management, 7(4), 38-48.

McAdam, R., & Reid, R. (2000). A comparison of public and private sector perceptions and use of knowledge management. *Journal of European Industrial Training,* 24(6), 317-329.

McDermott, R., & O'Dell, C. (2001). Overcoming cultural barriers to sharing knowledge. *Journal of Knowledge Management, 5(1),* 76-85.

Murray, S. (2001). *Motivating public sector employees.* Financial Times, 10.

Nonaka, I. (1994). A dynamic theory of organizational knowledge creation. *Organization Science, 5(1),* 14-37.

Nonaka, I. & Takeuchi, H. (1995). *The knowledge creating company: How Japanese companies create the dynamics of innovation.* New York: Oxford University Press.

Office of Security Defense (OSD). (2002). *Knowledge management: Maximizing human potential.* Retrieved June 20, 2006 at www.dod.mil/comptroller/icenter/learn/knowledgeman.htm.

Perrow, C. (1967). A framework for the comparative analysis of organizations. *American Sociological Review, 32,* 194-208.

Probst, G., Raub, S., & Rombhardt, K. (2000). *Managing Knowledge.* Chichester: John Wiley & Sons.

Riege, A. (2005). Three-dozen knowledge sharing barriers managers must consider. *Journal of Knowledge Management,* 9(3), 18-35.

Schein, E. (1985). *Organizational Culture and Leadership.* San Francisco, CA: Jossey-Bass.

Seidler-de Alwis, R., & Hartmann, E. (2004). *The significance of tacit knowledge on company's innovation capability.* In B. Bekavac, J. Herget & M. Rittberger (Eds.). Informationzwischen Kultur und Marktwirtschaft. Des 9. Internationalen Symposiums. Vol. 42 (pp.373-394), Retrieved April 7, 2006, from http://www.inf-wiss.uni-konstanz.de/infwiss/download/isi2004/cc-isi04-art21.pdf

Stenmark, D. (2000). Turning tacit knowledge tangible. *Paper presented at the 33rd Hawaii International Conference on System Sciences, Hawaii.* Retrieved April 12, 2006, from http://csdl2.computer.org/comp/proceedings/hicss/2000/0493/03/04933020.pdf

Svieby, K., & Simons, R. (2002). Collaborative climate and effective knowledge work: an empirical study. *Journal of Knowledge Management,* 6(5), 420-433.

Swarts, J., & Pye, A. (2002). Conceptualising organizational knowledge as collective tacit knowledge: a model of redescription. *Paper presented at the Third European Conference on Organizational Knowledge, Learning and Capabilities.* Athens, Greece. Retrieved April 12, 2006, from http://www.tacitknowing.com/papers/ID315.pdf

Syed-Ikhsan, S., & Rowland, F. (2004). Knowledge management in a public organization: a study on the relationship between organizational elements and the performance of knowledge transfer. *Journal of Knowledge Management,* 8(2), 95-111.

Tagger, B. (2005). *An enquiry into the extraction of tacit knowledge.* Retrieved April 30, 2006, from http://www.cs.ucl.ac.uk/staff/B.Tagger/FinalIMR.pdf

Taylor, W. A., & Wright, G. H. (2004). Organizational Readiness for Successful Knowledge Sharing: challenges for public sector managers. *Information Resources Management Journal,* 17(2), 22-37.

Van Beveren, J. (2003). *Does health care for knowledge management? Journal of Knowledge Management,* 7(1), 90-95.

von Hippel, E. (1994). "Sticky information" and the locus of problem solving: Implications for innovation. *Management Science, 40,* 429-430.

Von Krogh (2002). The communal resources and information systems. *The Journal of Strategic Information Systems. 11*(2), 85-107.

Weiss, L. (1999). Collection and connection: The anatomy of knowledge sharing in professional service. *Organizational Development Journal, 17*(4), 61-74.

Zeira, A., & Rosen, A. (2000). Unraveling "Tacit Knowledge": What social workers do and why they do it. *Social Services Review, 74(1),* 103-118.

Index

Page numbers in *italics* designate figures.